Herbs

for Pets

Second Edition

Herbs for Pets

i-5 PUBLISHING, LLC™
Chief Executive Officer: Mark Harris
Chief Financial Officer: Nicole Fabian
Vice President, Chief Content Officer: June Kikuchi
General Manager, i5 Press: Christopher Reggio
Editorial Director, i5 Press: Andrew DePrisco
Art Director, i5 Press: Mary Ann Kahn
Digital General Manager: Melissa Kauffman
Production Director: Laurie Panaggio
Production Manager: Jessica Jaensch
Marketing Director: Lisa MacDonald

Library of Congress Cataloging-in-Publication Data
Tilford, Gregory L.
  Herbs for pets : the natural way to enhance your pet's life / Gregory L. Tilford & Mary L. Wulff. — 2nd ed.
    p. cm.
  Rev. ed. of: All you ever wanted to know about herbs for pets / Mary L. Wulff-Tilford & Gregory L. Tilford. 1999.
  Includes bibliographical references and index.
  ISBN 978-1-933958-78-1
  I. Wulff-Tilford, Mary, 1955– II. Wulff-Tilford, Mary, 1955– All you ever wanted to know about herbs for pets.
III. Title.

SF745.5.W86 2008
636.089'5321—dc22
                    2008055534

This book has been published with the intent to provide accurate and authoritative information in regard to the
subject matter within. While every precaution has been taken in the preparation of this book, the author and publisher
expressly disclaim any responsibility for any errors, omissions, or adverse effects arising from the use or application of
the information contained herein. The techniques and suggestions are used at the reader's discretion and are not to be
considered a substitute for veterinary care. If you suspect a medical problem, consult your veterinarian.

i-5 Publishing, LLC™
3 Burroughs, Irvine, CA 92618
www.facebook.com/i5press
www.i5publishing.com

Printed and bound in China
14 15 16 17   3 5 7 9 8 6 4

Herbs
for Pets

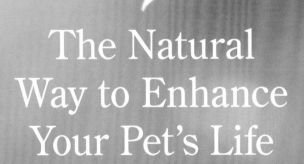

The Natural
Way to Enhance
Your Pet's Life

by Gregory L. Tilford &
Mary L. Wulff

Contents

Acknowledgments

It's funny how a book takes on a life of its own. This one began like most others—first as a compilation of research, expressed knowledge, and the inspiration and ideas of an author or two. But now after many years have passed and many thousands of people have read, shared, used, and reflected on the content from its pages, this book has grown into something much more—something far greater than anything I ever expected. For many, *Herbs for Pets* has become a gold standard—the definitive guide to herbs for pets. But it is not the authors, nor even the information contained in its pages, that stand at the forefront of this book's resounding success. It's the growing audiences of pet loving people who are realizing that the biggest rewards of animal companionship can come only after we learn to accept and respect the true nature of our animals. Without people like you, this latest edition would not exist. Thank you.

And once again—thank you to my now ex-wife and forever friend, Mary, who remains one of my foremost herbalist teachers. Thanks also go to Nancy Kerns, editor of *Whole Dog Journal* magazine, who throughout the years has been keeping the "holistic word" alive and visible to so many like-hearted animal lovers. And thanks to my dear friend Ikuko Kanada, who not only translated this tome into Japanese but also has been at the forefront of a new natural pet care revolution in Japan; your work brings renewed hope and inspiration to all who truly care about animal wellness. Thank you to Gail Pope and all of the incredible people at Brighthaven Sanctuary—a place where, because of you, miracles really do happen.

A special thanks to all of you who came to our rescue when my home burned in the Montana fires of 2000. There is absolutely nothing to describe the feelings of love coming from so many people.

And of course, thank you to all of the wonderful holistic veterinarians and natural pet-care providers who work on the front lines to bring the gifts of human intellect, love, and compassion to the true innocents of the world: the animals.

—Greg L. Tilford

I would like to thank and acknowledge my parents, George and Dixie Wulff for allowing me to be who I am and for letting Uncle Eldon give me my first puppy; Cindy Nicholls, a dear friend; Jan Newman, my cousin and friend: Jeanie Notti-Fullerton, a dear friend who shares a deep love and devotion for all creatures; to all of my animals past and present, for sharing their love and lives with me: Mister, Max, Mollie, Cedar, Willow, Stephanie, all gone but in my heart forever; Sage, the new Heeler in my life; Lili, the new cat in my life; and to Frog (the Doberman) and Kyra, the Shepherd; to my ex-husband, Greg, who made this book and many things possible, thank you for being a good friend.

—Mary L. Wulff

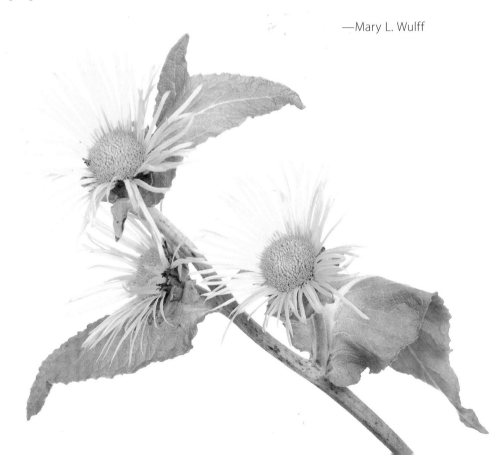

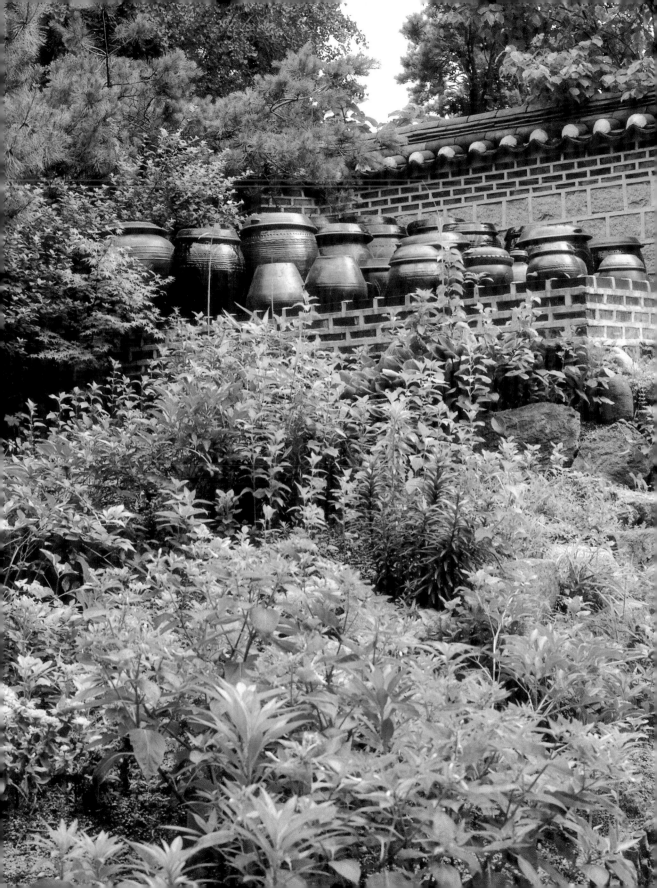

Introduction

Herbs and animals
have lived together
for a long, long time.

Millions of years before the first human walked the earth, creatures large and small were using plants as their primary source of healing. In fact, much of our modern medicine originates from what early humans learned through observation of wild animals and their instinctive uses of plants. For instance, we know that Indian tribes of the western United States learned of the powerful antimicrobial properties of *Ligusticum porteri* by observing bears ingest and roll in the plants to heal themselves. Even today, the plant is still known by many as "bear medicine."

In the face of diseases such as AIDS and cancer, modern-day pharmaceutical researchers continue to scour the remaining wilds of our planet in search of cures, and once again we are turning to the animals for answers. Zoopharmacognosy, a new discipline of science that investigates how animals use plants to heal themselves, is attracting attention at leading research universities throughout the world. At the forefront of the zoopharmacognosy effort are Dr. Eloy Rodriguez, a biochemist specializing in natural products and synthetic chemistry, and Harvard primatologist Richard Wrangham, who has been studying chimpanzees and gorillas in their native African habitats. Rodriguez and Wrangham have discovered that the apes have an innate ability to select specific plant species for use against internal parasites. In fact, not only can the animals select plants that possess specific medicinal compounds that are effective at expelling their parasites but somehow they know exactly how much plant material is needed to initiate a cure without causing toxic side effects.

As zoopharmacognosy recaptures our attention and as our respect toward the healing wisdom of animals grows, our quest for herbal curative answers is becoming more urgent. But we're faced with a problem. Strains of bacteria once thought to be conquered are reemerging despite our antibiotics, and healing resources are disappearing faster than we can discover them. Tens of thousands of acres of wild lands are lost each day to the effects of a growing human population and the relentless demands we place upon the planet. The Smithsonian Institution and fifteen other research organizations recently completed a twenty-year study

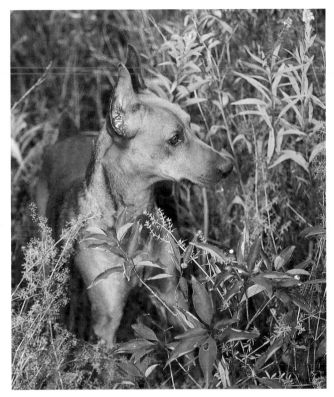

that concluded that at least one in every eight plant species worldwide are currently at risk of becoming extinct.

In North America alone, it is estimated that 29 percent of sixteen thousand plant species are on the verge of disappearing forever—and with each loss, a vital connecting link between earth and all the creatures who walk her ground is being broken forever.

As scientists struggle to find cures before plants are eliminated from the face of the planet, a tremendous "green revolution" is under way. A growing number of people are coming to realize that much of the healing wisdom we seek rests not in science and technology but within the ancient healing traditions of nature itself. To access this awareness, we find ourselves turning to the aboriginal peoples (who adopted healing ways from observing animals) to relearn ways of healing that have been passed down through hundreds of generations from humankind's oldest teachers—the animals.

Ancient cultures knew that healthful living, healing, and good medicine are not gauged by how effectively people can exploit the medicinal properties of natural resources. Instead, shamans and medicine women of the past saw human health as an integral part of the living celestial body we have since grown to know as Earth. They knew that our gravest ills emanate not from what nature bestows upon us but from what we bestow upon nature. This message is being repeated to us everywhere in the form of ancient bacteria, once thought to be conquered, that are mutating into stronger, more resistant, more aggressive strains of infectious disease. Vaccines that we once viewed as miracle medicines are now thought to debilitate the immune system they were designed to support and protect. Heart disease, cancer, arthritis, osteoporosis, and even psychosis-driven murder are being linked to the stresses of modern society and the nutrition-depleted foods we eat. Violent rainstorms of unprecedented ferocity wreak havoc as a by-product of air pollution and the effects of global warming. You may ask, how is all of this relevant to a book about herbal animal care? The answer: in the most fundamental ways imaginable.

This book introduces you to hundreds of plant medicines that can be used in the daily care of animals. In the first chapters, you learn the importance of feeding your companion a natural whole-foods diet. Then step by step you are guided into new levels of self-reliance as you learn to select, prepare, and apply natural remedies, many of which may be as accessible as your own backyard, on behalf of your companion animal. To help overcome possible skepticism, we have provided references to hundreds of cutting-edge scientific studies that support the effectiveness of herbs in animals. But even more significant to the purposes of this book, we share what herbalists and animals have learned in the absence of science (without the cruel inhumanities of animal testing) from thousands of years of continuously safe and effective herb use.

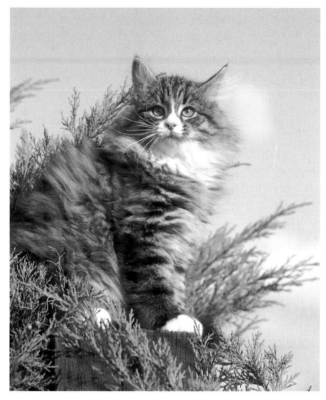

However, all of this represents the lesser side of what this book has to offer. Our deepest wish is to pass on the sense of interconnectedness that grows within the heart of the healer, as he or she learns and accepts ancient ways of healing that have been utilized by all life-forms on earth. This is not just a book about finding alternatives to conventional drugs; it is one about honoring and supporting a system of health care and healing that far exceeds the effectiveness of any medicine devised by humans—a system contained in and shared among the bodies of animals, plants, and Mother Earth herself.

In nature, plants represent much more than containers of active chemical constituents that have been identified and validated by the halls of human science. They are healing delegates of nature's design, here to serve the needs of all creatures who benefit from the nectar of their flowers, the shelter of their leaves, and the healing powers they hold. They are the critical link between what is alive and what is not, providing us and other organisms with the oxygen that is necessary for life and the base elements of the food chain—from macrobiotic soil nutrients to the vegetables on our dinner plates. Yet most people see plants as humanity's gift: insignificant by virtue of their silence but powerful and valuable when their secrets are revealed by science. Likewise, most of humanity still sees animals as expendable, lower forms of life that exist without intelligent consciousness or emotional pain and that offer no resistance when exploited.

In the minds of millions of people, plants and animals are here for the sole purpose of serving us, as fruits and beasts of burden without equal rights, in the pursuit of health and happiness. Whether it be a feedlot steer or a companion German shepherd dog, the needs of most animals become secondary concerns when we are buying pet food at the grocery store or when a chronic immune system disorder erupts into a household flea infestation. Instead of addressing their pet's real needs, many pet owners are predisposed to remain focused on themselves—the grocery bill dictates the quality of nutrition their animals receive, and fleas are approached as something that invades our homes, rather than as a symptom of a weakened animal host.

With *Herbs for Pets*, we hope to precipitate a change in this paradigm. The fact that you are reading this book implies that you are not like most people—in fact, you are part of a growing community of special human beings who are on a healing path that leads to something much more significant than the simple joy derived from opening up a can of cat food for the cat or giving the family dog rawhides to keep him busy. Like us, the authors of this book, you have probably discovered that caring for an animal brings about a very special and powerful type of healing.

When we provide our companion animals with considerations of health and healing that meet their needs and not just our own, we are in effect healing ourselves as well. In fact, we are healing one of the primary causes of earth's greatest ills: humanity's disconnection from nature.

Somewhere in the history of our species we have chosen a relationship of consumption and control rather than of coexistence with our planet, and it seems that our goal has been to defeat or defy nature at all costs. We defy nature's mechanisms of resisting disease by suppressing or bypassing the immune system with corticosteroid drugs, antibiotics, and vaccines. We ignore the natural requirements of good nutrition by supplementing an unhealthy diet with vitamin tablets. We dam rivers and drain swamps; we even try to change the duration of daylight by resetting the clocks for "daylight saving time." To compound all of this heady nonsense, we have placed our own self-imposed needs far above those of our earthly neighbors, and as a result the entire planet is suffering. For much too long, the human condition has prohibited us from living in harmony with the natural world that surrounds us.

The key to changing this trend rests not in the halls of science but in our willingness to see nature as nature is. Instead of studying the nature of plants from a mind-set that insists on picking their chemistries apart in an arrogant attempt to find singular compounds that may be exploited as drugs, we must learn to examine plants as they exist in nature, to discover and explore the intermingled relationships they share with the physical and nonphysical needs of all living things on earth. Likewise, instead of subjecting our animals, our most ancient teachers, to unthinkable pain and torture in a quest for rational answers to satisfy our scientific needs, we must learn to accept nature's medicines simply as nature presents them. The reality is that the need for scientific validation is shared only among humans—no other life-form on earth insists on analyzing and rationalizing nature's design, especially at the cold-hearted expense of animal suffering. In essence, science is merely striving to rationalize what has been known throughout the natural realm for eons.

This is a book about a level of healing that reaches far beyond that which can be provided by science. It is about holistic healing in its truest sense—a process that does not begin or end with the administration of a medicine but with our connection to nature. Holistic healing is not something that is given or received between caregiver and patient—it is part of a continuous circle that is shared among all entities involved in the maintenance of health. Our planet provides the elements from which plants are born and must reproduce. The animals and insects serve as stewards for the plants and in turn pass their intuitive wisdom to us. However, to access this wisdom, we must rethink our ways—we must relearn how to give for all that we receive from nature, and we must pay attention to the quiet lessons that surround us in the circle of life.

As someone who cares for a companion animal, you have taken a fundamental step back toward the circle of life by accepting a part of nature into your home. Now, as you investigate the healing power of nature's oldest medicines, and as you learn how to honor your companion's innate system of health maintenance, you will find yourself stepping into the circle. Here you will find that animals are not human property but are among our most valued teachers and healers. You will see that from the moment a puppy, a kitten, a baby bird, or another companion animal enters a human life, a special bond with nature begins. From this bond we can learn innocence, compassion, respect, unconditional love, and the tragedy of time wasted. And most important of all, we can finally realize that despite centuries of our abuses, animals and plants remain quietly waiting to reconnect humankind with the ways of nature.

In return for these offerings, and to assure that the circle remains unbroken by our presence, we must give something equally precious back to our beloved companions and teachers: we must listen to them and help serve their needs by providing the natural foods and medicines that have sustained their kind for millions of years.

Chapter 1

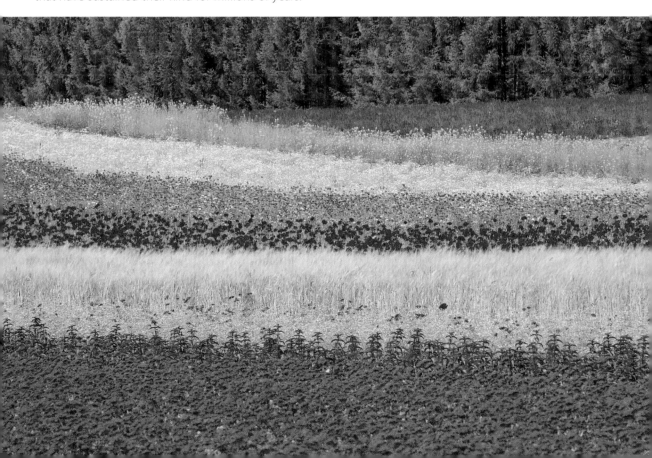

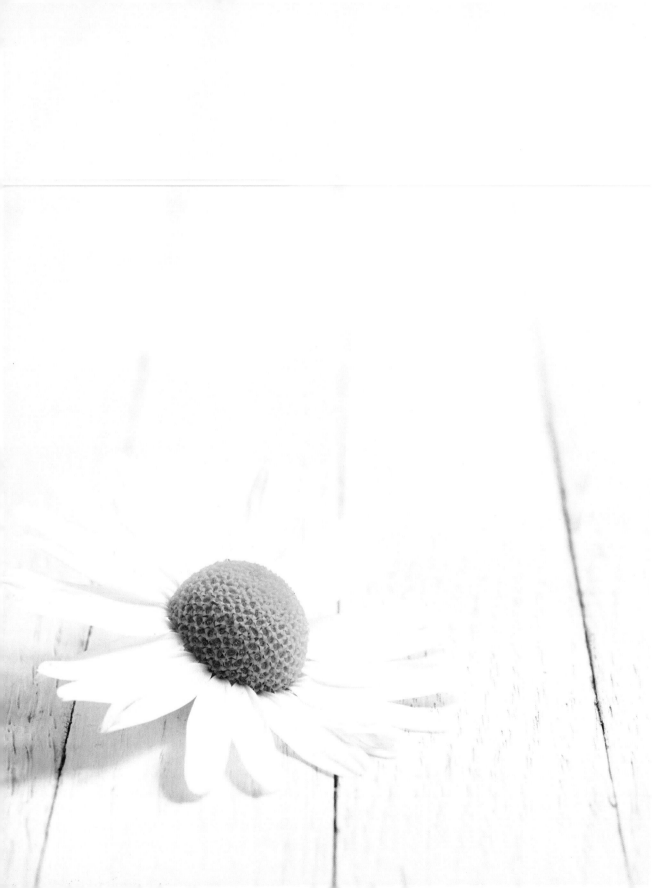

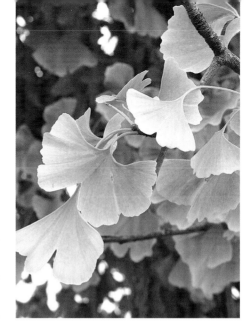

Principles and Practices of Herbalism

Using Herbs Naturally

Old ways die hard—especially when we have been raised with them. In our society, mainstream approaches to health maintenance focus on symptomatic intervention. Typically, when a person or animal gets sick, the conventional practitioner works to identify and suppress uncomfortable or unsightly symptoms in order to achieve immediate relief. As children, most of us are taught time and again to confront fever with pain relievers such as aspirin, acetaminophen, or ibuprofen; dandruff with shampoos; and constipation with laxatives.

But what about the causes of these discomforts? Are we really taking a curative approach toward a fever if we don't recognize its origin and its purpose? Why do we have dandruff anyway? Why are our animals suffering with chronic constipation? These are questions that are addressed by the holistic herbalist—one who looks at the body as an entire, intricately balanced biocommunity of countless organs, chemicals, microorganisms, and life energies. From a holistic perspective, the herbalist realizes that all body functions are interdependent and that physical or emotional discomforts do not represent the totality of a health crisis but only the body's conveyance of an underlying imbalance or crisis—a state of "dis-ease."

Unlike conventional Western medicine, the focus of holistic healing is not to kill or cut out disease as it occurs, but to reestablish and maintain holistic homeostasis, the state of harmonious balance and rhythm among mind, body, spirit, and environment. For most of us, this involves putting some old predispositions aside, revving up the imagination, and engaging in some open-minded observation. We don't need bioscience degrees to embrace the principles of effective herbalism, but we are required to view health and healing from a much deeper perspective—one that takes into account not only the discomforts of disease but also the totality

List of Abbreviations

AAFCO: Association of American Feed Control Officials

ACTH: adrenocorticotropic hormone

AIDS: acquired immune deficiency syndrome

ASPCA: American Society for the Prevention of Cruelty to Animals

AVMA: American Veterinary Medical Association

BHA: butylated hydroxyanisole

BHT: butylated hydroxytoluene

CHV: canine herpes virus

CoQ$_{10}$: coenzyme Q$_{10}$

CPR: cardiopulmonary resuscitation

DLE: discoid lupus erythematosus

EFA: essential fatty acid

FDA: Food and Drug Administration

FeLV: feline leukemia virus

FIP: feline infectious peritonitis

FIV: feline immunodeficiency virus (also known as feline AIDS)

FUS: feline urinary syndrome

FVR: feline viral rhinotracheitis

F: Fahrenheit

FLUTD: feline lower urinary tract disease

GABA: gamma-aminobutyric acid

GBE: ginkgo biloba extract

GI: gastrointestinal

GLA: gamma-linolenic acid

G6PD: glucose-6-phosphate dehydrogenase

GST: glutathione S-transferase

HCl: hydrochloride

HCM: hypertrophic cardiomyopathy

HSV: herpes simplex virus

IU: international unit

MAOI: monoamine oxidase inhibitor

NDGA: nordihydroguaiaretic acid

PABA: para-amino benzoic acid

PAF: platelet aggregating factor

PAs: pyrrolizidine alkaloids

PDA: patent ductus arteriosus

RDA: recommended daily allowance

sp.: species (singular/not specified)

spp.: species (plural)

TCM: traditional Chinese medicine

TSH: thyroid stimulating hormone

TTouch: Tellington Touch

of wellness. From this perspective, for example, smoking is not a cause of lung cancer but a by-product of whatever prompts us to smoke in the first place. Cigarettes are only a mechanism of cellular destruction, and the tumors they feed are the end products of something insidious that lies within the psyche of the host. It is that "something" that allows us to abandon our well-being in favor of an addictive habit we all know is bad for us, and it is from this level that the healing process must begin.

Although this bit of holistic philosophy may sound simple, it is fundamentally broader than Western orthodox medicine, which centers on intervention and subsequent suppression of disease symptoms. Western society is spoiled by the concept of making problems go away quickly so we can get on with life. Rather than taking the longer route toward finding a true cure, the conventional goal is to find a quick-fix solution to the inconveniences of a crisis. Herbs are often employed in much the same capacity. The greatest healing potential of herbs, however, emanates not from their uses as natural drug alternatives but from the holistic principles and philosophies that enable us to use them in support of the natural healing mechanisms of the body.

The holistic herbalist looks beyond the symptoms of disease to identify and correct their underlying causes. An herbalist strives to understand the harmonious checks and balances that are required among all physical and nonphysical aspects of mind, body, spirit, and environment.

At the core of this tightly orchestrated synergy, we find a continual need for complete nutrition because a body must have the fuel and tools it needs to build, maintain, and repair itself. In the absence of complete nutrition, necessary tools and building blocks are missing, and the body

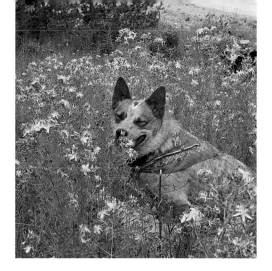

lacks the resources to make repairs and correct imbalances. In addition to complete nutrition, a body sometimes requires a specialized source of stimulation or systemic support in order to maintain a state of health and well-being. This is where herbs come in.

The holistic herbalist employs the chemical and energetic properties of plants to help bridge the gaps between what a body receives from complete nutrition and what it requires from time to time in terms of supplemental support. In this holistic context, herbs are used to stimulate, regulate, or adjust natural body functions back into healthy harmony with the rest of the body. The therapeutic effort is directed not at treating disease but at supporting the body in its efforts to correct the problem itself. In other words, herbs are used to assist the body naturally at what it is designed to do: stay healthy.

For many people, allowing the body to correct itself may not be easy because this requires trust in something that still baffles our greatest scientists: the body's remarkable, almost miraculous, ability to take care of itself. A living body, be it animal or human, represents a system of healing and health maintenance more efficient than anything devised by human intellect. To allow herbs to work at their optimum potential, the herb user must respect and honor the healing powers with which we were all born.

The Many Faces of Herbal Medicine

Many of the plants we use in Western herbalism are identical to those used in other modalities of herbal medicine. But the philosophies of how an herb interacts with the mind, body, or spirit tend to vary greatly from culture to culture. Here are some brief descriptions of three of the most popular forms of holistic medicine in which herbs are commonly employed.

• **Ayurvedic Medicine**
In India and adjacent areas of the Middle East, ayurveda has prevailed as the primary modality of healing for thousands of years. Ayurvedic medicine focuses on recognizing the doshas, the metabolic body type of an individual. The first step in ayurvedic healing is to identify the specific strengths, susceptibilities, and tendencies of the patient from a broad perspective and to take into account the entire constitution of the individual. Once these are identified, herbs, diet, meditation, or other mechanisms are used to bring the constitution of the individual back into harmonious balance with all elements of the mind, body, spirit, and environment.

• **Traditional Chinese Medicine**
Herbs have been used in traditional Chinese medicine (TCM) for at least seven thousand years. Many principles of TCM are similar to those of ayurvedic medicine. The primary

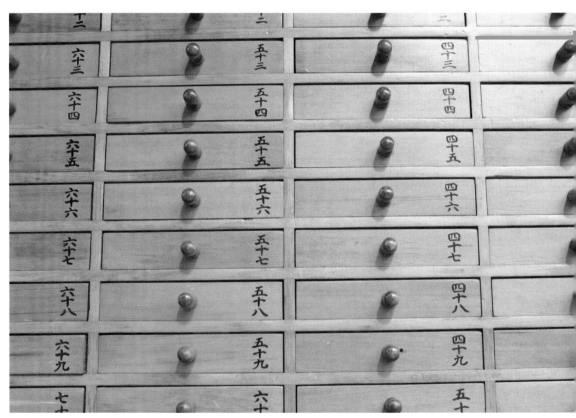

Traditional herbal cabinet at a Chinese pharmacy

difference is in how the body is viewed in terms of channels, rivers, winds, and energetic flows in TCM. In other words, the body is seen as a reflection of nature, and practitioners look for energetic blockages or disruptions—dampness, dryness, hot or cold winds, or bank breaches in the flow of *qi* (pronounced "chee"), the life force. The physical body is also viewed as a set of balanced polarities: yin, which generally refers to the tissues of the body organs, and yang, the activity of the organs. Yin and yang are opposites that cannot work independently of one another. If a yin deficiency occurs, it is because the body does not have proper nutrients or adequate physical structure to perform its functions. If a yang deficiency occurs, the body cannot react to metabolic stimuli. In TCM, herbs are used to assist and maintain proper energetic flows and polarities in the body.

• Western Herbalism

In contrast, Western herbalism seems almost superficial in nature. Western herbalism originates from ancient uses of medicinal plants in Europe. Many of the principles, philosophies, and certainly our validations of how herbs are used to effect healing are constantly evolving in this form of herbalism. For instance, the spirituality of the healer, the patient, and even the herb itself was once the primary focus of herbal medicine in ancient Europe. But today, Western herbalists incorporate many philosophies, including scientific validation of photochemical compounds, plant energetics, folkloric accounts and belief systems, and several other points of opinion.

As Western herbalists, we base our use of herbs on a balance of all philosophies. We respect and admire recent scientific validations of medicinal plant chemistries, but we also strongly believe that plants contain synergistic balances of chemical, energetic, and perhaps spiritual elements that make them unique and unexplainable. We see a great deal of value in much of the anecdotal evidence that has been handed down regarding the traditional uses of herbs over the past few millennia. Although scientific studies have failed to validate many of the claims that have been passed down through the ages, the fact that many of these customs have worked safely and effectively for thousands of people throughout several centuries is certainly convincing to us. But despite differences in opinion, most Western herbalists share a similar, holistic perspective when it comes to doing the actual work of healing.

The body is viewed from a biological perspective but with a focus that takes into account the totality of the individual. While mainstream modalities of Western medicine focus primarily on the treatment of disease and suppression of symptoms with little regard to cause, the herbalist works from the opposite direction. While working to promote health by addressing the underlying causes and providing aid to the body's efforts, the Western herbalist views the body as a tightly knit biosystem of organs, cooperative cells, microbes, enzymes, nutrients, and synergistic energies that must be maintained in a state of cooperative balance. During a disease crisis, herbs are utilized to strengthen or stimulate the body's natural functions at chemical and energetic levels so that a state of health can be reestablished quickly and efficiently. After the crisis is over, herbal tonics may then be used to strengthen body functions that are chronically deficient to avoid reoccurrence.

Herbs that are Frequently Used as Substitutes for Conventional Drugs

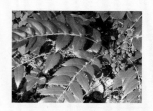

HERB	SUBSTITUTE USES
Licorice (*Glycyrrhiza glabra*)	Used as an anti-inflammatory alternative to yucca root (*Yucca schidigera*), steroidal,and nonsteroidal drugs
Black walnut (*Juglans nigra*) Wormwood (*Artemisia absinthium*)	Used in place of conventional wormers
Saint-John's-wort (*Hypericum* spp.)	Used as a natural substitute for Prozac (fluoxetine HCl)
Oregon grape (*Mahonia* spp.) Valerian (*Valeriana officinalis*)	Used as an antibiotic for eyes, ears, and mucous membranes
Skullcap (*Scutellaria laterifolia*) Passionflower (*Passiflora incarnata*) Hop (*Humulus lupulus*)	Used as alternatives to sedative drugs
Dandelion leaf (*Taraxacum officinale*)	Used in place of furosemide (Lasix)
Senna (*Cassia angustifolia*)	Used as a natural laxative

While the philosophies that lead people to the use of herbal medicines are variable worldwide, all modalities of herbal healing share two fundamental similarities. One is that the therapeutic focus is holistic, taking into account the totality of the individual instead of the symptoms of disease only. The other is that all good herbalists know that herbs work best in a proactive capacity when employed from a perspective that recognizes health maintenance as the paramount cure for disease.

HERBS AS ALTERNATIVES TO CONVENTIONAL MEDICINES

Many of us are introduced to the realm of herbal medicine by using herbs as direct replacements for over-the-counter or prescription drugs. Like drugs, herbs can be used to treat the symptoms of disease effectively. Unlike many drugs, herbs are relatively safe and gentle medicines—they are very forgiving, offering a much greater margin of error and fewer adverse side effects.

Most drugs are composed of specific chemical compounds that have been isolated from their source and concentrated to maximum potency. A medicinal plant, however, consists of dozens, sometimes thousands, of interactive or inert chemical components. Many skeptics argue that herbal medicines are less effective and unsafe because the concentrations of active constituents are too low and are variable from plant to plant.

To the herbalist, the presence of scientifically proven compounds is only part of what makes a plant useful. Instead of focusing on isolated chemical components, the herbalist accepts the inexplicable synergy that exists among all components of a plant's chemistry and all components of the physical and nonphysical recipient. In the mind of the herbalist, this is what makes herbal medicine safe, effective, and unique. The whole plant is always greater, and usually safer, than the sum of its parts.

For those who are trying to break away from conventional ways of thinking, this concept of holistic synergy can be difficult to grasp. Having been raised and trained in a science-based culture, accepting something that cannot be fully rationalized can be difficult. But to put things into a scientific perspective, let's look at thymol, the primary active constituent of thyme (*Thymus* spp.).

Thymol is potentially toxic when isolated from the rest of the thyme plant. But when employed as part of the whole plant in a tincture or tea, thymol serves as an active part of a safe and effective antimicrobial, dewormer, and cough suppressant medicine.

Anybody from any discipline of science can pick up a simple herbal remedy and use it for the purpose of treating illness. It's really very easy to substitute many of the favored conventional medicines with herbal remedies. But here are a few important things to remember.

• Keep in mind that herbs are slower acting than most drugs. Expectation of rapid results is perhaps the greatest cause of frustration and failure among would-be herbalists. The difference between a successful herbal therapy and resorting to a shot of, say, prednisolone often amounts to a day or two of patient waiting.
• When using herbs as direct replacements for allopathic medicines, don't expect results beyond those you would expect from the drugs you are replacing. The only difference in therapy when using herbs as drug substitutes is the medicinal device; the curative depth of the therapy remains the same.
• If you opt to use herbs symptomatically, it is important to remember that you will likely end up discouraged if you expect to find a cure. For example, when treating conjunctivitis that is secondary to bacterial infection, a combination eyewash of Oregon grape (*Mahonia aqui-folium*), raspberry leaf (*Rubus idaeus*), and sterile saline will effectively replace most conventional ophthalmic preparations—but just like a conventional preparation, the herbs won't address the underlying causes of a chronic problem.

HERB ACTIONS AND SPECIAL AFFINITIES

It is unrealistic to think a full conveyance of effective herbal wisdom can be contained in this book, but a large measure of awareness can be perpetuated by embracing a basic understanding of how each of these plants works within the body. In Western herbalism, the effects that plant materials have in or on the body are called "medicinal actions" or "active properties." By becoming familiar with the medicinal actions of the herbs to which you have access, you will have a good idea where to look for an appropriate course of therapy when a need for one arises. In addition to knowing the manner by which herbs work in the body, it is also important to begin learning each herb's specialty,

A Basic Start-up Apothecary
for Veterinary Applications

All of the herbs in this table are generally safe, well validated, and easy to use in a wide variety of veterinary applications. They are listed by medicinal activity, and brief comments about the areas of special usefulness are noted.

ALTERNATIVES

Herbs that gradually alter an existing condition in the body by strengthening or stimulating various systems and eliminating waste from the bloodstream. For skin and coat disorders, rheumatoid conditions, cancer, and other disorders where the body may benefit from improved elimination of toxic excess and systemic waste.

Herb	Condition
Alfalfa (*Medicago sativa*)	Arthritis, blood disorders
Burdock (*Arctium lappa*)	Seborrhea, pyoderma, rheumatoid diseases
Red clover (*Trifolium pratense*)	Tumors, blood disorders
Gotu kola (*Centella asiatica*)	Dermatitis

ANTI-INFLAMMATORIES

Herbs that help reduce inflammation

Herb	Condition
Licorice (*Glycyrrhiza glabra*)	A general anti-inflammatory for skin conditions such as arthritis
Oregon grape (*Mahonia aquifolium*)	Reduces inflammation of the eyes, mouth, and other mucous membranes
Devil's claw (*Harpagophytum procumbens*)	Arthritis and general uses
Yucca (*Yucca schidigera*)	Reduces inflammations of the joints

ANTIMICROBIALS

Herbs that inhibit reproduction and growth of harmful bacteria, fungi, or protozoa

Herb	Condition
Echinacea (*Echinacea* spp.)	Especially for the urinary tract
Oregon grape (*Mahonia aquifolium*)	General purpose (eye, nose, ear, throat, digestive, and urinary infections)
Sage (*Salvia officinalis*)	Skin and mouth infections, gingivitis
Marshmallow (*Althaea officinalis*)	Low-grade infections of the urinary tract, where inflammation is evident
Yarrow (*Achillea millefolium*)	External wounds, digestive, respiratory, and urinary tract infections

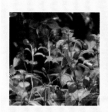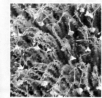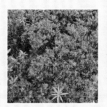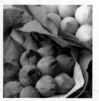

ASTRINGENTS

Herbs that reduce inflammations of the skin, eyes (conjunctivitis), and mucous membranes; treat diarrhea, irritable bowel, and colic; and tonify smooth muscles of the urinary tract and uterus

Herb	Condition
Raspberry leaf (*Rubus idaeus*)	Conjunctivitis, dermatitis, uterine tonic
Nettle (*Urtica* spp.)	Conjunctivitis, dermatitis
Plantain (*Plantago major*)	Dermatitis, gastrointestinal (GI) or urinary inflammation
Slippery elm (*Ulmus fulva*)	GI or urinary inflammation

CARDIOVASCULAR TONICS

Herbs that strengthen the physical integrity of the heart and blood vessels, moderate blood pressure, and increase circulation

Herb	Condition
Hawthorn (*Crataegus* spp.)	Strengthens cardiac output, moderates blood pressure, and increases circulation throughout the body
Ginkgo (*Ginkgo biloba*)	Improves circulation in the brain, extremities, and kidneys
Cayenne (*Capsicum* spp.)	Improves peripheral circulation and circulation in the joints
Yarrow (*Achillea millefolium*)	Improves circulation and strengthens vessel structure in the extremities

CARMINATIVES

Herbs that help relieve intestinal gas and indigestion, and are antispasmodic to the digestive tract

Herb	Condition
Fennel (*Foeniculum vulgare*)	Dyspepsia, flatulence, colic
Dill (*Anethum graveolens*)	Dyspepsia, flatulence, colic
Peppermint (*Mentha piperita*)	Dyspepsia, flatulence, colic
Chamomile (*Matricaria recutita*)	Dyspepsia, flatulence, colic

A Basic Start-up Apothecary for Veterinary Applications

DEMULCENTS

Herbs that provide a protective lubricating barrier in the digestive and urinary tracts for the passage of wastes and to help relieve irritation of mucous membranes

Herb	Condition
Marshmallow (*Althaea officinalis*)	Respiratory, digestive, and urinary irritations
Plantain (*Plantago major*)	Respiratory, digestive, and urinary irritations
Slippery elm (*Ulmus fulva*)	Respiratory, digestive, urinary irritations
Ginkgo (*Ginkgo biloba*)	Urinary irritations

DIURETICS

Herbs that stimulate diuresis in kidney disorders and water retention problems and help eliminate excess waste and superfluous materials from the body and urinary tract

Herb	Condition
Dandelion leaf (*Taraxacum officinale*)	The strongest herbal diuretic available
Corn silk (*Zea mays*)	For calculi
Shepherd's purse (*Capsella bursa-pastoris*)	Especially good for water retention secondary to rheumatoid conditions

IMMUNOTONICS

Herbs that stimulate and support immune system functions

Herb	Condition
Echinacea (*Echinacea* spp.)	For early onset of bacterial or viral infections
Astragalus (*Astragalus membranaceous*)	A better-tasting but general alternative to echinacea; especially good for problems involving weak kidney function

LYMPHATICS

Herbs that assist with lymph production and circulation; drain and heal lymph-engorged tissues and masses (tumors, cysts, ulcers); useful in the systemic treatment of chronic dermatitis

Herb	Condition
Cleavers (*Galium aparine*)	Digestive and urinary cysts, ulcers
Red clover (*Trifolium pratense*)	Cysts and tumors of the skin; swollen lymph nodes

NERVINES AND SEDATIVES

Herbs that suppress or moderate nervous tension and anxiety or that moderate or suppress activity in higher brain centers

Herb	Condition
Skullcap (*Scutellaria* spp.)	For jittery anxiety; to help reduce severity f seizures; to relieve pain
Valerian (*Valeriana officinalis*)	For acute anxiety and hyperactivity; to help reduce severity of seizures; to relieve pain
Passionflower (*Passiflora incarnata*)	A relaxing mood elevator; for fear, for posttraumatic depression, and as a good alternative for animals who respond unfavorably to valerian
Saint-John's-wort (*Hypericum* spp.)	For nerve injuries
Oat straw (*Avena sativa*)	An especially good nervous system tonic for older animals

NUTRITIVES

Herbs that lend rich nutritional values; especially good for anemia and mineral deficiencies

Herb	Condition
Nettle (*Urtica* spp.)	Broad-spectrum minerals, vitamins, and proteins
Alfalfa (*Medicago sativa*)	Broad-spectrum minerals, vitamins, and proteins
Flaxseed (*Linum* spp.)	Rich source of omega-3 essential fatty acids (EFAs)
Dandelion (*Taraxacum officinale*)	Broad-spectrum minerals (especially potassium), vitamins, and proteins

VULNERARIES

Herbs that promote healing, internally or externally

Herb	Condition
Aloe vera (*Aloe* spp.)	Externally for burns, wounds, dermatitis; internally for ulcers
Arnica (*Arnica* spp.)	For external treatment of closed-tissue injuries only
Comfrey (*Symphytum officinale*)	For external use on open- and closed-tissue injuries
Calendula (*Calendula officinalis*)	For dermatitis, burns, wounds
Saint-John's-wort (*Hypericum perforatum*)	For crushing soft-tissue injuries and any type of trauma where nerve damage is evident

or systemic affinity—its special kinship with certain portions of the anatomy. For instance, we may know that slippery elm has a general astringent action (meaning that it shrinks tissues), but its effective usefulness can be really pronounced when we know that it has a special affinity to the digestive tract, where its astringent actions are particularly well suited to shrinking the inner wall of the small intestine to relieve diarrhea and other discomforts.

DOSAGE AND DURATION OF THERAPY

The dosage suggestions provided in this book represent what we feel are safe and conservative starting points for use in most animals. The exact dosage and duration of an herb therapy that your companion may need depends on the animal's specific needs, tolerances, and metabolism. In other words, the answers to how much and for how long may vary from animal to animal. Some animals respond favorably to very small doses—perhaps just a drop or two of tincture. Others require larger doses or may not respond to certain herbs at all (as you know, such is the case with drugs too). Therefore, a conservative starting point for administration of herb extracts, infusions, or dried herbs in dogs, cats, and herbivores is to use only one or two herbs at a time and to proportion the dosage based on the animal's body weight compared to the recommended human dosage. For example, a 30-pound dog would receive one-fifth of that which is recommended for a 150-pound human. Also to be considered is your veterinarian's opinion, a reputable reference book, or the product manufacturer's recommendations.

Remember, this is just a starting point. Dogs, cats, and other carnivores have much faster metabolic rates than we do; therefore, initial dosages might have to be increased later to achieve the results you are looking for. The biggest mistake is to think of dosing in terms of absolutes. Instead, watch the animal you are treating; read up on the side effects, contraindications, and active nature of the herbs you are using; and don't hesitate to change dosages. If you need to increase a dosage, do so in 10 percent increments to a maximum of 50 percent above the starting dose. In other words, if you have determined that the starting dose for "Max" is 20 drops of burdock, twice daily, then you can increase the dose 2 drops at a time until you reach 30 drops, if necessary. If a dosage needs to be decreased (if, for example, valerian causes acute vomiting in your cat), cut the dose in half. If you feel it's necessary, stop the therapy altogether for a day or two, and let the animal's body readjust before proceeding with the reduced dosage. Most animals require a dose two to three times daily.

The duration of an herbal therapy also depends on the specific animal and varies according to the disease you are confronting. Generally, it is best to take at least a two-day break from herbal therapies each week (five days on, two days off). This allows you to monitor the animal's responses to the herbs and to alleviate any tolerance or toxicity problems she may otherwise develop as a result of long-term use. The duration required to see results varies greatly and is dependent on the nature of the herb, the animal, and the severity of the imbalance you are confronting. If results don't begin to materialize after you have maintained a maximum dosage schedule for more than seven days, it may be time to try another herb or to consult your holistic veterinarian. In any case, keep detailed records of your successes, failures, and observations. Exactly how long to maintain an herbal therapy can be determined only through experience and familiarity with your animal, and good record keeping is instrumental to becoming an effective herbalist.

A Few Words About Toxicity

Serious adverse reactions are rare, but when used outside the parameters of common sense and moderation, any plant can be toxic.

Toxicity is dose dependent, relative to the rate of absorption and the individual's ability to assimilate or eliminate an excess. If a body receives a substance in quantities or concentrations that cannot be effectively dealt with by its natural functions, the excess must be dealt with by emergency means. Vomiting, diarrhea, and other purgative functions are then triggered to eliminate the invasive substance(s). If this fails, systemic shutdown or damage may occur.

Most herbs that are commonly used in veterinary medicine are safe and forgiving—in most cases in which an animal is hypersensitive to an herb or has received too much, she will vomit shortly after administration. Other common indicators of toxicity include itching, photosensitivity, and diarrhea.

The key word in the avoidance of toxic reactions is moderation. Although herbs are generally weaker and gentler medicines than most drugs, they still demand respect. "More" is not necessarily "better," even in the employment of nutritive "food-medicine" herbs such as nettle (*Urtica* spp.), alfalfa (*Medicago* sativa), or flaxseed (*Linum* spp.). All of these herbs may cause digestive upset

and dermatological reactions if fed to the animal in large quantities.

Aside from the issues of overdose and prolonged use, it is important to remember that some animals may have allergies to certain herbs; a few are especially sensitive to certain plant substances; and some have preexisting conditions. Therefore, to be safe, it's always a good idea to proceed with caution. Start with a small dose, and watch the animal for any signs of adverse reaction.

When to Take Your Pet to the Vet

This book is aimed at enabling you to be somewhat self-sufficient in ensuring the health and welfare of your companion animals. However, there are some problems that caregivers should not attempt to treat on their own at home. Some of these include life-threatening situations such as poisonings; major traumas such as those caused by being hit by a car; bleeding; broken bones; instances when the condition you're treating at home doesn't get better in a few days; and cases in which there are questions or other avenues of treatment to be taken.

Most of us believe that our animals must be seen by a vet in order to get treatment. In many cases this is true. But holistic vets can't be found in all areas of the U.S., so it becomes necessary for some of us to consult

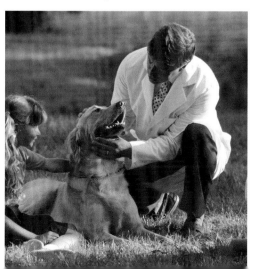

Cautions, Contraindications, and Potential Side Effects

The following chart lists a few of the most common types of problematic plant compounds to be aware of in the natural care of animals. This list is intended for the purpose of cautious awareness. It is by no means complete, and the presence of one or more of these compounds in a specific herb does not necessarily exclude that herb from safe use.

ANTHRAQUINONES

Anthraquinones, including dianthrone glycosides, sennosides, aloe-emoden, chysophanol, among others, are the active laxative constituents that are present in aloe (certain preparations), senna (*Cassia senna*), cascara sagrada, and turkey rhubarb (*Rheum palmatum*). Anthraquinones act as laxatives by stimulating intestinal peristalsis and may cause cramping and severe diarrhea if misused. These compounds are hard on the liver and kidneys, and extended use of anthraquinone-bearing herbs may lead to dependency.

COUMARINS

Coumarins include coumarin, medicagol, furanocoumarins, among others. Most coumarin-bearing plants do not contain enough coumarins to represent a risk in normal therapeutic doses. Large doses of coumarins, however, can cause photosensitivity. Coumarins are known to thin the blood and may potentiate the effects of anticoagulant drugs. Coumarin-rich herbs such as red clover (*Trifolium pratense*) and alfalfa (*Medicago sativa*) should not be given to animals with clotting disorders.

OXALIC ACID AND OXALATES

Oxalic acid and oxalates are present in many plants (a small amount is even present in fresh spinach), but can be found especially in members of the Polygonaceae and Cruciferae families. Oxalic acid is characterized by a tart, lemony flavor and is especially evident in the leaves of sheep sorrel (*Rumex acetosella*) and French sorrel (*Rumex scutatus*). Oxalic acid can cause urinary tract irritation, can deplete the body of vitamin B_1, and is known to bind with calcium in the urine—thus potentially causing stones. Although the oxalic acid content of most herbs, such as yellow dock root (*Rumex crispus*), is generally small and usually will not cause a problem with moderately dosed, short-term use (up to fourteen days), it is best to avoid such herbs in cases of preexisting kidney or urinary disease.

PYRROLIZIDINE ALKALOIDS

Pyrrolizidine alkaloids are present in many plants but most notably in comfrey (*Symphytum officinale*). Most PA-bearing plants have received an undeserved bad name; it takes doses that are dozens of times in excess of a therapeutic quantity to cause hepatotoxic effects—especially in a healthy liver. Nonetheless, there are documented cases of liver damage (in both human and animal modalities) as a result of comfrey overuse.

There are hundreds of different alkaloid compounds present in thousands of medicinal plant species—many are generally safe; some present a risk of toxicity. Many present themselves as the primary active constituent of a plant. Perhaps the most frequently employed alkaloid in Western herbal medicine is berberine, the bitter yellow substance that is found in Oregon grape (*Mahonia* spp.), goldenseal (*Hydrastis canadensis*), and a few other plants. Berberine is generally safe, but overuse of berberine-rich plants may overstimulate bile production (especially in cats), resulting in vomiting. Berberine is contraindicated in pregnant or lactating animals.

SALICYLATES

Salicylates, including salicylaldehyde, salicin, methyl salicylate, salicylic acid, among others, are the precursors to acetylsalicylate (aspirin). This means that herbs such as willow bark (*Salix* spp.), meadowsweet (*Filipendula ulmaria*), poplar (*Populus* spp.), and others must be used with extreme caution in felines or other animals who are sensitive to aspirin.

SAPONINS

There are hundreds of different saponin (soaplike) constituents in various plants. Most notably, saponins are among the primary active constituents in valerian (*Valeriana officinalis*), licorice (*Glycyrrhiza* spp.), sarsaparilla (*Smilax* spp.), and yucca root (*Yucca* spp.). Saponins are characterized by their foaming, soapy nature. Although they seldom present any problems, excessive or extended use of saponin-rich herbs can produce GI irritation and vomiting, and some may eventually interfere with the absorption of fat-soluble vitamins.

STEROLS

Sterols include ß-sitosterol, stigmasterol, ampesterol, among others. Some plants, such as licorice, that contain large concentrations of phytosterols or steroidal saponins can cause problems, such as water retention and hypertension, similar to those presented by steroidal drugs but only if used excessively or over an extended period. The side effects of phytosterols are much harder to procure, and can be largely avoided by occasional breaks in the therapy (for example, five days on, two off) and with concurrent use of diuretic herbs such as dandelion leaf and alterative herbs such as dandelion root and burdock.

TANNINS

Tannins such as corilagin pyranoside, ellagic acid, and gallic acid are found in the bark and leaves of many herbs and are the most frequently employed astringents of the plant world. Herbs that are especially tannin rich include uva ursi (*Arctostaph los uva-ursi*), any part of the juniper (*Juniperis* spp.) plant, black walnut hulls (*Juglans nigra*), and white oak bark (*Quercus* sp.). Tannins are typically used to reduce inflammations of mucous membranes in the digestive and urinary tracts, but if used excessively they can have a reverse effect, causing mucosal irritation. Herbs that contain tannins should not be used in animals with inflammatory kidney disease. Some tannins are labor inducing (oxytocic) and may cause abortion in pregnant animals.

Cautions, Contraindications, and Potential Side Effects (continued)

VOLATILE OILS

Volatile oils include myristicin, apiole, terpineol, sesquiterpenes, menthone, pulegone, piperidinone, thujone, jugulone, 3-octanol, among others. There are hundreds of volatile oil compounds, many of which make up the aromatic principles of a plant, present in thousands of plant species. Menthol, for example, is a volatile oil found in members of the mint family. The medicinal activities and toxicology of volatile oils are widely variable, but most have an effect on the genitourinary and digestive tracts, causing irritation to the kidneys and urinary passages when used in large quantities. Others, such as the pulegone found in pennyroyal (*Mentha pulegium*) or the myristicin and apiole found in parsley seed (*Petroselinum crispum*) and nutmeg seed (*Myristica fragrans*), are potentially hepatotoxic and nephrotoxic if used in overabundance. Volatile oils have been shown to cross the placenta barrier to adversely affect the fetus of pregnant animals.

The s-methyl cysteine sulfoxide and n-propyl disuldhide contained in garlic has been shown to produce Heinz-body anemia, a serious blood disorder, if the cloves are consumed in excess of 0.5 percent of the subject animal's body weight. This means that a healthy 60-pound dog would have to eat several cloves of garlic just to start the Heinz-body process. The problem is dose dependent, meaning that blood structure quickly normalizes when garlic use is reduced or discontinued.

with a vet over the telephone. Some holistic veterinarians do provide telephone consultations, but many don't. No matter, it's wise to have a local vet to whom you can take your animals in case of a major trauma or if surgery is needed.

Basics of Herbal Preparations

The manner in which an herb is used is determined by a holistic assessment of the particular circumstances at hand and the overall nature of the animal. Once you have investigated the origins of the symptoms that have caught your attention, you can select the medicinal actions you need to confront the problem. This leads you to one or more herbs that have a specific affinity to the body systems that are involved.

Choosing the correct herb to fit therapeutic circumstances is critical not only to the effective treatment of disease but also to the conservation of botanical resources. Many plant species are currently at risk of extinction because they have been touted as "curative silver bullets." But in reality, there are no cure-all herbs. In fact, no single herb serves as a definitive cure for anything. For an herb to be used effectively and responsibly, it should be used only within the true confines of its therapeutic capacity. It also must be used in a form or preparation that is complementary to its medicinal attributes and the task at hand.

Each herb's physical and chemical structures determine how the herb should be prepared and subsequently administered. For instance, many herbs are very water soluble, which means that if you pour hot water over them, their medicinal constituents quickly and completely infuse into the water, making their desired chemical attributes freely available for the body to absorb and use. Many other herbs, however, are poorly water soluble, which means that if you pour hot water over them to make an infusion, little or nothing of medicinal value is drawn from the plant's tissues.

Following is an introduction to the basic how-tos of making herbal preparations. Those of you who collect books will find that compared to other books on herbal medicines, the guidelines we offer here are loose. We have done this for the sake of practicality and simplicity. While exact measurements and strict procedures are necessary measures of quality control in the commercial production of herbal products, the self-reliant herbalist really doesn't have to worry so much about precision. As long as there's enough herb, a strong- enough solvent, and the correct type of preparation, you will be rewarded with a good, strong herbal medicine.

DRIED BULK HERB MATERIAL
Dried bulk herbs are handy to have around because they allow for a great deal of diversity in how they can be prepared and applied. In addition to being used in various herb preparations, some dried herbs can be sprinkled directly onto an animal's food. As a general rule, roots keep two to three times longer than dried leaf material. But don't stock up on more than you can use within one year, and be sure to store your herbs in airtight containers that are kept away from sunlight. Regardless of proper storage methods, dried herbs eventually oxidize and lose their potency. A few herbs lose much of their medicinal and nutritive value within days of drying. Buy herbs from an honest, knowledgeable herbalist who knows the origin of his or her merchandise, or grow your own herbs to assure optimum potency and shelf life.

FRESH HERBS
Fresh herbs, clipped, dug, or plucked directly from a garden, are rich in nutrients and medicinal constituents. Provided that their physical nature allows for the form of preparation you need, fresh herbs are without compare in terms of medicinal potency. While most herbs are strong when used fresh, others require at least partial drying before they impart their active components into a useful medium. Cascara sagrada (*Rhamnus purshiana*) bark is one example. This herbal laxative is far too strong if used fresh and should be dried for at least a full year to mellow it before use. It is also poorly water soluble when fresh, and until it dries it will not infuse adequately in water for a good tea.

HERB CAPSULES
Because dogs and cats have short digestive tracts, encapsulated herbs tend to pass right through them. Even if they don't, you may find some difficulty in getting a large enough dose into your animal. In horses, sheep, llamas, goats, and other herbivores, capsules work fine—but plan on feeding the animals dozens of them. In these animals, you are often better off feeding the bulk herb or using an extract.

ALCOHOL EXTRACTS, OR TINCTURES
With few exceptions, an alcohol tincture is by far the most versatile, strongest, and most readily usable form of herb

preparation. It can be administered orally; used in topical applications; diluted with water; or used as part of an eye, hair, or skin rinse.

A tincture is prepared by soaking a measured quantity of fresh or dried herb in a certain proportion of alcohol and water, using a specific formula for each herb. The alcohol serves as a solvent that breaks down the plant material and releases the active ingredients into a liquid base called a menstruum. After two days to two weeks (depending on the method used) the menstruum is then strained and pressed from the plant material (called the marc), to produce the finished liquid product. Alcohol tinctures offer the advantages of maximum potency and unlimited shelf life provided they are stored properly.

The concentrated liquid nature of tincture preparations allows for their quick and complete absorption into the body, even in the short digestive tracts of dogs and cats. When kept in 1-ounce dropper bottles, they can be carried anywhere and are easy to use. The biggest problem with alcohol tinctures is getting them into an animal. These preparations are typically 30–70 percent grain alcohol, and while typical dosages do not present any alcohol-toxicity problems, animals truly hate the way they taste.

There are two basic methods for making tinctures: one is a process called percolation, the other, simpler method, is called maceration. The percolation method entails using a specially designed, cone-shaped glass vessel. Herb material is placed into the cone, then the menstruum is poured over it, left to stand for a short while, and eventually allowed to trickle (or percolate) through the plant material and out a tube at the bottom end of the vessel.

Making herb tinctures by maceration takes more time, but it is much simpler and requires no specialized equipment. To make a macerated tincture, herb material is placed into a glass jar, plastic container, or other nonmetallic container. The menstruum is poured over the herb and the entire mixture is covered with an airtight lid and allowed to soak for a period of two weeks. The menstruum is then strained from the plant material (the marc), to produce the finished liquid product.

The proportions of alcohol and water needed to make an herb tincture vary according to the solubility of the herb itself. Some herbs, such as milk thistle seed, require a high percentage of alcohol to extract optimum quantities of active constituents from their cell structures. Other herbs, such as raspberry leaf, require little or no alcohol to extract their useful compounds. Fortunately, knowing what percentage of alcohol you need is easy because these determinations have already been done for you. Most of the formulas used in contemporary herbal practice are from the *U.S. Pharmacopoeia*

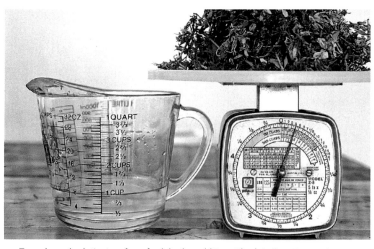

To make an herb tincture from fresh herbs, add 1 part herb to 2 parts menstruum.

and other standard references that have been used in the pharmaceutical production of simple herb extracts throughout most of the twentieth century. This information is still used by herbalists and laboratories throughout the world and can be found in several books about herbs and herbalism.

The amount of menstruum needed to extract the active constituents from a plant also varies. With most fresh (un-dried) herbs, you will need a 1:2 ratio of herbs to menstruum. Most dried herb materials require a 1:5 ratio. This means that to make a tincture from the fresh root of dandelion, you need one part of chopped herb material (by weight) to two parts of menstruum (by liquid volume). For example, 16 ounces of fresh root must be covered with 32 fluid ounces of menstruum to make a tincture (and the menstruum must be at least 40 percent alcohol). If you are using dried root, 16 ounces of dried root material will require 80 fluid ounces of menstruum to make a tincture. Make sense? Don't worry if it doesn't; we'll simplify in a moment. So how does one make a menstruum?

The most accurate and inexpensive way to make a menstruum is to buy pure grain alcohol (brand named Everclear) at a liquor store. Everclear is 95 percent pure grain alcohol (190 proof). For simplicity, let's just call it a pure, 100 percent alcohol. To make a 70 percent alcohol menstruum, we would add 30 percent water to its volume (i.e., add 3 parts water to 7 parts alcohol). If it's a 50 percent menstruum we need, then all we have to do is add an equal (50/50) amount of water. It's that simple. Unfortunately, Everclear isn't available in some portions of the U.S., so a medicine maker may have to do some liquor shopping. For tinctures that require 70 percent alcohol, uncut 151 proof rum works fine (it's 75 percent alcohol). For a 50 percent menstruum, you can use 100 proof vodka (it's 50 percent alcohol), and so forth.

Now here's the simplified version of medicine making we promised. Get some fresh or dried herb, chop it up or grind it as fine as possible, put it in a container, then add enough menstruum (of the appropriate strength) to just barely cover the herb. Cover the container, then let it sit for two weeks, strain the mixture through a cloth, and store the liquid in an airtight glass jar. Amber glass is best because it blocks ultraviolet rays that may damage your tincture. You now have an herb tincture. The primary rule in this simplified method of making tincture is always to use the correct percentage of alcohol in your menstruum. If you do, you will always end up with a nice tincture by covering a maximum amount of chopped or ground herb with a minimum amount of menstruum.

GLYCERIN-BASED HERB EXTRACTS, OR GLYCERITES

Glycerites are made essentially the same way as alcohol extracts, but a solution of 60 percent vegetable glycerin and 40 percent water is used in place of alcohol. The big advantage of glycerites in animal care is their palatability—glycerin tastes sweet, with a flavor and consistency similar to light corn syrup. While some glycerin-based extracts are not as potent as their alcohol counterparts, they allow pet owners to get the herbs into their animals in the first place—hence, half the battle is won. Potency can then be adjusted by increasing the dosage. Vegetable glycerin is refined from coconut oils, and despite its syrupy-sweet flavor, it is metabolized in a manner similar to that of triglycerides, not sugar. This means it can be used safely in animals with alcohol sensitivity or in those with diabetes. Glycerites do not keep indefinitely but remain viable for at least two years if refrigerated.

The biggest disadvantages of glycerites are their limited shelf life (one to two years) and, in many cases, their strength. Glycerin is not as strong a solvent as alcohol, and many herbs are not taken up well into a glycerin menstruum, especially if they are of a resinous nature. However, some herbs, especially those that are highly water soluble, release their active ingredients into glycerin very well. To find out if a particular herb that interests you is good for making glycerites, refer to one or more of the books we recommend at the end of this section.

WATER INFUSIONS (HERB TEAS)

Infusions are made by steeping a specific quantity of plant material in hot water. The disadvantages of using teas internally for animals are twofold: many animals don't like tea, and it can be difficult to feed an animal enough tea to bring about therapeutic results. Unlike tinctures, which provide a plant's active constituents in a highly concentrated, fully assimilable form, teas generally amount to a weaker medicine, and plant compounds that are not water soluble are not imparted to the animal.

Infusions are especially useful for skin and coat rinses and as vitamin- and mineral-rich tonic food supplements. When mixed into an animal's food, an herb tea provides most of what a dried or fresh herb offers in a form that is quickly and more easily absorbed into the body. Herb teas also offer the advantage of melding with the flavor of an animal's diet without adding a new texture to the food— an important attribute for those who wish to feed nutritive herbs to a finicky feline.

DECOCTIONS

A decoction is an infusion that requires some gentle simmering to make a strong enough preparation for therapeutic use. Decoction is required of many roots when the plant material is too insoluble in water to allow a

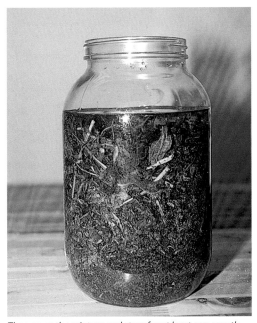

Completely cover the herb with olive oil to make an oil infusion.

Then cover the mixture and store for at least one month.

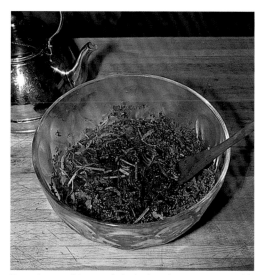

To make a poultice, mash the herb with water or vegetable oil until it forms a paste.

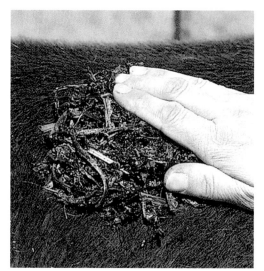

Then you can apply the poultice directly to your animal's skin or fur.

strong enough infusion. Decoctions should be prepared using a minimum of heat. Simmer the herb for about fifteen minutes at a temperature that is only slightly above the boiling point. Too much heat destroys many of the plant constituents you wish to employ. Decoctions are used in the same manner as water infusions, but they tend to be strong in comparison.

OIL INFUSIONS

An oil infusion is produced by completely covering an herb with olive oil and allowing it to steep in a covered nonmetallic container in a warm location for at least one month. The oil is then pressed out and stored in the refrigerator for up to one year. Although several choices of oil can be used, olive oil possesses its own preservative qualities, is relatively affordable, and is nourishing to the body, both internally and externally. Oil infusions are excellent for topical applications, acting to soothe and protect the affected area while holding the herb

constituents at the site where they are applied. Extra caution should be used when applying oil to burns or infected areas because it may seal in heat and bacteria.

In these cases, make sure that the possibility of infection has been addressed with a good, clean antimicrobial preparation and the burn has entirely cooled before anything is applied.

POULTICES

A poultice is made by mashing plant material (usually dried foliage) with enough water or vegetable oil to make a wet, pesto-like paste. Poultices are good in topical field applications when other preparations are impossible to make. A simple poultice can be applied directly to an animal's skin, or it can be made into a compress that can be secured onto the animal. To make a compress, wrap the wet poultice in a piece of clean cloth, allowing the liquid to freely soak through the cloth. Wrap the compress onto the affected body part and secure with knots.

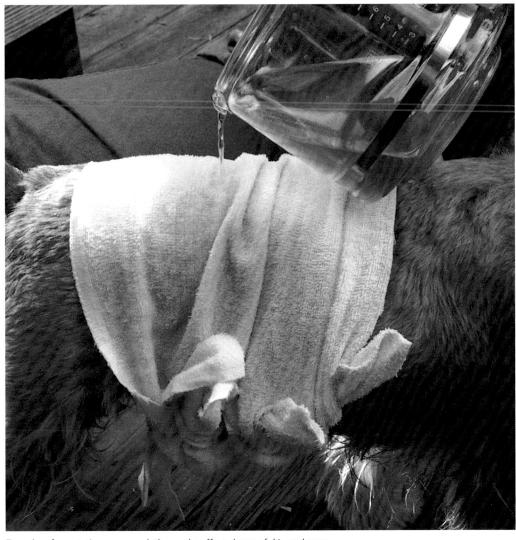

To make a fomentation, secure a cloth over the affected area of skin and pour the infusion over it until the cloth is soaked.

SALVES AND OINTMENTS

Salves and ointments are simply thickened oil infusions. In making salves, beeswax is frequently used as the thickening agent. The thinner ointment preparations typically employ coconut butter, particularly if the ointments are to be used in suppository applications. The oil infusion is gently heated, and the beeswax or coconut butter is melted into the liquid until the cooled product yields the consistency that is desired.

For salves, use a ratio of 1 ounce of beeswax or cocoa butter to 8 ounces of oil. If the salve or ointment turns out to be too thick or thin when it has cooled, gently reheat it and adjust the proportion of beeswax or cocoa butter. Suppository molds and salve tins are available through herb catalogs and at some drugstores.

As with oil infusions, extra caution should be used when applying salves or ointments to areas of the body that are burned or infected. In these cases, make sure that a good, clean antimicrobial preparation is used and that the burn has cooled completely before applying any kind of topical treatment to the area.

FOMENTATIONS

A fomentation is used for topical applications where a water or oil infusion must remain on a particular body site for a specific period. Gauze or another cloth material is placed over the area, and the infusion is poured onto the dressing until it is soaked. Mustard packs, castor oil packs, and other traditional remedies employ this method. This is a good approach for horses with fungal infections of the skin or other animals who don't mind "wearing" an herbal ornament for a while.

STANDARDIZED EXTRACTS

A standardized extract is more of a plant drug than an herbal medicine. These preparations are made by scientifically increasing the content of certain active ingredients in order to bring about specific therapeutic effects. This is done by removing a desired active ingredient from the chemistry of a particular plant species, then adding it back to the extract at much higher concentration. For example, in nature, milk thistle seeds contain anywhere from 2 percent to 6 percent silymarin, the most medicinally active component of the plant. In cases of severe liver damage or toxicity, a much higher percentage of silymarin may be needed to quickly bring about a therapeutic effect. A milk thistle extract that has been "standardized" to as much as 80 percent

silymarin can be used in such cases.

On the surface, standardized extracts may seem like a superior form of herbal medicine. In the aforementioned example in which milk thistle is indicated, this is absolutely true. However, it's important to remember that when we standardize an herb we alter its physical and energetic nature. Our manipulation of its nature is based on our scientific understanding of only one or a few of its chemical components. In its natural form, each herb is composed of hundreds of chemical components that are arranged in a unique, synergistic manner that cannot be replicated by science. It is this synergy that makes herbs a mysteriously effective form of medicine. Every time that we alter the chemistry of an herb, we change everything that the herb represents in terms of a natural and holistic medicine. To the holistic herbalist, the question is not so much what can be gained by standardizing an herb but rather how much is lost in the process.

The bottom line is that standardized extracts are best reserved only for specific indications—they do not represent a complete form of herbal medicine.

The Connection between Herbs and Diet

To use herbs to the best of their potential, we must take on a holistic perspective of health and healing that views all components of mind, body, spirit, and environment as equal parts of an individual's well-being. At the core of this "whole body" perspective is a good diet. Without balanced nutrition, the use of herbal medicines in the holistic care of your animal is a waste of time, money, and plants.

The food that your animal eats should provide all of the nutritional components that are necessary for all organs and systems of a healthy body to perform in

A General Herbal Dietary Adjunct

Combine equal parts of the following:

spirulina
nettle
dandelion leaf
alfalfa
powdered flaxseed

This formula can be fed at a rate of 1 teaspoon per pound of food fed daily (½ teaspoon daily for cats) as an adjunct to a natural diet. While it may not fill all of an animal's supplemental nutrition needs, it will complement his diet with foodlike concentrations of fully assimilable protein, vitamin C, B complex (including B$_{12}$), vitamin A (beta-carotene), vitamin E, vitamin K, iron, potassium, calcium, phosphorus, magnesium, and omega-3 fatty acids.

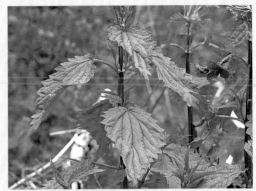

Nettle is a good source of potassium.

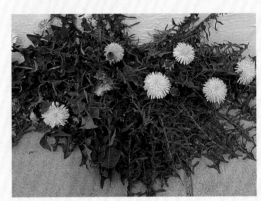

Dandelion flowers are rich in lecithin.

harmonious unison. A properly functioning body does an amazing job of preventing disease and healing itself, and to do this it requires the energies and nutrients of a well-balanced diet. However, sometimes the body needs special measures of outside support to optimize its healing efforts to assist the body at working harder, faster, longer, or more efficiently toward reestablishing a balanced state of holistic health. Enter herbs.

In the holistic context in which they are used most effectively, herbs serve as functional adjuncts to good nutrition by helping the body to use its innate and acquired resources more effectively. For example, echinacea does not act as a substitute for the body's immune system but serves to stimulate the body's natural defenses into working harder, thus boosting the body's abilities to resist infection. Likewise, herbs such as dandelion root, Oregon grape, and burdock assist in the elimination of waste from the body by stimulating the liver and gallbladder into working more efficiently. These supportive functions are diet dependent: in order for an herb to call upon the body to do something extraordinary, there must be an adequate store of energy and building materials with which the body can work.

Many people use herbs only for treating the symptoms of a disease in the absence of adequate nutrition and without considering the whole being. For instance, if we use an herbal ear oil externally to treat a chronic ear infection without addressing why the body is unable to fight the infection by itself, we are not using a holistic approach toward healing. Instead, we are treating only the symptoms of a disorder that emanates from the body's inability to defend itself. While the ear oil may inhibit the external microbial cause of the infection, it is really doing nothing more than serving as a natural alternative to any number of pharmaceutical preparations that may be able to alleviate symptoms more quickly. However, if our goals are to reach beyond the symptoms to affect the underlying causes of disease, the healing effort must begin by ensuring that the body is afforded everything it needs to heal itself. In other words, we must provide the body with the foundation of holistic health—complete nutrition—before our healing efforts with herbal medicines can begin to approach curative results.

Using Nutritive Herbs as Dietary Supplements

Many herbs are foods, and some provide nutritional qualities in such abundance that they can be used as nutritional medicines or dietary supplements. Herbs provide minerals, vitamins, fatty acids, and other nutritional components in a form that a body can fully utilize without becoming burdened with excess. Dandelion leaves, for instance, contain impressive amounts of potassium and iron but not so much as to present a risk of toxicity. With nutritive herbs, the body is given the chance to take the nutrients it needs and easily eliminate what it does not, unlike many highly concentrated vitamin supplements that force the liver, kidneys, and digestive tract to work overtime at their jobs of eliminating the excess. On the other hand, the nutritional content of herbs may vary considerably from plant to plant, and in therapeutic or dietary situations where high concentrations of specific vitamins or minerals must be guaranteed, herbs usually prove to be inadequate.

Many herbs can be used as nutritional adjuncts to a good diet. Finding which nutritive herbs are best for the needs of an individual animal comes from the one-on-one experience of the caregiver with his or her animal, but a simple dried herb formula that can be used for most dogs, cats, horses, ferrets, and other animals can be found in the box on page 38.

The Ethical Use of Herbs

We are living in a time when millions of people are turning away from anything they perceive as artificial, unhealthy, or forced upon them. A huge natural health care industry has arisen, fueled by people who are eager to embrace products, healing methods, and lifestyles that offer a healing step back toward nature. On the surface of this "green revolution," more people are becoming aware of the curative possibilities that exist beneath the trees, and a renewed sense of hope for a healthy environment has been born. But in many ways, this scenario also brings about a whole new level of environmental crisis. While a great deal of promise may exist in our growing awareness of earth's natural treasures, our journey toward "getting back to basics" is consuming resources faster than we can learn to replace

Basic Ethical Guidelines
for the Harvesting of Wild Plants

Follow these ethical guidelines if you wish to have the least impact on our earth while harvesting medicinal plants from wild areas.

• Never gather endangered or environmentally sensitive species. Many plants are abundant in certain areas but relatively rare in others. Learn to recognize and use plant species in your home bioregion that are abundant and resilient to human impact, while taking into account that the ecological niche you see is a small, unique part of a much larger environmental picture. Get to know the general status of the plants you are interested in from a global perspective. You may find that as an "ecoherbalist," your role among certain plants around your home is strictly that of guardian.

• Be absolutely certain of plant identification before you harvest. Gathering the wrong plants not only may be harmful to you and your pets but may be wasteful and potentially damaging to the ecosystem as well.

• Collect a small amount of plant material from several different stands to minimize your impact. Never gather so much from a stand of plants that you can see a difference after your harvest. Remember, mathematical solutions to the number of plants that can be ethically harvested do not apply in the natural realm. The only way to determine how much is ethically acceptable is to begin learning about the ecology of your bioregion before you harvest. Observe your impact over a long period of time, and always gather conservatively.

• Never gather from a group of plants until you have thoroughly investigated the health, welfare, sustainability, and interdependent elements of the entire area. Is there a healthier stand nearby? Is the stand large enough to sustain your impact? Do you know the ecosystem well enough to harvest plants in a manner that is conducive to its health? What may seem to be a lush, healthy stand of plants may in fact be a biocommunity in trouble. Walk, look, listen, feel, and, most important, learn as much as you can about the ways of the land before you begin your harvest.

• Never gather more than you can conservatively use, bearing in mind that many herbs lose their potency quickly after harvest. Unless you plan to make alcohol tinctures, expect no more than six months to a year of shelf life for properly dried and stored herbs.

• Always ask permission before entering private lands, even if you are doing the landowner a favor by pulling a few weeds. Check with your local land management agencies for permit requirements before you begin gathering herbs from public lands.

- Keep a journal of your observations during each visit to a harvest site and learn to work within nature's capacity. Remember, you will always be a student in nature, and there are no absolutes in how an ecosystem operates. Maintain a set of wildcrafting site records, and keep a detailed log for each wildcrafting venture. From these records, you can monitor your long-term impacts while enriching your awareness of nature.

- Gather only from areas that are endemic to the plants you are looking for. Learn the typical elevation, habitat, soil composition, exposure, and climatic requirements of each plant you wish to harvest, then harvest from areas that match these criteria. Small, isolated stands of plants that have adapted to an unusual set of environmental circumstances are particularly vulnerable to human impact and should be used for learning, not for medicine making.

- Learn the environmental issues of your area, and familiarize yourself with other people who have an interest in the wild lands you will be working within, including other herbalists, the logging and mining communities, developers, environmentalist groups, and government agencies. Learn about their plans for the land, and adjust your activities. Plan ahead for the possibility of future impact.

- Find opportunities to salvage or transplant useful plants from areas that are scheduled to be heavily impacted by human activities such as areas where trail or road construction is planned. Many areas have ongoing native plant restoration projects under way. In these instances, you might be able to assist with the survival of native species by "weeding out" the invasive, nonnative species.

- Find ideal stands that are representative of how a plant community should look, then don't harvest from them. Instead, preserve them for use as models from which to base your observations and stewardship efforts at the sites from which you will be harvesting.

- Always use the correct tools and wear the right clothing to get your job done. Digging long taproots from a steep, rocky hillside with a soupspoon while wearing penny loafers will result not only in physical trauma to the herbalist but will tear apart the hillside as well. Be considerate of the environment by acknowledging that the human body is poorly adapted to many of the tasks we perform there.

- Never gather from stands that are wilted or otherwise unhealthy. Not only may sick plants have altered chemistries but they may be covered with poison as well. Contact your county, state, or federal weed abatement officials and learn about weed control programs in your area before you harvest anything. Check your local noxious weed list, and see if there is an opportunity to reduce the distribution of toxic herbicides by offering to hand-pull the plants for healing purposes. Many homeowners and farmers will welcome you onto their land to gather plants such as dandelion, Saint-John's-wort, mullein, burdock, or countless others. By focusing your wildcrafting efforts toward plants that people generally hate, you will be giving a precious gift of healing back to the environment by reducing the use of toxic herbicides.

Basic Ethical Guidelines for the Harvesting of Wild Plants (continued)

• Be as quiet as possible and plan every step when you enter a wild area. Stop frequently to look, listen, and feel the earth; and don't forget to look behind you to monitor the impact you may be causing while en route to that special patch.

• When gathering from a stand of plants, work at a deliberate pace that allows you to remain conscious of your surroundings and of the task at hand. Harvest carefully and thoughtfully. Don't attack the plants; work as the loving caretaker you are.

• Always be careful to use the proper processing and storage methods for the herbs you gather. Spoilage equates to waste—one of the worst types of vicarious human impact. Good wildcrafting ethics are not exclusive to your time in the field—take care of the plants all the way from earth to medicine.

• Stay obscure during your harvest and field studies. If you attract uninvited attention to a stand of plants, the result might be added impact from curious onlookers. A good rule is to always focus your efforts in areas where you will remain out of the view of other people.

• Be critical of your human shortcomings. We are foreigners in wild areas. Strive to deepen your awareness to understand that even the simplest organisms of nature serve complex roles in the environment, and that we are all just beginning to learn the ways of the wild. Nothing is insignificant, and virtually every organism in an ecosystem is interdependent with the plants we harvest.

• Never reseed a stand of plants to an extent that exceeds the natural density that existed prior to your harvest. A human-engineered overpopulation of plants can be as devastating to an ecosystem as careless overharvesting. Watch the bioregion from which you are harvesting over a period of several years, and take note of how each species reseeds itself. Then try to replicate what nature would do in your absence. Many plants compete with one another. Propagating an overabundance of a species may be satisfactory to our conscience but may also pass a death sentence to dozens of noncompeting plants and interdependent organisms.

• Accept your personal weaknesses, identify your chronic mistakes, then add to this list your own personal set of wildcrafting guidelines.

To learn more about the earth-conscious harvest, use, and preservation of wild medicinal plants, pick up a copy of *From Earth to Herbalist* by Gregory L. Tilford (Mountain Press Publishing, 1998).

them. It seems that a great many of us have become so intoxicated by the freedom-based premise of using self-prescribed natural alternatives, we have forgotten where they come from.

Many plant species are disappearing not so much because they are overharvested but because they are misrepresented in the marketplace. Goldenseal (*Hydrastis canadensis*), for example, has been one of the most popular North American herbs of commerce for centuries, but it is also one of the most misused. Like many other herbs, goldenseal continues to be heralded as some sort of miracle medicine that is effective against virtually any microbe that terrifies us enough to try something "alternative." Indeed, the popularity of this and many other herbs has arisen from therapeutic success stories and promising scientific studies, but most of their appeal is attributable to marketing savvy and no small measure of consumer hysteria. In truth, most plant medicines work within narrow parameters of therapeutic usefulness. Goldenseal is not a systemic antibiotic that courses through the body to fight infection like a shot of penicillin; instead, it works only to inhibit microbes it comes in direct contact with on the surface membranes of the digestive tract, eyes, and nasal passages.

We must also take into account that many medicinal plants are at risk of disappearing because of factors totally unrelated to their uses as medicines. Pipsissewa (*Chimaphila* spp.), for instance, is used as a "secret ingredient" in certain brands of soft drinks, and the habitat destruction associated with its harvest may be more devastating than the loss of the plants themselves. Another example is goldthread (*Coptis* spp.), which is an old-growth forest inhabitant that is quickly running out of places to live in the Pacific Northwest. Goldthread is not

a popular plant of commerce in North America, but the old-growth firs and cedars it lives beneath are.

And then there's all the hype. Newsstands are packed with the latest word about scientific herbal breakthroughs, even about the same medicines that just yesterday were considered "snake oil" in the eyes of science. Some herbs are becoming as fashionable as the fastest computer: if you haven't tried the latest herbal craze, then your life is unnecessarily difficult. *Don't take Prozac—we've got Saint-John's-wort, the herbal alternative for chronic depression. Too busy to slow down? Don't worry. The latest double-blind studies say that we can boost the body's immune system with echinacea, cat's claw, astragalus, and ginseng.*

Herbs are touching the far reaches of our society at an unprecedented rate. Much of what drives this green revolution is born from solid scientific discovery and consumers' independent desire to take charge of their health and well-being. Certainly, these are good goals, but where do herbs come from? Is there something we should know about their natural environment? What do these plants contribute to their ecosystems? Do they really work the way that we are led to believe? What makes herbs different from

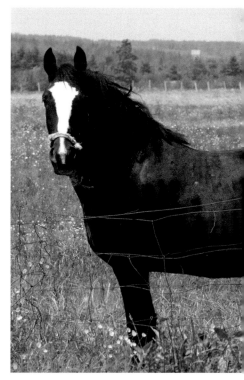

conventional medicines? What effect is our consumption having upon plant populations and their environments?

Our point is this: We have to be careful. If we wish to use and sustain our botanical resources into the future, we must step away from all the hoopla long enough to find healthful solutions for the plants themselves. The answers to all of the above questions rest within our willingness to look beyond the sensational advertising to see what herbs really are and what they represent in the larger global scheme of things. Until we do, our herbal heritage will continue to disappear under the pressures of ignorance, waste, and greed.

Many North American medicinal plants of commerce are now being cultivated, but sadly, many of them continue to disappear from the wild. While part of the problem stems from unethical wildcrafting practices, the demise for plants such as goldenseal and American ginseng originates from a complexity of economic and environmental causes. As herbalists, we could easily point an accusatory finger at the herb industry, but this would not be fair. Many herbalists have chosen to exclude wild plants such as goldenseal, American ginseng, black cohosh, and osha from their personal medicine cabinets as a gesture, if not a preventive measure against their demise. But in sad reality, such measures provide only a bandage treatment for a global problem. The painful truth is that too many people are impacting too much of the planet for too

many reasons. Indeed, consumer demands are taking a serious toll on plants such as goldenseal and American ginseng, but these and thousands of other plant species are also disappearing under the combined pressures of logging, grazing, mining, weed abatement, urban development, farming, pollution, recreational impact, and several other human-centered factors.

So then, what can we do to save medicinal plants? On a community level, we can share what we learn from books such as this one by educating others on the curative possibilities that may exist beneath the trees around their homes. Show your neighbor a medicinal plant that grows on the roadside—such as mullein, dandelion, licorice, Saint-John's-wort, or milkweed— and raise the question of whether a weed is really just a weed. Tell people about the plight of goldenseal, and remind them that the greatest curative gifts of this plant may yet to be discovered. Then tell them they can use Oregon grape as a substitute.

On a personal level, you can accomplish even more. Join organizations such as United Plant Savers, become involved with native plant clubs in your area, or become actively involved in land restoration efforts. If you use herbs, learn as much as you can about the plants and the ecosystems they live in.

Above all, take time to evaluate and improve yourself as a consumer of our planet's resources, and learn how to give something back for everything you consume.

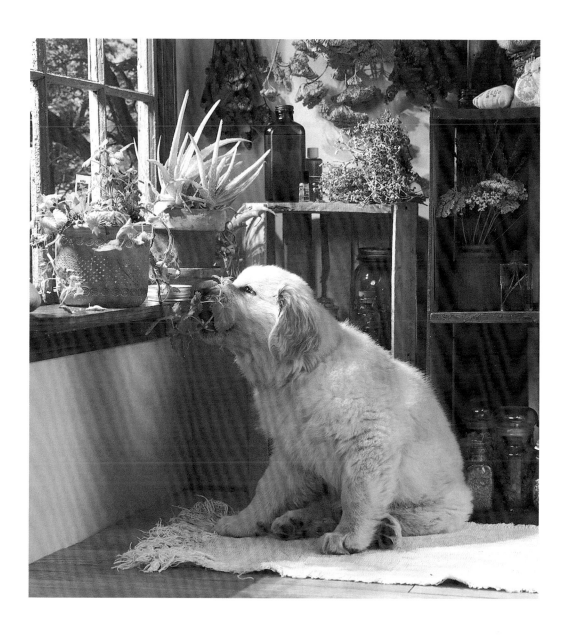

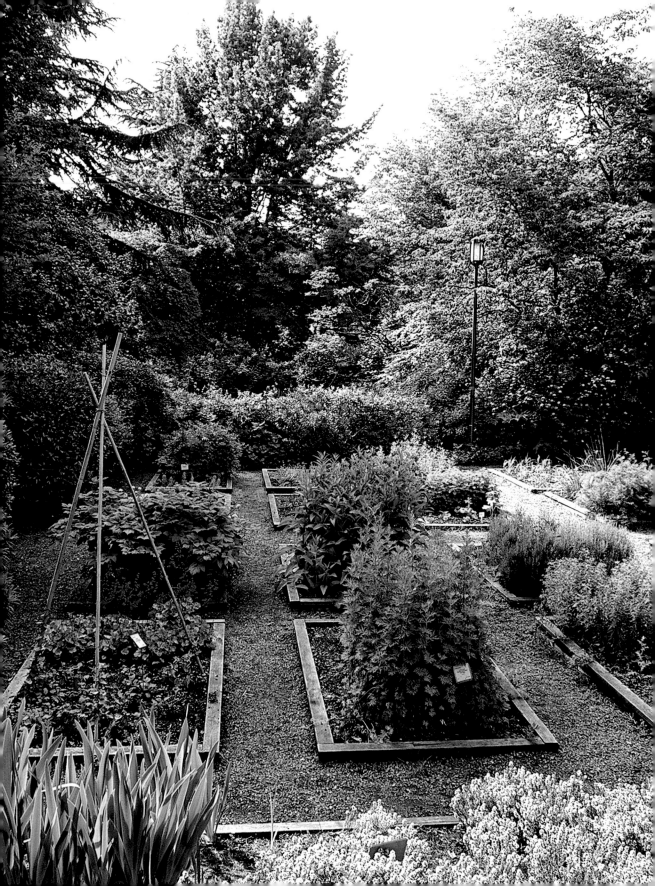

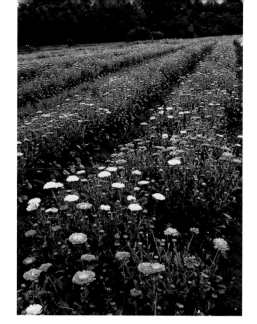

Chapter 2

Materia Medica: An A-Z Guide to Herbs for Animals

hese detailed monographs are specific to the identification, harvest, preparation, and applications of the herbs we most frequently find useful in the care of animals. Please keep in mind that this is not an exhaustive list of the herb resources that are available to you and your pet; it represents only a few that are most familiar to us and other herbalists who find themselves involved in the care of animals. To list and describe the hundreds of other potentially useful herbs that exist worldwide would be time and space prohibitive, if not impossible.

Despite all measures of scientific study or clinical success that may be in place to validate and substantiate the efficacy and safety of an herb (or for that matter any medicine), it is important to remember that a golden rule must never be forgotten: There are no absolutes in nature. Each individual animal is unique so no single herb can be relied upon to work at the same level of effectiveness in each and every animal.

With this rule in mind, we have also included a supplemental herb list at the end of this chapter where you will find general information about several other herbs you may find useful in the care of your companion. The herbs in this list should not be overlooked as lesser or secondary options but as resources worthy of further investigation. Following is an explanation of the subheads:

Appearance: Under this subheading is a brief physical description of the subject plant. Please keep in mind that the plant descriptions we provide here are intended only to give you a general idea of what a specific plant looks like. This book is not intended to serve as a definitive means of plant identification. The process of accurately identifying a plant involves the use of a highly scientific botanical plant key that enables the user to systematically recognize or rule out characteristics that are unique to a species. To obtain a botanical key that is specific to plants in your area, visit your local library or obtain one from a bookstore. To learn how to use a botanical key, consider taking an introductory botany class at your local college.

Habitat and Range: Under this subheading we tell you where you can expect to find the subject plant growing in the wild. We may also mention which climatic regions are best suited to the cultivation of the plant.

Cycle and Bloom Season: Here we inform you of the reproductive characteristics of the plant.

Parts Used: Under this subheading we have listed the plant parts (leaves, root, etc.) that are most commonly used by herbalists.

Primary Medicinal Activities: This is not an exhaustive list—most herbs offer dozens of medicinal activities, many of which may be too weak to be of therapeutic value. Here we have listed the strongest and most predictable effects the herb is likely to produce when used in a healing context with most animals.

Strongest Affinities: Under this subheading we have listed the body structures or systems that are likely to benefit the most from the medicinal activities of the herb.

Preparation: Here we have listed which types of medicinal preparation (infusion, alcohol tincture, glycerin tincture, decoction, etc.) are best suited to the use of the herb.

Common Uses: Under this subheading you will find the "meat" of the monograph. Here we identify and explain what we feel are the best applications for the herb. This information is a mix of personal opinion, hands-on experience, clinical observations, and scientific and anecdotal evidence.

We've included information about scientific studies that we feel are especially relevant to the use of herbs in animals. We vehemently oppose any form of experimentation that imposes discomfort, disease, or a reduced quality of life upon an animal. Such experimentation violates the foundations

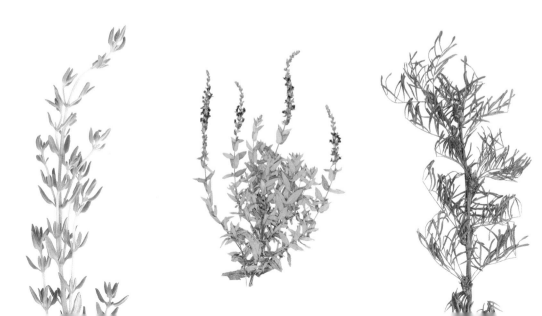

of holistic healing—wellness cannot be sustained from induced suffering. However, we also feel responsible to the animals who have already suffered or died at the hands of human science. We must do our best to assure that the knowledge we have gained from their past suffering is not wasted, and that every shred of useful knowledge that humanity has gained through their sacrifices is used for other animals in the form of better care and better understanding. In the realm of holistic healing, there is no need or justification for future animal experimentation—but there is also no point in denying ourselves or our pets the understanding we have already attained, even if by dark, arrogant means.

Availability: Here you will find information specific to where you can access the herb.

Propagation and Harvest: Under this subheading is information about how to grow your own plants or how to harvest and handle the herb in the wild. If harvesting wild plants interests you, please keep these three important rules in mind before embarking on any wildcrafting ventures: 1) Do not pick any plants that are endangered or scarce. 2) Beware of pesticides. Never gather plants from roadsides, cultivated fields, irrigation ditches, or other areas where weed control efforts may have taken place. 3) You must be 100 percent certain of the identity of the plant you are picking—before you pick it!

Alternatives and Adjuncts: Under this subheading we list and categorize herbs that serve especially well as alternatives or as complementary additions to the herb we have been discussing throughout the monograph.

Cautions and Comments: Here you will find any contraindications or side effects that we are aware of. You will also find our comments and opinions relative to the overall safety or potential misuses of the herb.

References: Most of the scientific studies used to research each monograph can be accessed through the Internet at the Medline Web site: www.medline.gov.

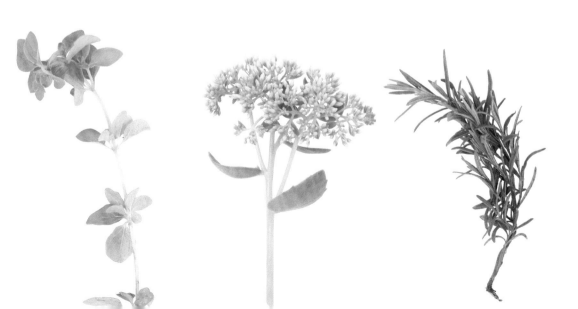

ALFALFA

Medicago sativa   Pea Family

Appearance: Alfalfa is a sprawling member of the pea family (Leguminosae) with small, tightly arranged blue or sometimes pink or white flowers; small, prickly, seed-bearing pods; and cloverlike leaves.

Habitat and Range: Widely cultivated throughout the world

Cycle and Bloom Season: A perennial that first blooms in early summer, alfalfa continues to bloom after successive harvests throughout the growing season as long as the climate permits vigorous regrowth.

Parts Used: Dried leaves, stems, unopened flowers

Primary Medicinal Activities: Nutritive, anti-inflammatory, antioxidant, stimulates urination (diuretic)

Strongest Affinities: Musculoskeletal system, digestive tract, liver

Preparation: Capsules, infusion, liquid extract, or dried bulk herb sprinkled onto food

Common Uses: Alfalfa contains a broad spectrum of nutrients, including considerable quantities of protein (up to 50 percent by weight), trace minerals, dietary fiber, and vitamins A, B_1, B_{12}, C, D, E, and K. It is also high in chlorophyll, which serves as an antioxidant in the bloodstream. All of this makes alfalfa particularly attractive as a livestock feed. In addition to being highly nutritive, alfalfa is traditionally known as one of the best herbal treatments for arthritis, rheumatism, and gout. Clinical research of

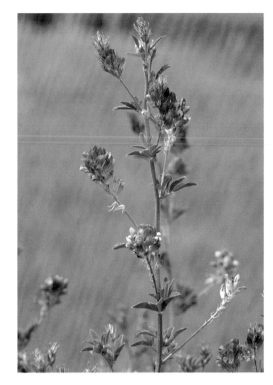

Medicago sativa

the use of alfalfa in treating these diseases has shown that at least 10 to 20 percent of human subjects experience dramatic reduction of painful symptoms. Traditional uses in animals have commonly led to similar results. For arthritis and other inflammatory diseases of the joints, alfalfa can bring long-term relief to dogs, cats, rodents, and horses and various other herbivores who receive it as a daily food supplement. By now you probably see the value of this herb in the care of older animals. For use in therapeutic doses, it works well when combined with dandelion, yucca, and licorice.

Alfalfa possesses cancer-preventive qualities as well. It is believed that alfalfa induces complex cellular activities that serve to inactivate chemical carcinogens in the liver and small intestine before they can cause damage, thus helping to reduce the risk of cancerous growths.

Alfalfa's considerable vitamin K content has been shown to be beneficial in remedying bleeding disorders that may result from long-term use of antibiotics, anticoagulants, aspirin, and anticonvulsant drugs. The coumarin constituent of alfalfa is also well known for its anticoagulant qualities, and in fact many anticlotting drugs were derived from this compound. Excessive doses of fresh alfalfa or concentrated extracts may be contraindicated in animals with anemia, but moderate dietary supplementation may be useful in some types of this disease.

The various saponin constituents of alfalfa are known to help with the absorption of fat-soluble nutrients in the small intestine and may act to stimulate the body's natural production of growth hormones— yet another reason for its popularity as a livestock feed. In this capacity, alfalfa works by mechanisms very similar to those of yucca, but it is much less irritating to the stomach and intestines than yucca and therefore can be used over longer periods without adverse side effects. It may be especially useful in animals with debilitating diseases who need to gain weight but cannot afford added stress upon compromised body systems.

In the urinary tract, alfalfa has an alkalinizing effect, making it useful in treating ailments that involve overly acidic urine, especially where there is bladder irritation and crystal formation. This nutritional plant also helps an animal adjust to a new diet.

For the brain, alfalfa is said to help improve mental vigor. This is likely due to alfalfa's broad spectrum of nutrients, many of which are critical to proper nerve and brain functions.

Availability: Health food stores; can be propagated in a home garden

Propagation and Harvest: Alfalfa is extremely easy to grow just about anywhere. In fact, if allowed to spread, it quickly becomes competitive with everything else in the garden. Being a legume, alfalfa changes nitrogen into a usable form within its extensive root system, making it a valuable soil-building ingredient when the plants are tilled in. Unfortunately, the weedlike character of this plant overshadows its value as a soil builder. Digging the roots is like pulling crabgrass, and tilling often results in even greater proliferation from the subsequent root cuttings. In other words, buy certified organic alfalfa at an herb store, unless you wish to delegate a portion (or perhaps all) of your garden to it. (A word of caution to the insistent gardener: If you plant alfalfa and then have second thoughts about keeping it, remove it before it goes to seed. Once it does, it's yours for life!)

Gather alfalfa before it comes into bloom. Cut (or mow) the plants during dry weather, cutting the stems at about 1 inch above ground level. Allow the herb to dry in an airy, moisture-free place that is away from direct sunlight until it is completely dry, or make a tincture from the freshly cut greens.

Alternatives and Adjuncts: Dandelion, garlic, licorice, red clover, and yucca

Cautions and Comments: Alfalfa is regarded as safe by the U.S. Food and Drug Administration (FDA). Although adverse side effects are rare, many horse owners testify that consumption of too much fresh alfalfa may lead to colic, a condition that can be serious in animals. This is due in large part to alfalfa's saponin constituents. Although these soaplike compounds are medicinally valuable, used in excess they may irritate the stomach lining and intestinal mucosa, resulting in nausea and gastritis. Horses and rabbits cannot vomit, which greatly compounds the seriousness of this side effect. The risk of colic occurring is greatly reduced by feeding only dried greens.

The seeds of alfalfa have been found to contain a toxic amino acid, l-canavanine, which has caused blood disorders in humans and in animals. Use alfalfa only during its prebloom stages of growth. Alfalfa can trigger allergic responses in animals who are especially sensitive to pollens.

ALOE

Aloe spp.   Lily Family

Appearance: Aloes are cactuslike members of the lily family (Liliaceae), having narrow, tapering, proportionately thick, succulent leaves with spiny margins. There are perhaps five hundred species of aloe, but the most common aloe of commerce is Aloe barbadensis, which we commonly know as aloe vera. This species produces its leaves directly from a stout central stalk, in a rosette fashion, while several other varieties of aloe are branched, almost bushlike. Aside from these variations, all aloes share a similar appearance and can grow very large. In some areas of southwestern Africa, aloes are seen in excess of 25 feet tall with stems more than 10 feet in circumference. Flowers are small, tubular, characteristically lilylike in appearance, and are produced in leafless, terminal spikes.

Habitat and Range: Aloes are indigenous to southern and eastern Africa and have been introduced to the West Indies, where a great deal of commercial cultivation takes place. In areas of North America and Europe

with Mediterranean climates, aloes are used as landscape and garden plants. They are popular indoor plants throughout much of the world.

Cycle and Bloom Season: Aloes are perennials that bloom opportunistically when mature. In other words, if they receive all of the elements they require to thrive, they will likely remain in bloom throughout each year of their lives.

Parts Used: Primarily the gel-like juice of the inner leaf or the yellowish latex contained immediately beneath the skin of the leaves

Primary Medicinal Activities: Wound healing (vulnerary), soothes skin (emollient), anti-bacterial, antioxidant, stimulates the immune system (immunostimulant), anticancer, antitumor, cooling to the skin.

Strongest Affinities: Skin, digestive system, lymph system

Preparation: Freshly pressed juice or stabilized (commercial) aloe gel preparations are the most commonly used forms of aloe. Using this plant at home is as easy as cutting a mature leaf from the lower part of the plant and squeezing out the juice. Intravenous formulations of aloe ingredients have been FDA-approved and are available for use by veterinarians. Acemannan, a chemical compound found in aloe vera juice, is a powerful immunostimulant.

Common Uses: Aloe's great claim to fame is from its use as a topical skin dressing. Fresh aloe juice or commercially prepared gel contains dozens of minerals, proteins, enzymes, polysaccharides, and other elements that help soften and soothe the skin and promote the rapid healing of minor burns and wounds. Topical application of aloe gel will likely bring immediate, cooling relief to fleabites, poison ivy, and sunburns. It is also excellent for reducing the itch and tightening of postsurgical incisions. Applied after sutures are removed, the gel reduces much of the irritation that so often leads to persistent chewing or scratching and may result in inflammation and infection. In any external application, apply enough juice to lightly cover the affected area and allow it to dry. If possible, keep the animal from licking it off—the idea is to leave the juice on as long as possible. Unless your animal has an adverse reaction to the juice (such as reddening or an allergy rash), aloe can be applied liberally once or twice per day until the healing process is progressing well.

Internally, a small dose of aloe juice may be useful for healing minor injuries and irritations of the digestive tract, such as those that may occur when Bowser swallows a jagged bone.

Scientists have recently found that acemannan acts as a strong immunostimulant in animals, particularly in cats. It has been found to be especially effective in the treatment of fibrosarcoma and feline leukemia virus (FeLV). It is theorized that acemannan triggers an increase in the autoimmune attack upon the viruses believed to cause these usually fatal diseases. Typically, over 70 percent of cats who become ill with FeLV die within ten weeks of the onset of disease. But in a recent study, forty-four cats with confirmed FeLV were injected with 2 milligrams per kilogram of acemannan weekly for six weeks and reexamined six weeks after the treatment ended. At the end of the twelve-week study, 71 percent of the cats were alive and in good health. Acemannan has also been shown to be effective against cancerous

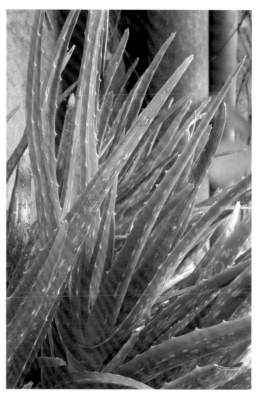

Aloe barbadensis

tumors in rodents and dogs. It has been FDA approved for veterinary use and will undoubtedly be tested in humans.

Other chemical compounds found in aloe juice have been shown to have antioxidant actions in the body.

Availability: Aloe gel or juice (the difference being consistency) is available at health food stores. Any good nursery has the plants.

Propagation and Harvest: Aloe is easy to grow as a houseplant. It requires well-drained, sandy soil and should be watered only once or twice a month. Avoid using potting soil—it retains too much moisture and may cause rot problems. Ordinary garden soil will do fine. A happy aloe that receives plenty of sunlight will bloom

A

Materia Medica

continuously and reproduce aggressively from side-shoots. These shoots are easily transplanted into separate pots. If you live in an area where frost is rare, aloe can be planted in a garden. Again, just give it plenty of sun, don't overwater it, and it will be yours forever.

Alternatives and Adjuncts: Nothing really compares with aloe, but if you don't have it around, look toward chickweed, plantain, self-heal, and comfrey as topical alternatives. Internally, ginger, cayenne, red clover, cleavers, dandelion, yarrow, garlic, and burdock are worth considering to complement the activity of aloe.

Cautions and Comments: Aloe juice, although bitter, is generally safe for internal or external uses in dogs, cats and most other animal types. However, be cautious of any products containing "Aloes." Aloes consists of a sticky latex that is extracted from the inner skin of aloe leaves. This latex possesses strong purgative qualities that may result in digestive distress and severe diarrhea. Although several commercial laxative preparations use aloe latex in their formulas, we strongly discourage their use in animals. It is believed that aloe components may be passed in mother's milk to nursing infants, so it should not be used in such circumstances.

ARNICA

Arnica spp.   Sunflower Family

Appearance: Arnica is a classic sunflower with bright yellow daisylike flowers. Leaves oppose one another on the stem and range from narrowly lance shaped to broadly heart shaped (depending on species). The leaves and stems of most species are at least partially covered with fine hairs. Most arnicas are aromatic, particularly when the leaves are bruised, with a distinctive pinelike odor. Arnicas are small plants, seldom exceeding 12 inches in height.

Habitat and Range: Arnica is a mountain plant that occurs in coniferous subalpine and alpine regions of western North America from Alaska to the mountains of southern California, where it grows only above 9,000 feet in elevation.

Cycle and Bloom Season: Arnica is a perennial that blooms during its second year of growth and every year thereafter. It is among the first flowers to bloom in early spring and is often one of the first to die back in early summer. During dry years, arnica may not bloom at all.

Parts Used: The entire flowering plant

Primary Medicinal Activities: Heals wounds, dilates blood vessels

Strongest Affinities: Muscles and subdermal capillaries

Preparation: Oil infusion, water infusion, fresh poultice, or commercially prepared gel

Common Uses: Arnica is used for closed-tissue injuries, including fractures, sprains, and contusions. It is perhaps the best-known herbal sports medicine. Used topically, preparations of arnica act to open up peripheral capillaries and lymph ducts and increase circulation in tissues that are engorged with fluids as a result of injury. When used immediately after an injury occurs, results can be dramatic. In essence, arnica helps to speed the healing process by moving waste-bound fluids out and moving cleansing fluids and platelets into the affected area. Arnica is especially valuable for treatment of horses and other large animals who are subjected to rigorous exercise and an occasional twist or strain of the leg or hip joints. Arnica can be used on dogs as well, but special measures must be taken to prohibit the animal from licking it off because arnica can be toxic if taken internally in improper dosages. Cats are not excluded from the use of arnica, but they are more sensitive to arnica's volatile oils and are more prone to allergic reactions with this herb as they are with so many other substances. Test a small portion of your cat's skin before using arnica for an injury. Look for development of redness or other signs of irritation.

To use arnica on a dog or cat, apply enough of the infusion or gel to wet the skin of the animal (not just the fur), then wrap the area with gauze or a piece of cloth and secure it so the animal cannot easily remove it. The idea is to keep the preparation on the animal as long as possible. Arnica can be applied this way twice daily for up to three days. Long-term applications should not be necessary and are not recommended because a rash is likely to develop from overuse.

When used internally in carefully measured doses, arnica is said to act as a neurological device in cases of chronic urinary incontinence that cannot be attributed to physiological pathologies. While use of arnica in this capacity holds a great deal of promise for many animals suffering from urinary incontinence, the toxicity of this plant limits such use to the advanced professional. Talk with a holistic veterinarian if you are interested in this use.

Although this book focuses on herbal remedies, the value of arnica in homeopathic preparations should not be overlooked. In a homeopathic capacity,

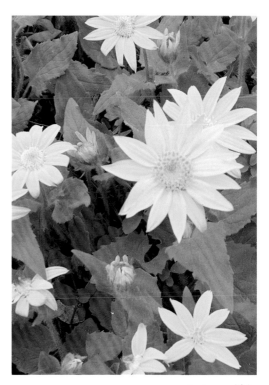

Arnica cordifolia

arnica can be used internally with a great margin of safety. We have seen amazing results with the use of homeopathic arnica at the onset of traumatic injury in animals, and keeping homeopathic arnica on hand is as simple as purchasing a small vial of the tiny white pellets and slipping it into your pocket, purse, or first aid kit. To learn more about using homeopathic arnica, we highly recommend Dr. Pitcairn's *Complete Guide to Natural Health for Dogs & Cats*.

Availability: Arnica gels and tinctures are readily available from herb retailers. Seeds are available from specialty seed catalogs.

Propagation and Harvest: Arnica requires soil with plenty of organic matter and does best when its root system can crawl around under a blanket of pine needles. Given that it is seldom found at altitudes under 3,000 feet except in Canada, it likely has some specialized light- or air-quality requirements that prohibit it from flourishing in urban areas. If you live in the mountains, arnica can be grown from seeds or root cuttings. But beware—the roots will quickly consume your garden.

To harvest arnica from the wild, grasp the stem of the flowering herb just above ground level, then snap it off, taking only what you need. Take care not to damage the roots by pulling on the plant or stepping into a patch of plants—the roots crawl horizontally, and the pressure of a human foot can injure them.

After gathering what you need, you have the option of processing them fresh or allowing them to dry in a dark place. Fresh plants yield a more potent infusion but spoil quickly in the refrigerator because of their water content. Regardless, we opt for the use of fresh arnica. To learn how to make an oil infusion, refer to chapter 1.

Another option for the use of arnica in emergency situations is to make a simple poultice by mashing a flowering plant with some water to make a pestolike paste. The poultice can then be applied to the injury as a crude ointment. It can really work wonders when you're out on the trail—just bear in mind that animals (or people) should not ingest the poultice in any quantity.

Alternative and Adjunct Herbs: Saint-John's-wort, ginger, cayenne, and yarrow are good choices as internal adjunct therapies here. Saint-John's-wort can be used topically as well and is especially useful if nerve trauma is suspected.

Cautions and Comments: Arnica can be toxic if ingested in anything but homeopathic or minute quantities and may cause internal bleeding if ingested in large enough quantities. Because arnica works quickly to stimulate dilation and circulation of peripheral blood vessels, it should not be applied to open, bleeding wounds. To do so might actually increase bleeding and slow the coagulation process. Animals generally dislike the taste, but extra measures are warranted to prohibit dogs and cats from licking arnica-treated areas.

ASTRAGALUS

Astragalus membranaceous   Pea Family

Appearance: A typical member of the pea family, astragalus has finely divided leaves, small pealike flowers and seed pods, and a sprawling, vinelike stature that brings to mind any of the hundreds of wild vetches that inhabit much of the globe. *Astragalus membranaceous*, the species of commerce, may grow as tall as 6 feet, which gives it an appearance that is similar to licorice (*Glycyrrhiza* spp.), yet another member of the pea family. There is a growing belief among herbalists, botanists, and medical researchers that North American milk vetch (*A. americana*), a common weed, may have similar medicinal attributes and may even be the same plant as *A. membranaceous*, the medicinal astragalus of commerce. The *Astragalus* genus is large, consisting of hundreds of species, which in many cases are difficult to differentiate even by trained botanists. Some varieties of *Astragalus* are toxic, and to compound this mystery even more, these plants often cross-pollinate and hybridize. For now, no one knows whether or not we have a wild, medicinal *Astragalus* in North America.

Habitat and Range: An import from China, Astragalus has been cultivated throughout much of the world as an important herb of commerce.

Cycle and Bloom Season: A perennial that blooms from spring to early summer

Parts Used: Mature (at least three years old) roots

Primary Medicinal Activities: Immuno-stimulant, anti-inflammatory, antiviral, mildly depresses thyroid function (hypothyroid), lowers blood pressure (hypotensive), aids blood cleansing (alterative), strengthens digestion

Strongest Affinities: Immune system, lungs, liver, heart, kidneys, thyroid, digestive tract

Preparation: Tincture or infusion

Common Uses: One of the best known and widely used herbs in Chinese medicine (where the herb is known as *huang qi*), astragalus has found its way into Western herbalism by virtue of its widely versatile immune-strengthening qualities. In Chinese medicine, astragalus root is considered sweet and mildly warm, tonifying the qi (pronounced "chee") and hoisting the yang. (Sweet and warm are terms used in Chinese medicine to describe an herb's relation to the body's energy flows and do not relate to flavor.) Astragalus root is commonly used for spleen and lung qi deficiency, including symptoms of emaciation, weariness, shortness of breath, loss of appetite, diarrhea, and prolapse of the uterus or anus.

Astragalus is especially useful for strengthening the body against viral infections of the respiratory tract and heart through stimulation of killer-cell activity and interferon production in the body. It imparts direct antibacterial and anti-inflammatory qualities to this effort as well. Astragalus is a viable option for early treatment of various forms of respiratory infection, including

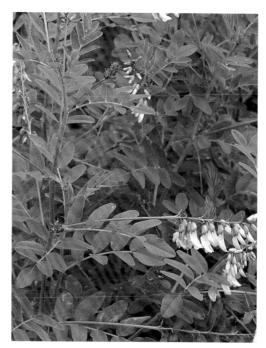

Astragalus membranaceous

kennel cough (*Bordetella bronchiseptica*), a condition that theoretically involves this bacterium's opportunistic cooperation with various forms of virus. While astragalus works to stimulate T cell activity and helps to raise white blood cell counts, it also boosts the body's defenses through its liver-strengthening attributes. In a study involving rats, saponin constituents were shown to enhance DNA synthesis in the liver—a process believed to be a major factor in the strengthening of cell structures against infection or the introduction of toxins. Other studies suggest that astragalus may be useful for helping the body protect itself and speed recovery from the damaging effects of long-term steroid therapies. Astragalus is known to strengthen kidney circulation, making it useful in early stages of kidney infection or renal failure.

For any of the aforementioned purposes, up to 20 drops of the extract can be administered for each 20 pounds of your animal's body weight, up to twice daily.

In addition to its broad-spectrum ability to boost resistance to disease, astragalus is traditionally used to boost energy levels in debilitated people and animals, which adds to its promise as a candidate in the treatment of various cancers, especially those compounded by depressed immune functions. For pet owners who are going through the horrors of chemotherapy or radiation treatments for their animals, astragalus may offer a foothold in maintaining some functional balance in an immune system that is stressed by both a disease and toxic intervention. To use astragalus in this capacity, first consult a holistic veterinarian.

Astragalus is also known to have antiviral qualities that are specific to infections of the heart. Again, if you suspect a problem of this serious nature, talk to a holistic veterinarian.

Availability: Astragalus is available through many herb retailers. The seed can be purchased from specialty seed catalogs.

Propagation and Harvest: Astragalus is easy to grow from seed—some rich soil, full sun, and ample watering are all it requires to thrive. If you decide to grow this plant in your garden, however, choose a place where it can remain for quite some time. Astragalus roots require three or more years to reach their full medicinal potential, and during this time, the plants will likely spread throughout the area where they were planted. Do not plant astragalus unless you are certain that the seed you have is in fact A. membranaceous, and do not plant astragalus if you live in an area where soils have a high selenium (a nonmetallic element) content.

Alternatives and Adjuncts: For respiratory infections, astragalus combines well with coltsfoot, grindelia, or mullein leaf. For kidney infections or dysfunction, couch grass, corn silk, pipsissewa, and goldenrod are noteworthy adjuncts. For use in situations involving liver toxicity, cancer, or depressed immune functions, gentle tonic herbs with diuretic, alterative, and nutritive qualities are indicated to help remove toxins and excess waste from the body. Dandelion, burdock, red clover, licorice, and alfalfa are excellent herbs to investigate.

For an overactive thyroid, Astragalus works well by itself, but if you don't have access to any, an alternative choice might be bugleweed.

Cautions and Comments: While *A. membranaceous*, the medicinal variety of *Astragalus*, is among the safest of medicinal herbs for both humans and animals, many other species of *Astragalus* are toxic, especially to grazing animals. Buy astragalus roots, preparations, and seeds only from reputable sources. Also, astragalus is known to accumulate selenium in its tissues in areas where a high selenium content is present in the soil. Selenium can be toxic in high doses. Check with your county extension agent before planting this herb.

In Chinese medicine, astragalus is contraindicated in "excess heat" and "yin deficiency" patterns.

BEE BALM

Monarda spp.   Mint Family

Appearance: This pungent genus of dry land mints is known by many common names: wild bergamot, purple bee balm, horsemint, wild oregano, Oswego tea, and sweet leaf. Leaves are lance shaped, oppose one another on the stem, and have a tendency to curve backward toward the ground. Leaf margins are sometimes, but not always, toothed. Like most members of the mint family, the stems of bee balm are distinctively square (four-sided). Flowers are presented in clusters at the top of the plant, each containing dozens of tiny, rose- to purple-colored blossoms. Perhaps the most distinguishing characteristic of this plant is its strong but pleasant odor, which ranges from sweetly sagelike to that which leads many to believe they have discovered a wild strain of oregano. The plant can grow to 3 feet on its sturdy stems, but most are found in the range of 6 to 18 inches tall.

Habitat and Range: Wild bee balm likes meadows and slopes that are predominantly dry and sunny. Unlike most mints, bee balm is drought tolerant and prefers dry land habitats. Bee balm (*M. fistulosa*) is generally found at elevations below 4,000 feet. Other varieties of *Monarda*, such as *M. menthaefolia*, grow at higher elevations in shady, moist soils.

The range of this plant remains largely undefined, but in the U.S. it seems to be spreading westward from the east. Livestock enjoy grazing on this plant and have undoubtedly served as a vehicle in the expansion of bee balm's range.

Cycle and Bloom Season: A perennial that blooms by midsummer and often continues to bloom until the first frost

Parts Used: Leaves plucked from the plant; the entire aerial plant if the stem is taken

Primary Medicinal Activities: promotes sweating (diaphoretic), expels intestinal gas (carminative), antiseptic, reduces pain (analgesic), antifungal

Strongest Affinities: Skin, mouth, digestive tract, kidneys, urinary tract

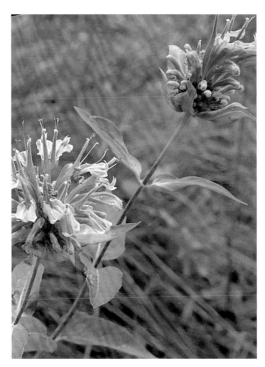

Monarda fistulosa

Preparation: Unlike most leafy herbs, which begin to break down and lose their potency after about six months, bee balm can be dried and stored for up to two years. The fresh or dried leaf, stem, and flower material can be made into an alcohol or glycerin tincture. The dried plant can be infused for use in skin and eyewashes.

Common Uses: Although this plant is widely available and infinitely useful, it is often overlooked by herbalists, and it has not received the clinical study that it deserves as a healing ally. Despite an overall lack of scientific validation, bee balm is a safe herb to use in both animals and humans. Many North American Indian tribes used this plant extensively for healing and in spiritual ceremonies.

Like most mints, bee balm has a special affinity toward the digestive tract, where it is useful for relieving gastritis and spastic colon. However, it does not taste good, and most herbivores abandon it in favor of less pungent forage. Therefore, for use as a digestive aid in animals, the best form of administering bee balm is gelatin capsules (gel capsules) or a glycerin extract.

Bee balm has excellent antibacterial qualities and is especially useful for mouth and gum infections. Two methods of application work here: a poultice can be made from the dried or fresh herb and applied directly to the affected area, or a strong infusion or tincture can be used the same way. The poultice or infusion can also be effective as an antifungal agent. Dogs, cats, and horses and other large animals with fungal infections of the skin are likely to benefit from a generous topical application of bee balm poultice or salve or from twice-daily skin rinses with cooled bee balm tea (also see "Calendula"). To make the tea, cover a generous handful of the herb with hot water and allow it to steep until the water has thoroughly cooled. Don't worry about straining the herb—just pour the entire mixture over the affected areas of the animal. In dry weather, or in cases where the animal chooses to lick the rinse off before it can be effective, you might consider applying the tea as a fomentation (see chapter 1). Bee balm skin rinses also can bring soothing relief to itchy skin that has resulted from infected fleabites or spontaneous dermatitis (commonly caused by poison ivy, nettle stings, or contact allergic reactions) and help to relieve pain while reducing scarring from minor burns. The rinse also imparts a pleasant odor to your pet.

In large animals, bee balm tea can be used as a douche or enema to treat fungal or bacterial infections, or to treat irritations of the rectum or vagina.

A dilute infusion can be used as a gentle antiseptic and anti-inflammatory eyewash or ear wash, especially if a fungal or bacterial infection is suspected. For application in the eye, don't make the infusion too strong—it should be only light yellow in color. Rinse the eye and surrounding tissues with the use of an irrigation syringe. To add stronger antimicrobial activity to the rinse, a pinch of dried Oregon grape root or certified organic goldenseal can be added to the infusion while it is steeping. Just remember to keep the eye rinse very weak. Ear rinses can be made much stronger.

Bee balm works well for low-grade urinary tract infections, and you might find it useful for kidney infections as well. Unless you can get your animal to drink the tea, a glycerin-based tincture is probably your best bet: administer 12–25 drops per 20 pounds of animal weight two to three times per day.

Availability: Wild harvested or organically grown bee balm is available through herb retailers, as is the tincture. Seeds and plants can be purchased through specialty catalogs and nurseries.

Propagation and Harvest: Bee balm reseeds readily and transplants well. This is an excellent plant to introduce into your herb garden. No stratification or other special treatment is required, and the plant is adaptable to almost any soil. Gather the upper parts of this plant when it is in full bloom (May through September, depending on location), which is when the parts are the most potent. Pluck individual leaves to minimize impact, or gather the stem and leaves after the plant has bloomed and gone to seed. If the latter is your choice, clip the stems about 1 inch above ground level to allow for perennial regrowth and root protection. When gathering while the plant is in bloom, always be sure to leave plenty of flowers intact for pollination and seed development.

Alternatives and Adjuncts: Combines well with catnip, chamomile, or fennel for digestive upsets and gas. Works well as an infusion with echinacea, couch grass, raspberry leaf, or goldenrod for urinary or kidney disorders. As a skin rinse, bee balm serves as a good base infusion to which feverfew flowers can be added for control of fleas.

Cautions and Comments: Bee balm is a safe herb, but it often grows in areas that are heavily grazed by livestock, where the presence of neighboring weeds may have led to the introduction of herbicides. Always check or ask for evidence of spraying before you harvest.

BLACK WALNUT

Juglans nigra   Walnut Family

Appearance: A large tree that may grow to 120 feet, black walnut is characterized by its 6-inch- to 2-foot-long leaves, which are each divided several times into twelve to twenty-four, lance-shaped and toothed leaflets. Fruits are presented as green orbs with fleshy outer husks that later dry into very hard dark-brown nuts.

Habitat and Range: Common throughout eastern North America; sporadically distributed throughout the Dakotas, Nebraska, and Kansas; introduced as an ornamental tree in most other regions of the U.S. and southern Canada

Cycle and Bloom Season: Blooms in spring; bears fruit beginning in early summer

Parts Used: Primarily the green (un-ripe) outer fruit hulls

Primary Medicinal Activities: expels worms (anthelmintic), tightens skin and mucous

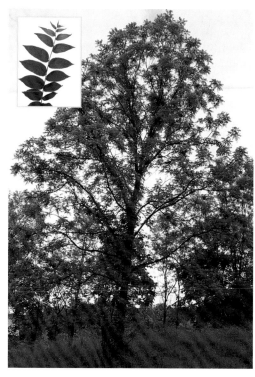

Juglans nigra

membranes (astringent), may induce vomiting (emetic), laxative

Strongest Affinities: Digestive tract, skin

Preparation: Extract of the green, unripe hulls

Common Uses: Our purpose for in-cluding black walnut in this herbal repertory for animals is as much to discourage its misuse as it is to express its medicinal attributes. Black walnut hull extract is unquestionably one of the best and safest worming agents offered by the plant world. But like many substances that can actually make a tapeworm hate life, it can be toxic to the host if not used with proper care, caution, and training. Black walnut offers symptomatic worm intervention that is generally safer and kinder to the host animal than most other herbal wormers. The holistically minded pet owner should also take into account that such intervention is actually contrary to the holistic principles of using herbs in a natural context. Black walnut kills and expels tapeworms, but the underlying reasons an animal is infested with an overpopulation of these opportunity-seeking parasites in the first place is not addressed. For more on the principles we are referring to, and our recommended approaches to parasite control, please read the section "Parasite-Related Problems" in chapter 3. For now, we must tell you that black walnut, although safe and effective when used in the correct dose and where indicated by specific circumstances, is an herb best reserved for use by experienced practitioners.

Availability: Black walnut is available in the form of an alcohol tincture from several human-oriented herb product companies. Black walnut is also used in several over-the-counter wormers, most of which we do not recommend by virtue of holistic principles.

Propagation and Harvest: Black walnut is a beautiful, full-sized shade tree that can be purchased from many landscape nurseries and fruit tree catalogs. The green, unripe fruit hulls are harvested while they remain fleshy, in early to late spring.

Alternatives and Adjuncts: Garlic and raw pumpkin seeds, added to a good natural diet, are the better choices for worm control in the majority of circumstances.

Cautions and Comments: Black walnut can be toxic to horses and may cause laminitis, severe gastritis, and breathing problems in these animals. These problems are believed to be caused not by the hulls themselves but by a fungus that attacks the green fruit hulls shortly after they fall to the ground. While this suggests that the properly harvested, fungus-free hulls may be safe for use in horses, we are often left with an unanswerable question of whether or not the hulls we are using are in fact clean of this fungus. Problems have been recorded in cases where horses had merely used black walnut shavings as part of their bedding! Concentrations of strong tannins, volatile oils, and various alkaloid ingredients contained in the bark, leaves, stems, and hulls of black walnut may lead to vomiting, diarrhea, and gastritis in dogs and cats if ingested in excessive quantities. Remember, anything that can kill a tapeworm has the potential of being harmful to your animal.

BORAGE

Borago officinalis   Borage Family

Appearance: Borage looks similar to its relative comfrey except borage has a more unruly stature. Plants may grow to 3 feet tall and quickly sprawl all over a flower bed shortly after rocketing skyward from their emergence as flattened, well-mannered little rosettes of basal leaves. The unique, 2- to 6-inch-long broadly lance-shaped or narrowly oval leaves have wrinkled, prickly haired surfaces that bring to mind two-day-old beard stubble. Flowers are brilliant blue, with five petals and a black-tipped conelike structure at the center of each flower. Flowers are borne in drooping clusters at the upper branches of the plant.

Habitat and Range: Native to many parts of Europe and Asia, borage has been widely introduced as a garden plant in North America. It grows just about anywhere that has a long enough bloom season to allow for seed development—basically, from the midlatitudes of Canada southward.

Cycle and Bloom Season: Borage is a self-seeding annual that blooms from spring to midsummer in most areas.

Parts Used: Leaves, flowers, and the oil extracted from seeds

Primary Medicinal Activities: Stimulates milk production (galactagogue), stimulates mucous secretions in the bronchi (expectorant), astringent, anti-inflammatory, diuretic, mildly calming to the nerves, adrenal stimulant

Strongest Affinities: Adrenal glands

Preparation: The most common uses of this plant require extracting oil from the seed—a process that is impractical for the do-it-yourself herbalist. The leaves can be dried and used within three months for infusions, in capsules, or in bulk form powdered and added to your pet's food. Dried leaves lose their medicinal qualities rather quickly, so use this herb as early after drying as possible.

Fresh leaves can be scraped of their prickly hairs and made into a poultice or briefly steamed in their entire form for use as a warm cover dressing for overexerted muscles and minor skin inflammations. Although fresh borage can be fed to horses and other herbivores, most animals dislike the prickly texture of the foliage.

Common Uses: Borage is one of many herbs that have been in traditional use for many centuries but nonetheless has not received the scientific attention it deserves. What we do know about borage is that its seeds contain impressive amounts of EFAs, especially gamma-linolenic acid (GLA), a

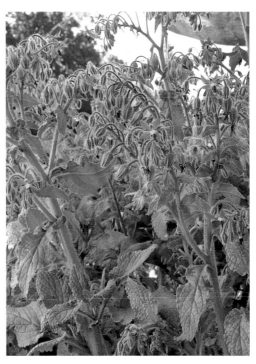

Borago officinalis

compound that has proven to be extremely useful in the treatment of various liver, cardiovascular, and metabolic disorders. In fact, borage seed oil may contain twice the GLA offered by the oil of evening primrose (*Oenothera biennis*) seeds. The use of evening primrose should be avoided in subjects with blood-clotting disorders. Some scientists claim that the GLA in evening primrose oil can decrease blood cholesterol and blood pressure and cure rheumatoid arthritis.

Recent studies suggest that EFA deficiencies may be strongly associated with many chronic diseases in both people and animals, including atopic eczema, diabetes, and various inflammatory disorders. In dogs and cats, fatty acid disorders are characterized in the early phases by a dull coat, itchy skin, and excessive shedding. Gamma-linolenic acid is important in the production of prostaglandins, compounds that are critical to the healthy performance of countless metabolic functions—from breakdown of carbohydrates, fats, and other essential nutrients into usable forms, to maintenance of cellular integrity and proper functioning of smooth-muscle tissues (including the heart, uterus, and vascular system) throughout the body. In other words, animals cannot survive without a proper balance of fatty acids, including GLA, in their bodies.

The body does not produce GLA, and therefore it must be received through dietary sources. The problem is that GLA is relatively rare in nature—it occurs in only a few vegetable sources. Borage seed oil is one of the richest GLA supplements available and can be easily administered by breaking a gel capsule onto your pet's food each day. Ask your holistic veterinarian for recommendations on how much of the oil your animal may need.

Borage leaf has also received attention from herbalists who believe that it may be useful for gently strengthening adrenal function, particularly in subjects who have recently undergone extended steroid therapies. The adrenal cortex (the outer tissues of the adrenal glands) is chiefly responsible for the body's production of corticosteroids, the hormones responsible for natural reduction of inflammation. When synthetic corticosteroids are introduced into the body, natural adrenal functions are replaced and the adrenal cortex often begins to shut down its natural production. As a result, many animals who are ending prednisolone or other steroid therapies have depressed adrenal function. Fat metabolism and mineral balances may also be affected if this happens. While borage is by no means as powerful as licorice (*Glycyrrhiza* spp.) in its adrenal-stimulatory actions, it is believed by many herbalists to gently stimulate adrenal function that is slightly depressed, especially when used over an extended period. It may be particularly useful in cases where

water retention and high blood pressure are prevalent in an animal's holistic condition. In these situations, the stronger herb licorice may be contraindicated because of its potential side effects. While the use of borage in this capacity lacks scientific validation, it has nonetheless been used safely and effectively for hundreds of years. The dried leaves may be tinctured (12 drops per 20 pounds of body weight, twice daily) or fed in bulk form (½ teaspoon sprinkled onto each pound of your animal's food). Borage also has a folkloric reputation for increasing milk production in nursing mothers (both human and otherwise)—an action that may be attributable to increased hormone production by the adrenal gland.

Topically, borage leaves can be applied as a soothing poultice or compress for minor skin irritations. To sum up its potential for topical use, consider borage as a limited alternative to comfrey.

Availability: Virtually any nursery or seed catalog that sells herbs is likely to have borage.

Propagation and Harvest: Borage prefers dry soil and full sun. Aside from these requirements, it is extremely easy to grow from seed or nursery-raised transplants. If you choose to transplant borage from one part of a garden to another, do it while the plants are young because the taproot grows straight down and is easily damaged when removed from the soil.

Borage is a successful self-seeding annual that drops thousands of tiny seeds almost immediately after blooming. Give the plant plenty of room to sprawl, and consider planting it with other annuals because it may become a nuisance when dozens of young plants emerge beneath your perennials during the second year.

Harvest the mature leaves while the plant is in full bloom. Borage leaves are especially susceptible to mold while they are drying, so never harvest when the leaves are wet and never stack the leaves on top of each other. Dry them in an area that is away from direct sunlight and has plenty of air circulation. Spread the leaves on clean newspapers or a nonmetallic screen and turn them once or twice daily to assure quick, even drying. The dried leaves can then be crumbled and stored in a glass jar for up to three months before they begin to lose their usefulness.

Alternatives and Adjuncts: For similar topical applications, look toward comfrey, which is perhaps a more effective alternative when indicated. For anti-inflammatory applications and situations involving depressed adrenal function, such as with Addison's disease, look toward licorice and astragalus as stronger alternatives.

Cautions and Comments: The leaves of this plant contain small amounts of PAs, a potentially toxic group of compounds that may lead to liver damage. Although the presence of these alkaloids in borage is very low (much lower than in comfrey) and require ingestion of large and sustained quantities to become harmful in most animals, borage has nonetheless been banned from human use in Germany.

BUGLEWEED

Lycopus spp.   Mint Family

Appearance: Bugleweed also goes by the name of water horehound. The deeply and irregularly lobed leaves of *Lycopus americanus* differentiate it from other mints (and even other species of *Lycopus*). Other species of bugleweed (such as the less common *L. uniflorus* and *L. asper*) have leaves that are not deep-ly lobed but are

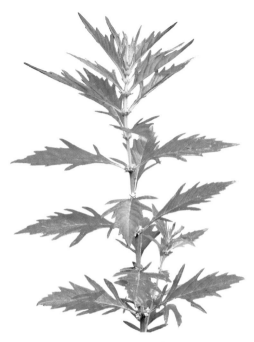

Lycopus americanus

simple and coarsely toothed, making them difficult to differentiate from other mints such as skullcap. The easily identified *L. americanus* remains by far the most common and conspicuous variety in North America, making it the bugleweed to remember. Bugleweed, unlike many other mints, does not have a minty odor. Small whitish to pink flowers are whorled in the leaf axils (the point at which the leaf meets the stem). Stems may be lightly to moderately hairy, especially toward the base of the plant.

Habitat and Range: An inhabitant of stream banks and marshes, bugleweed is typically found in the shade beneath willows and other shrubs. Several species of Lycopus are widespread throughout most of North America.

Cycle and Bloom Season: Perennial, blooming from early to midsummer

Parts Used: Leaves, stems, flowers

Primary Medicinal Activities: Slows thyroid function, mild cardiac sedative, calms nerves, diuretic, constricts subcutaneous blood vessels, astringent, cough suppressant

Strongest Affinities: Thyroid glands, heart, nervous system

Preparation: Although this herb may be useful in dried bulk form or in capsules, it doesn't taste very good, and it may be difficult to administer to a dog or cat in an appreciable quantity that doesn't just pass through the short digestive tract. An alcohol or glycerin tincture is your best choice here.

Common Uses: Although relatively little research has been done to validate bugleweed's usefulness in animal subjects, it may prove useful in dogs and cats with hyperthyroid conditions. While bugleweed cannot physically correct a diseased thyroid gland and does not work as quickly as synthetic drugs, human studies have confirmed that bugleweed slows the release of the hormone thyroxine in the thyroid, making it useful in the treatment of mild forms of hyperthyroidism. Specifically, it should help ease abnormal excitability, relieve acute hyperventilation, slow a rapid heart rate, and relieve spastic coughing in dogs and cats who suffer from spontaneous hyperthyroidism. It should be noted, though, that small, frequent doses of the herb extract must be given for a period of at least a few days before results are seen. Giving 2–6 drops per 20 pounds of the animal's body weight three times daily is a good starting point.

Bugleweed is also useful in many heart and vascular system disorders. It is believed to work in the cardiovascular system in a way that is similar to the drug digitalis—by strengthening the heartbeat while slowing a rapid pulse. But unlike digitalis and other such drugs that are used primarily in humans, bugleweed is virtually free of dangerous side effects.

Adding to bugleweed's usefulness in cardiovascular disorders is its ability to help expel water from the body. This makes it useful in animals with lung fluid associated with weak, rapid pulse and unproductive coughing. However, some extra caution is advised here: bugleweed is believed to suppress the cough response even if such suppression is not conducive to the healing process. In respiratory disorders such as *Bordetella* or pneumonia, cough suppression may be contradictory to the holistic principles of using herbs in the first place and may even be dangerous to the animal. Remember, the primary goal of herbal therapies is to assist the body in its capacity to heal itself, not to interfere with its efforts to do so. If the animal is successful at expelling mucus as a result of persistent coughing, the body is doing its job, and the use of bugleweed is probably contraindicated. See a holistic vet.

The nerve-calming and vasoconstrictor actions of bugleweed make it useful for pain relief in situations that involve irritability and tension. This is true especially when circumstances are compounded by injured nerves such as in posttraumatic circumstances where an animal is in pain from a crushing injury, is jumpy and cannot get comfortable, and just paces, whines, and pants. Bugleweed does not contain salicylates, so it can be used for posttraumatic pain relief in cats. It is especially useful in cats with preexisting functional thyroid adenoma or other forms of disease that may contribute to an overactive thyroid. In humans, bugleweed is often used by herbalists in the treatment of migraine headaches.

Availability: Seeds are available from specialty seed catalogs. Bugleweed herb and herb tinctures are available through natural products retailers.

Propagation and Harvest: This herb requires consistently moist soil and at least 50 percent shade cover. For the best results, sow the seeds indoors in February or March then transplant them to an area that gets plenty of shade and water throughout the summer. Plants are ready to harvest when the flowers are just beginning to bloom. The freshly cut herb is the best choice for making your own medicine, but if this isn't possible, cut the stems at about 3 inches above ground level during a period when the foliage is completely dry. Hang them in small bunches of four to six stems apiece in an airy location away from direct sunlight. When properly stored, the dried herb retains its medicinal potency for at least six months.

Alternatives and Adjuncts: For use in hyperthyroidism, bugleweed combines especially well with lemon balm (Melissa officinalis). For use in heart and vascular disorders associated with a rapid, erratic pulse, ginkgo and motherwort serve as substitutes in many cases, and skullcap, hawthorn, garlic, and astragalus should all be investigated as adjuncts. For nervousness associated with abnormal irritability, pain, or rapid heartbeat, bugleweed will combine nicely with valerian, skullcap, hop, or chamomile. When water retention is an associated factor in any of the above conditions, try adding dandelion leaf to the formula as a diuretic aid.

Cautions and Comments: Like all members of the mint family, bugleweed is a safe herb with no known toxicity when used sensibly. However, since bugleweed constricts blood vessels and may have hormonal properties, common sense dictates that it should not be used in pregnant or nursing animals. For obvious reasons, bugleweed should not be used in animals with depressed thyroid function. Another point to consider before using bugleweed in your pet is that very little research has been done into the attributes and side effects of bugleweed in some animals. Although it can be safely used in most dogs, cats, and horses, its effects in birds, rodents, and other animals are largely unknown. If in doubt, contact a professional who is familiar with the specific applications of this herb.

BURDOCK

Arctium lappa   Sunflower Family
or *A. minor*

Appearance: In its first year of growth, burdock appears as a rosette of large heart-shaped leaves up to 12 inches long. During the second year, the plant continues skyward, often reaching 6–8 feet, while branching out to produce multitudes of thistlelike, light lavender to purple-flowered seed-bearing burrs at the upper reaches of the plant. Each burr contains several small black seeds and is covered by reverse-hooked spines that enable them to stick to anything that brushes by. The entire plant is covered with tiny hairs that give the leaves and the stems a tacky texture similar to that of ultrafine grit sandpaper. The light-brown taproot may weigh 2–3 pounds and extend 2 or more feet below a second-year plant. This sturdy taproot, combined with the annoying and extremely efficient reproductive qualities of the burrs, has earned burdock a hated reputation as a farm and garden enemy.

Habitat and Range: Burdock is a Eurasian import that has made its home throughout most of North America. It prefers rich, deep, consistently moist soil and is frequently found in profuse abundance along the edges of cultivated fields and at roadsides (particularly where human or livestock traffic can cooperate with the hitchhiking burrs).

Cycle and Bloom Season: A biennial that blooms in mid- to late summer

Parts Used: Root

Primary Medicinal Activities: Blood cleansing, liver and gallbladder stimulant, diuretic, nutritive

Strongest Affinities: Liver, skin

Preparation: Although all preparations of this herb are useful, the active constituents of this plant must be given in relatively large doses to be of therapeutic advantage. Since most animals don't like eating it, a strong tincture of fresh or dried root is the most effective preparation. The medicinal ingredients of burdock root are extracted well in a glycerin menstruum (solvent), and the flavor of the resulting liquid, or glycerite, is sweet and agreeable to most animals. The fresh roots have a high water content, which is imparted to the finished tincture. A tincture that contains more than 40 percent water spoils quickly. Therefore, it is best to use 100 percent undiluted vegetable glycerin in your mixture. Fresh or dried burdock root can be decocted, as well, and poured over your animal's food. Be liberal with the quantity—burdock is a healthy food.

Common Uses: We cannot emphasize the value of this herb enough in the long-term care of companion animals. Burdock has an ancient and respected reputation as a nutritive liver tonic that helps to clean and build the blood. Just 2.5 ounces of fresh burdock root contains up to 61 milligrams of calcium, 77 milligrams of phosphorus, 1.4 milligrams of iron, 0.03 milligrams of thiamine, and 0.05 milligrams of riboflavin.

Burdock root is a specific treatment for chronic or acute psoriasis or eczema; it has a strong affinity toward the treatment of flaky, oily, or inflammatory skin disorders that can be traced back to liver deficiencies or a general overload of toxic substances in the body (usually the result of a poor diet). It is also useful in the holistic treatment of arthritis, rheumatoid disorders, inflammatory kidney and bladder diseases, and virtually any other type of metabolic disorder that may be the result of poor waste elimination. Adding to all of this is a diuretic action that helps in the elimination of waste materials from the body. In simple terms, burdock helps clean the body from the inside out.

Burdock contains chemical elements that have been shown to be effective in preventing disease that may result from environmental toxicity. Specifically, burdock helps to remove mutagenic substances such as pesticides and airborne pollutants from the bloodstream before they cause harm to the body. Animal studies have indicated that burdock extract has free-radical scavenging qualities in the liver, thus weeding out carcinogenic elements before cellular damage can occur.

Virtually every living creature is continually subjected to the harmful effects of human society—our companion animals are no exception. The liver is the organ that begins the cleansing process. The liver not only filters the blood but contributes bile and numerous enzymes to the digestive tract that are essential to the breakdown and absorption of essential nutrients. By assisting liver function and prompting the efficient removal of systemic waste, absorbed or ingested toxins, and allergens from the body, imbalances such as arthritis, kidney stones, bladder infections, and eczema can be avoided. By helping the liver do its job, we are also relieving pressure from secondary immune functions that need to remain unencumbered in their fight against viruses and other microbes that may have bypassed the liver. Furthermore, if the liver can work at optimum efficiency, less solid or toxic waste will reach the kidneys—a set of delicate organs that are vulnerable to the liver's deficiencies.

Burdock is an excellent long-term liver tonic, and it is gentle enough to use in cases of preexisting liver or kidney disease. It is an excellent choice for animals suffering as a result of a poor diet. Just remember, diet is where the road to a long, healthy life begins. Burdock will not replace a good natural diet, but it can help tremendously in allowing the body to utilize the good nutrition it receives.

Availability: Fresh organically grown burdock root is available at many health food stores. Dried burdock root and root tincture are available through most herb retailers. Seeds are available through specialty seed catalogs.

Propagation and Harvest: Provided you have deep, rich soil for taproots that can penetrate the earth 3 feet, burdock is easy to grow. Burdock likes moist (but not wet) soil, and it prefers to have at least a couple of hours of shade each day. Sow the seeds as you would carrots, in early spring. The roots are ready after the leaves die back in the fall of the first year. Second-year roots can

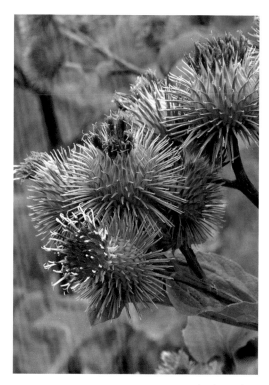

Arctium minor

be used if dug in the spring, but remember that biennials die after their second year of growth and the roots lose potency as they approach their demise.

Burdock roots can be refrigerated for several weeks after harvest, or they can be chopped and dried, made into tincture, or decocted for immediate use.

Alternatives and Adjuncts: Dandelion root serves well as an alternative to burdock. For treatment of flaky or itchy skin problems, burdock can be supplemented with licorice, red clover, dandelion, or yellow dock. As a liver aid in conditions associated with chronic constipation, burdock can be supplemented with dandelion, chicory, turkey rhubarb, yellow dock, or Oregon grape. In cases of preexisting liver damage resulting from chemical toxicity or vaccinosis, use the burdock with milk thistle or licorice. As an adjunct to an immune-support formula, combine burdock with echinacea or astragalus.

Cautions and Comments: This is one of the safest herbs available to humans and animals. In essence, burdock is a nutraceutical, a food that also offers medicinal attributes. No toxicity has been noted with this herb.

CALENDULA
Calendula officinalis   Sunflower Family

Appearance: This herb is also known as pot marigold. The bright yellow, orange, or red-orange flowers of calendula are a familiar sight in gardens and landscape designs found everywhere. *Calendula officinalis* is a small plant that seldom exceeds 18 inches in height. The lance-shaped or oblong alternate leaves have coarse surfaces and are borne on sturdy branching stems. Calendula should not be confused with other marigolds, namely French marigolds, and other members of the *Tagetes* genus of the sunflower family, which have a pungent odor and much different leaf characteristics.

Habitat and Range: Originally a native of Europe and Africa, calendula is a cultivated plant throughout most of the world.

Cycle and Bloom Season: The word *calendula* is derived from *calends* (the first day of the Roman month) because the plant was thought to bloom on the new moon of each month. While calendula really doesn't keep such an accurate calendar, it does remain in a constant and generous state of bloom throughout most of its annual life span.

Parts Used: Flowers

Primary Medicinal Activities: Anti-inflammatory, increases lymph circulation, heals wounds, astringent, antibacterial, antifungal, anti-tumor, liver stimulant, promotes menstruation (emmenagogue)

Strongest Affinities: Skin and mucous membranes

Preparation: Water or oil infusion, tincture, poultice, salve, ointment

Common Uses: Calendula is among the first herbs to consider in minor first aid situations. A broad array of medicinal compounds in the flowers of the plant (various essential oils, flavonoids, saponins, triterpene alcohols, carotenes, and others) combine to help speed cell reproduction and inhibit bacteria and fungi at the site of injury.

For minor cuts, insect bites, abrasions, and postsurgical incisions, a calendula salve applied externally brings quick, soothing relief to pain and swelling, while lending wound-healing, antimicrobial properties to the body's healing effort. Infusions of the flowers are effective as a soothing and healing skin wash for various forms of inflammatory dermatitis, such as those caused by fleabites, poison ivy, eczema, and sunburn. The infection-fighting, skin-healing nature of this plant makes it useful for treating burns as well. A cooled water infusion may be used as an eyewash for conjunctivitis, where the mild but predictable astringency of the plant combines with its bacteria-fighting properties to reduce irritation and infection. To make an eyewash or skin rinse, refer to chapter 1.

Internally, an infusion or tincture of the flower may be used in treating inflammation or ulceration of the digestive or urinary tracts, where it serves in the drainage of lymph-engorged tissues and reduces inflammation. It may also prove beneficial in the treatment of candidiasis, a fungal infection of the mucous membranes in the mouths and digestive tracts of birds, cats, horses, and sometimes dogs. The antifungal qualities of this herb also make it a possible option for topical treatment of chromomycosis, a fungal infection of the skin in cows, horses, dogs, cats, and amphibians, or for the treatment of entomophthoromycosis, a fungal infection of the nostrils, mouth, or lips of horses. While virtually no scientific data exist to validate the effectiveness of calendula against these three forms of disease, calendula's safety and reputed effectiveness as a broad-spectrum antifungal agent make it an option worth trying.

Preparations containing calendula have been shown to be effective in the treatment of chronic colitis. And animal studies have shown that the saponin constituents in calendula may possess antitumor activities.

Availability: Over thirty varieties of calendula are available at nurseries everywhere.

Propagation and Harvest: Sow seeds in early spring or transplant the starts after the danger of frost is past. Calendula likes moderately rich soil and full sun. It is not picky about pH—as long as the soil is not excessively alkaline or acidic, calendula will do just fine. Once established, plants self-sow from their prolific seed production. Seedlings that emerge each spring should be thinned to about 6 inches apart, so you can have a continuous, relatively carefree supply of calendula. Harvest the flowers whenever they are in full bloom. They can then be made into an herbal preparation

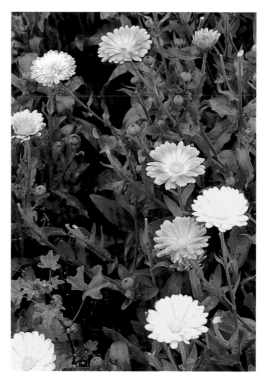

Calendula officinalis

while they are fresh, or you can dry them indoors for use in the near future.

Alternatives and Adjuncts: For use in first aid salves, calendula combines especially well with comfrey and Saint-John's-wort. To increase its effectiveness in antifungal uses (internally or externally), try adding bee balm, Oregon grape, or licorice. For urinary or digestive tract inflammations, calendula can be coupled with corn silk, marshmallow, or plantain.

Cautions and Comments: Although calendula is without question one of the safest herbs, it does have a reputation for stimulating menstruation. In some studies it has been shown to possess abortifacient (abortion-causing) activities in rodents, so it should be avoided during early pregnancy. Calendula may contain a very small measure of salicylic acid, a constituent that is potentially toxic to cats. Although this compound is likely confined to the leaves and stems of the plant and does not occur in quantities that are likely to be of immediate danger to cats, its presence should be taken into account prior to long-term internal use.

CATNIP

Nepeta cataria Mint Family

Appearance: Wild catnip is always a wonderful discovery. Its pungent tangy-mint aroma wafts to the nose with the slightest disturbance of the plant. And the flavor and soothing effects of the tea are likely to please even the most discriminating palate. Characteristically a mint, catnip has square stems and opposite leaves. Leaves are petiolate (stemmed), coarsely but often bluntly toothed, and nearly heart shaped to broadly lance shaped. Once one has become familiar with this plant, the aroma is a sure giveaway. The entire plant is distinctively fuzzy with an almost flannel-like texture. Unlike most other mints, which bloom in whorls at the upper leaf axils or in terminate clusters or spires, catnip blooms at both the upper leaf axils and in spikelike terminate clusters.

Habitat and Range: Catnip is a Eurasian import that is now widespread in North America. It likes full sun and rich, moist soil, and is most frequently found in disturbed areas such as along irrigation channels and at the edges of cultivated fields. Unfortunately, this characteristic often makes it difficult for the herbalist or wild food forager to find uncontaminated plants. Fortunately, catnip can be found at many nurseries.

Cycle and Bloom Season: A perennial that blooms from late spring to midsummer

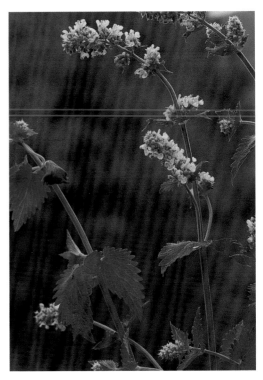

Nepeta cataria

Parts Used: Leaves, stems, and flowers are collected before seeds begin to develop.

Primary Medicinal Activities: Expels intestinal gas, sedative, antispasmodic, helps alleviate vomiting (antiemetic), feline-euphoric, diuretic

Strongest Affinities: Digestive and nervous systems

Preparation: Fresh or dried chopped herb, water infusion, tincture, or, of course, stuffed in a catnip toy

Common Uses: Catnip is a gentle gas reliever and antispasmodic for easing flatulence and stomach upsets. It also acts as a mild sedative to help calm the nerves and promote restful sleep in most animals.

Due to an ingredient called nepetalactone, cats become intoxicated when they sniff this plant. The effect of the herb when ingested is relaxing in a different way, calming to the stomach and relaxing to the nerves but without feline-erotic visions of candy-coated mice. Interestingly, about 20 percent of our feline friends do not experience a euphoric response to catnip. This is an excellent herb to consider for a high-strung animal with a nervous stomach, especially if episodes of vomiting are precipitated by stressful events such as running the vacuum cleaner, having the neighbors and their screaming child over for dinner, or—worse yet—bringing another kitten into the "royal palace." You can administer 12–20 drops (0.25 to 0.5 milliliter) of a glycerin-based catnip tincture for every 20 pounds of an animal's body weight, ten to twenty minutes prior to being subjected to stressful circumstances. For travel or other prolonged periods of stress, the tincture can be added to the animal's drinking water—12 drops per 8 ounces of water is a good starting dose. If the animal does not respond, try adding 6 drops at a time, until the desired calming effect is evident. Dropping a few fresh leaves into the animal's drinking water may work as well. You can also try feeding dried catnip to your pet by putting it onto her food at a dose of ⅛ to ½ teaspoon per pound of food fed. Just remember that this might make kitty roll around in her dinner!

Availability: Catnip has become a roadside weed in many areas. If you are not so fortunate, the plants or seeds are available through many nurseries.

Propagation and Harvest: Gather the leaves, stems, and flowers before the plant goes to seed. The herb can then be dried indoors. Spread the herb loosely on a clean sheet of paper, rearranging it frequently to prevent mold. The herb is ready for storage when it is crispy dry.

Alternatives and Adjuncts: To help settle an upset stomach and to prevent nervous vomiting, catnip combines well with fennel. Chamomile serves as an effective adjunct or alternative in these circumstances. For motion sickness, a pinch of ginger can be added to a teaspoon of dried, powdered catnip. The combination can then be given to a dog or cat in a small gel capsule. One capsule should do for a cat; a dog may require two or three, depending on her size.

Cautions and Comments: The herb is safe, but use it sparingly in pregnant animals, as it has been theorized that the volatile oils it contains may be passed on to the fetus, the result of which is unknown.

CAYENNE

Capsicum spp.   Nightshade Family

Appearance: Like many common names, the words capsicum and cayenne are used as generic terms for a broad range of small, very hot chili peppers. Most of these peppers are genetically engineered variations of two species of the *Capsicum* genus: *C. frutescens* and *C. annuum*. There are dozens of varieties, but they all share a similar appearance: shiny oval to lance-shaped, 1- to 5-inch-long leaves; small, white, star-shaped flowers; and sturdy, sometimes vinelike stems that reach anywhere from 1 to 3 feet tall when mature.

Habitat and Range: Originally a native of tropical regions of South and Central America, virtually all of the capsicums are now cultivated in areas throughout the world with long growing seasons. In northern climes, capsicum can be grown as an attractive houseplant.

Cycle and Bloom Season: Wild South American capsicums are perennial plants that can reach 7 feet in height, but in North America most capsicums are cultivated as annuals. Most capsicums bloom in early summer and produce ripe fruit by mid-August.

Parts Used: Fruits

Primary Medicinal Activities: Warms and reddens the skin (rubefacient), dilates blood vessels (vasodilator), stops bleeding (hemostatic), counterirritant, anti-inflammatory, analgesic, strengthens tissues (tonic)

Strongest Affinities: Skin and circulatory system

Preparation: For internal uses, the dried and powdered fruits are most commonly contained in gel capsules. The whole or powdered fruits may be used in oil infusions, salves, ointments, or tinctures. Various brands of capsaicin creams and ointments are commercially available at drugstores for topical treatment of arthritis, muscle aches, stiffness, and other conditions.

Common Uses: Capsicum is reliable in its activity as a peripheral vasodilator. Used internally, it acts to warm the body by quickly dilating small capillaries and increasing circulation to the skin and extremities. (This is why sweating and flushed skin is experienced when we eat foods containing cayenne.) Because of this activity, capsicum is commonly used in the systemic treatment of impaired blood circulation, and because it triggers the outward movement of blood throughout the body, it is often added as a "carrier" for the active components of other herbs. Its effect in this capacity can be quite dramatic, especially when it is combined with herbs that have an affinity toward the skin or extremities. By itself, capsicum is useful for opening capillary occlusions that are the by-product of a crushing injury, and it is considered a specific remedy for chronically deficient peripheral circulation—situations characterized by continuously cold paws, hands, or feet. Capsicum is also regarded as a circulatory stimulant for the lungs and may be useful for improving pulmonary efficiency in animals with hypostatic pneumonia (a condition arising from poor blood circulation through vascular structures of the lungs) or other conditions where edema or other factors are interfering with proper blood circulation in pulmonary tissues.

In most internal applications, capsicum is administered once per day in the form of a gel capsule. For a dog or a cat, the capsule would contain a small pinch of the powder. For horses and other large animals, several full large capsules may be needed to bring about desired results. Finding the correct dose is contingent upon the specifics of the individual animal and the situation at hand.

Topically, capsicum works as a contact rubefacient, serving to quickly open subcutaneous capillaries while acting as a nerve block and reducing pain at the site of application. These topical attributes make capsicum especially useful for therapies that are to be confined to a specific portion of the body, such as those for stiff or arthritic knees that may benefit from the herb's instantaneous warming effect. The compound chiefly responsible for this activity is called capsaicin, and in addition to its capacity to block pain and increase circulation, capsaicin has been shown to activate the body's own anti-inflammatory mediators at the site where it is applied. It not only helps to reduce pain and congestion in arthritic joints but also acts as an assistant to the body's internal anti-inflammatory mechanisms. These combined actions make topical preparations of capsicum useful for safely relieving the symptoms of rheumatoid arthritis and osteoarthritis.

On the top of our list of uses for capsicum, though, is its effectiveness at stopping bleeding. It's interesting to note that while capsicum has such a profound ability to increase blood circulation when taken internally or applied onto the skin, its effects are quite opposite when applied to the site of internal or external bleeding. To stop the bleeding of a barbed wire cut, a claw that was clipped too short, or any other minor to moderate wound where profuse bleeding does not coagulate readily on its own, capsicum powder, or ground cayenne from the kitchen cabinet, can be liberally applied directly to the site of injury. Unless bleeding is emanating from a fairly large vessel, the result is likely to be instantaneous, and believe it or not, capsicum really doesn't hurt much when applied to an open wound.

Availability: Readily available wherever culinary spices are sold. Capsicum plants are available through virtually any nursery that stocks vegetable plants.

Propagation and Harvest: Capsicum is often slow to start from seed, so it is best to purchase young plants. Like most peppers, capsicums that are planted outdoors require warm, sunny days and nighttime temperatures that seldom fall below 55 degrees Fahrenheit (F) in order to produce fruit. Many varieties are quite suitable as houseplants.

Alternatives and Adjuncts: To stop bleeding, capsicum combines well with yarrow. For circulatory problems, hawthorn,

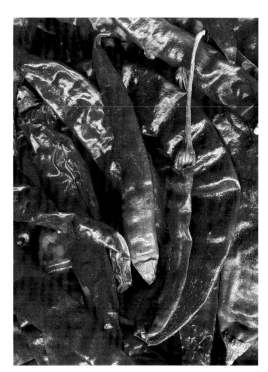

Capsicum sp.

ginkgo, ginger, and yarrow should all be considered as well.

Cautions and Comments: Contrary to what may seem obvious, capsicum does not cause irritation to the digestive tract when consumed in moderate quantities, but the key word here is *moderate*. You should not feed capsicum to animals who have a sensitive digestive tract or inflammatory digestive or urinary system disease unless you have a full understanding of all underlying conditions. When used properly and in moderation, capsicum is a safe herb, but extra care and attention are needed to assure that capsicum is truly indicated. No two animals are identical, and where capsicum may serve to benefit one, it can cause painful irritation to another. In other words, it is best to have your animal examined by a holistic veterinarian before proceeding with any internal therapy that includes capsicum. Cap-sicum is a strong irritant to mucous membranes and should always be kept away from the eyes and nose. This is the stuff that bear-defense pepper spray is made from. Its topical use should be avoided with animals who have hypersensitive skin. Although capsicum is generally considered safe during pregnancy, we recommend that its use be limited to topical applications. In our opinion, strong urinary tract irritants should not be used in pregnant or lactating animals.

Be sure to wash your hands with soap and water after handling any form of this herb, and don't touch your eyes, lips, or any other mucous membranes for about thirty minutes after.

CHAMOMILE

Matricaria recutita   Sunflower Family

Appearance: German chamomile is characterized by its ½- to 1-inch flowers, each with a yellow disk surrounded by ten to twenty white rays (petals). The common name *chamomile* is used in reference to dozens of related species, but most of the medicinal uses are isolated to two genera, *M. recutita* (German chamomile) and *Chamaemelum nobile* (Roman chamomile), and their respective subspecies. The differences between these two groups of chamomile rest in their life cycles, the number of flowers they produce, and their overall size. German chamomile is an annual plant that can grow to 2 feet tall, producing numerous flowers on each of its many stems. Roman chamomile, on the other hand, is a creeping perennial that seldom exceeds 1 foot in height and produces fewer but larger (1-inch-wide) flowers. Both German and Roman chamomiles share a nearly identical range of therapeutic usefulness, but German chamomile is by far the more

popular medicine because it has received much more research attention and has long been regarded by herbalists as a more potent medicine than Roman chamomile. For the purposes of this book, our primary focus is on German chamomile; there is, however, a generally overlooked wild relative of cultivated varieties of chamomile that also deserves a place in the animal herbalist's repertory: pineapple weed (*M. matricarioides*).

Pineapple weed looks, smells, and even tastes much like its cultivated cousins, but its flowers have no petals. This small wayside weed is often found growing in inconspicuous ground-hugging mats in vacant lots, on road margins, and sometimes right in the middle of a driveway!

Habitat and Range: A Native of Europe and western Asia, chamomile is cultivated worldwide.

Cycle and Bloom Season: Chamomile is notorious for its continuous bloom. In areas where the occurrence of frost is rare, chamomile often produces flowers throughout the year.

Parts Used: Flowers

Primary Medicinal Activities: Antispasmodic, expels intestinal gas, anti-inflammatory, sedative, antimicrobial, stimulates digestion (bitter), heals wounds, expels worms

Strongest Affinities: Skin, digestive tract, liver, nervous system, mucous membranes, smooth-muscle tissues

Preparation: Water or oil infusion, tincture, salve, ointment, fomentation

Common Uses: Chamomile is a mild sedative, antispasmodic, and digestive tonic that is safe, gentle, and effective in a broad spectrum of applications. The herb tea or tincture is helpful for indigestion, gas, and vomiting. Chamomile is perhaps the first herb to reach for in cases of digestive upset that arises from nervousness and hyperexcitability. The chemistry of chamomile is complex, and its medicinal activities are not attributable to any single class of constituents but rather to a synergistic sum of all its parts. However, dozens of scientific studies (using both animals and humans) have given us solid information about which of chamomile's chemical compounds contribute to its effectiveness as a holistic healing device. For example, apegenin, chamazulene (and its precursor, matricin) and other volatile oil constituents of the flowers have been shown to be strong antispasmodic agents both in and on the body, as have several of chamomile's flavonoid constituents. In the digestive tract, chamomile serves to ease nervous spasms, helps to expel gas, aids in the production of bile to improve digestion, and reduces inflammation. All of these activities amount to an excellent remedy for chronic or acute gastric disorders, including various forms of inflammatory bowel disease.

For inflammations of the skin, including those caused by fleabites, contact allergies, and various bacterial or fungal infections, a cooled water infusion of the flowers can be used as a soothing, healing, antimicrobial rinse. For conjunctivitis, whether it be from bacterial infection or the result of airborne irritants or allergies, the cooled infusion can be carefully strained through a paper coffee filter, diluted with saline solution (the end product should be transparent and light yellow), and used as an anti-inflammatory and antimicrobial eyewash that can be applied liberally several times per day until the inflammation subsides.

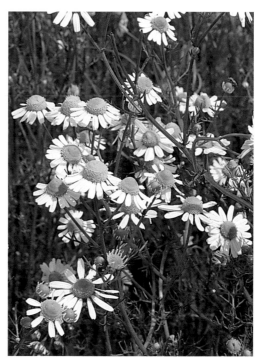

Matricaria recutita

Chamomile has also been shown to have a tonic (constricting and strengthening) effect on smooth-muscle tissues throughout the body, including the heart, bladder, and especially the uterus. While uterine tonics may be beneficial before pregnancy and during late-term pregnancy, herbs that constrict uterine tissues are generally contraindicated during early pregnancy.

In our experiences chamomile serves as a general-purpose calming herb that can be fed to animals as a "first try" remedy for any variety of spasmodic or anxiety-related problems. Because it tastes good, is soluble in water, and is safe for most animals, its use should be considered before stronger, less-palatable antispasmodics or sedatives are employed.

Chamomile's usefulness in expelling worms is often overlooked in favor of faster acting herbs (such as wormwood, black walnut hulls, or garlic), but it should not be. Chamomile is relatively nontoxic when compared to most other "herbal wormers." While it doesn't work as quickly as the other anthelmintics, it does work, especially for roundworms and whipworms, and it offers anti-inflammatory activities that help counteract the effect parasites often have on intestinal mucosa. Pineapple weed (*M. matricarioides*) is even more pronounced in its worm-expelling activities.

For internal uses, we prefer a glycerin tincture of the herb because it can be administered in small, easy-to-feed doses of 0.25–0.50 milliliter per 20 pounds of the animal's body weight, twice daily as needed to suppress symptoms. The sweet-tasting glycerin tincture can be administered directly into the animal's mouth, or it can be added to the animal's drinking water. The glycerite is also useful in treating gingivitis, especially when small proportions of stronger antimicrobial herb extracts (such as thyme, rosemary, bee balm, Oregon grape, or echinacea) are added. To use chamomile in this capacity, the tincture can be applied directly to the gums of the animal with a cotton swab.

Chamomile extract can also be used in a vaporizer or steamed from boiling water for inhalation treatment of asthma, allergies, bronchitis, and the like. In homeopathic form, chamomile is used for teething puppies to keep them from chewing everything in sight.

Availability: Chamomile can be purchased from any health food retailer and is available at most supermarkets. The plants are available through most nurseries, as are the seeds.

Propagation and Harvest: Chamomile is easy to grow in all climates, and once established its promiscuous, free-seeding character yields abundant growth year after year. If left to its unruly self, it is likely to find its way out of flower beds and into pathways and beyond.

Chamomile blooms continuously throughout the growing season. The flowers can be plucked off at any time and dried indoors on a piece of clean paper or a nonmetallic screen. Fresh flowers are useful, too, and in fact are a stronger option for use in skin rinses and against intestinal parasites, but the dried flowers have a much more pleasant flavor.

Alternatives and Adjuncts: In cases of nervous stomach problems and gas, look to catnip, fennel, and bee balm. Chamomile combines well with calendula, juniper leaves, or uva ursi in anti-inflammatory skin rinses. For irritable bowel, diarrhea, and other gastric disorders, consider plantain, slippery elm, and marshmallow. For inflammatory urinary tract problems, chamomile combines with corn silk, plantain, uva ursi, white oak bark, couch grass, and marshmallow. For use against worms, chamomile can be combined at a 4:1 ratio (four parts chamomile to one part other herb) with garlic, Oregon grape, organically raised goldenseal, wormwood, or black walnut hulls.

Cautions and Comments: Chamomile is, without doubt, one of the safest herbs in existence, but some animals (and humans too) are extremely allergic to this plant and its relatives. Always check for sensitivity before feeding this herb by applying a small amount of the preparation to an animal's skin. Then if no reactions are observed, feed just a drop or two and watch for any changes in your animal.

Studies suggest that excessive use of chamomile during pregnancy may increase fetus reabsorption and inhibit fetus growth in some animals.

CHAPARRAL

Larrea tridentata   Caltrop Family

Appearance: Chaparral (also commonly known as creosote bush) is the predominant low-desert shrub of the U.S. Southwest. The abundance of this shrub almost makes a description of it unnecessary, as many who live or travel between the Pacific Ocean and inland states of the Southwest invariably find themselves within what seems to be an endless expanse of these ancient plants. But, for those who are unfamiliar with the plant, chaparral is the chest-high to 10-feet-tall dark green bush with spindly wind-whipped branches, which contributes to the highway hypnosis we all suffer while driving to and from Las Vegas. The leaves are tiny (1/8 inch long) and have a greasy-leathery texture. The bark is reddish brown toward the base of the plant and progressively lighter (to almost white) on the smaller limbs. Flowers are minute and yellow, developing into oddly fuzzy seed-bearing capsules. Chaparral is one of the oldest living inhabitants of our planet, with some individual plants estimated to be over ten thousand years old!

Habitat and Range: Profusely abundant from the deserts of central Texas westward through the southern half of New Mexico and Arizona to the deserts of southern California and Nevada.

Cycle and Bloom Season: Chaparral often blooms according to precipitation. Generally, this occurs any time from March through May.

Parts Used: Leaves, flowers, fruits

Primary Medicinal Activities: Inhibits bacterial reproduction (bacteriostatic), antifungal,

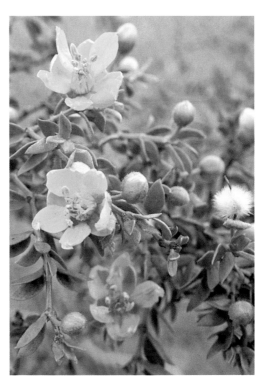

Larrea tridentata

kills certain types of amoeba (amoebicidal), antioxidant, helps with blood cleansing

Strongest Affinities: Skin, blood, liver

Preparation: A decoction is used externally as a skin and coat rinse or as an ingredient in salves and ointments. For small animals, the fomentation method of application is strongly advised (see chapter 1) because this form of preparation allows the active constituents of the herb to remain on the body longer and prohibits the animal from licking off the decoction. Salves or ointments that contain a large percentage of chaparral should also be kept out of the mouth of the animal. For horses or other large animals, this is less of an issue, especially if the decoction is applied to portions of the body that are beyond reach of the animal's mouth.

Because this plant is naturally designed to resist harsh desert elements, it is poorly soluble in water. Therefore, decoctions and alcohol-based tinctures are the best methods of extraction for this plant.

Common Uses: American Indians of the Southwest have used this plant for centuries—for everything from the internal treatment of tumors and hepatic (liver) diseases to topical skin treatments, including sunscreen, for themselves and their animals. Today, herbalists use the plant as a strong bacteriostatic and antioxidant agent in the treatment of blood and liver disorders. However, recent scientific research and documented incidents have raised both hope and concern.

Some studies have shown that chemical constituents in chaparral may inhibit the growth of cancerous cells, while others have shown exactly the opposite. And recently, a few accounts of serious liver damage (in humans) have been attributed to this herb. Many theories as to why this plant may suddenly be harming us after hundreds of years of safe medicinal use. One theory is that perhaps humanity and chaparral are evolving away from one another. Nevertheless, thousands of people still use chaparral on a daily basis, and it remains a popular herbal medicine in natural products markets worldwide.

In animals, chaparral has been shown to have strong antifungal, antibacterial, and, remarkably, amoebicidal properties. The constituent believed to be responsible for most of chaparral's medicinal activity is a lignan compound known as nordihydroguaiaretic acid (NDGA). Nordihydroguaiaretic acid may be effective in treating various forms of amebiasis, including *Entamoeba histolytica*, an amoeba that can be passed from humans to the digestive tracts of dogs (but rarely to other animals) and causes acute or chronic colitis characterized by persistent diarrhea. It has also been proven effective against *Salmonella, Streptococcus, Phylococcus aureus, Bacillus subtilis*, and various other pathogens and molds. Unfortunately, chaparral's toxicity prohibits it from most internal uses. But its remarkable antimicrobial properties make it an excellent broad-spectrum topical agent that is as useful for the animal handler as it is for the animal receiving care.

Used as a hand rinse before and after handling animals who may be carrying *Salmonella* or other transmittable pathogens or as a rinse applied prior to handling animals who are prone to infection from human-carried pathogens, a decoction of chaparral serves an effective two-way adjunct to soap and water. For external treatment of fungal infections of the hooves, nails, or skins of various large and small animals, chaparral is among the first herbs to try. Just remember, keep chaparral from going into the animal's digestive tract.

Availability: Available through herb retailers; profusely available in the low desert regions of the southwestern U.S. and Mexico.

Propagation and Harvest: In arid regions, chaparral can be transplanted into the garden as a slow-growing landscape shrub. The leaves, twigs, and flowers can be harvested any time.

Alternatives and Adjuncts: For antibacterial skin rinses, bee balm, chamomile, sage, thyme, or rosemary can be used. For treatment of psoriasis and other inflammatory skin disorders, chaparral combines well with calendula or aloe.

Cautions and Comments: Ingestion of any form of this plant in large enough quantities may lead to liver damage. For this reason, it is a good idea to take extra measures to assure that your animal does not lick off external applications of chaparral after they are applied. Therefore, we recommend that you wrap dogs, cats, and other small animals in a towel after a skin rinse has been applied.

CHICKWEED

Stellaria media   Pink Family

Appearance: Common chickweed is a weak-stemmed sprawling annual that is commonly found in lush, low-growing mats or entangled in other growth (oftentimes in rose beds). Chickweed exhibits a unique characteristic that makes it easy to differentiate from all look-alikes: a line of minute hairs runs up only one side of the stem; switching sides at each pair of leaves. Opposite leaves may grow to 1½ inches and range in shape from broadly lance shaped to oval but always have distinct points at their tips. Flowers are small (¼ inch across) and white with five petals that are clefted at their tips to give the false appearance of ten petals. Chickweed blooms continuously, each time dropping its seeds as it continues its sprawl.

Habitat and Range: Chickweed inhabits moist meadows, ravines, and disturbed areas throughout all of North America, from the Brooks Range of Alaska to all points southward.

Cycle and Bloom Season: An annual that blooms and free-seeds itself continuously throughout growth

Parts Used: Freshly harvested leaves, flowers, and stems

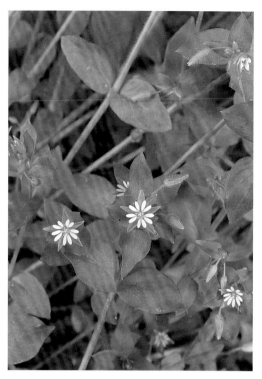

Stellaria media

Primary Medicinal Activities: Soothing to the skin; lubricates, soothes, and protects internal mucous membranes (demulcent), diuretic, tonic

Strongest Affinities: Skin and digestive tract

Preparation: Fresh whole plant, fresh juice of the plant, water or oil infusion, salves, ointments. If you have access to a juicer, try this: Juice enough of the fresh plants to fill an ice-cube tray (preferably a stainless steel one), then freeze it. If the tray is stored in a resealable bag and kept in a freezer, the frozen juice cubes keeps for about three months. Individual cubes can be thawed and the juice used as needed, internally or externally.

Common Uses: Whether for human or animal purposes, chickweed is a safe, delicious resource for providing soothing, cooling relief for virtually any form of minor irritation. Internally, chickweed acts to soothe, protect, and mildly lubricate the upper digestive tract. Fed in its entire fresh form, it is useful for relieving minor esophageal irritations, such as those caused by something Rover ate that had rough edges, or even a minor bite or sting that Godzilla the iguana suffered from snapping at an insect with bad manners. Chickweed can also be fed to dogs or cats as a source of lubrication and light roughage that may assist in the expulsion of hair balls. For mild cases of stomach upset that are believed to be the result of an irritated stomach lining or for a mild case of colitis, fresh chickweed or chickweed juice is indicated as a mild first aid tonic for dogs, cats, and horses or any other herbivore. If chickweed is not astringent or mucilaginous enough to bring relief, the therapy can be progressively "upgraded" by using stronger herbs. Chickweed is nutritious and an excellent nutritive and digestive tonic for birds. Chickweed poultices are useful for cooling and soothing minor burns and skin irritations, particularly when associated with itching and dryness.

Availability: Chickweed grows just about everywhere in the world. If you cannot find a wild source, many specialty seed catalogs now carry the seed. Don't bother with the dried herb you are likely to find in the marketplace—it just isn't the same!

Propagation and Harvest: Because chickweed is a vigorous free-seeder, transplanting it into the garden is as easy as grabbing a handful of the plants and spreading them on a moist flower bed. Give your chickweed plenty of water, rich soil, and at least four hours of shade each day, and it will likely be at your service forever.

Although this plant likes to sprawl, its delicate (and delicious) nature seldom poses a problem to the weed-weary gardener.

Alternatives and Adjuncts: Aloe juice or gel is a better option for burns and irritations of the skin. In salves and ointments, chickweed combines nicely with calendula or Saint-John's-wort. For cases of gastrointestinal irritation that will not respond to chickweed's gentle nature, slippery elm, plantain, or marshmallow should be considered.

Cautions and Comments: Generally, chickweed is considered to be a safe medicinal food plant—it can be fed to most animals in whatever quantities they desire. Large quantities of chickweed, however, can have a laxative effect. Always keep in mind that some animals may be allergic to chickweed. Perhaps the most important thing to consider with the use of this plant is that it often lives among hated weeds that have been subjected to herbicides, and it is frequently found in waste areas that are subject to various contaminants.

CLEAVERS

Galium aparine   Madder Family

Appearance: The *Galium* genus is large and widespread, with no fewer than thirteen species in the Pacific Northwest alone. Species can be divided into two general groups: perennial and annual. In essence, the annual varieties are sprawlers and climbers, often forming ground-covering mats with much weaker taproots and more delicate stems and leaves than perennial species. All Galium plants have square stems and slender leaves that grow in whorled clusters like bicycle spokes of two to eight leaves, depending on the species. Flowers are small and white to greenish in color. *Galium aparine* (see photo) is a widely distributed annual variety that has earned most of the attention of the herb market because of its delicate, aromatic, and readily water soluble nature. It has earned the common names of "cleavers" and "tangleweed" because of the thousands of infinitesimal, reversed hooks on the angles of its stems. These tiny hooks enable the plant to cling to just about anything in a fashion similar to the way static-charged hair clings to clothing. This allows cleavers to reproduce effectively because the delicate seed-bearing foliage is easily uprooted and carried away by passersby. Perennial varieties such as northern bedstraw (*G. boreale*) do not share this unique characteristic.

Habitat and Range: Cleavers (*G. aparine*) and most other annual varieties prefer moist habitats and are commonly found growing in shaded ravines and along streams. Northern bedstraw (*G. boreale*) and other perennial species can tolerate a much wider diversity of habitats and are commonly found along road margins and in dry, sunny areas. Both cleavers and northern bedstraw are common throughout North America and most of the Northern Hemisphere, up to about 6,000 feet in elevation.

Cycle and Bloom Season: Annual or perennial (depending on species). Most *Galium* spp. bloom in early to midsummer.

Parts Used: Entire fresh plant

Primary Medicinal Activities: Tonic, helps with blood cleansing, diuretic, astringent, anti-inflammatory, heals wounds

Strongest Affinities: Lymph system, urinary tract, skin

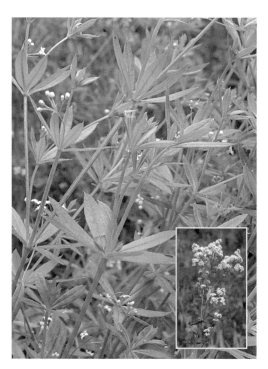

Galium aparine

Preparation: Juice, tincture, or tea of the fresh plant

Common Uses: Herbalists have long regarded cleavers as a valuable lymphatic tonic. In essence, the lymph system is responsible for "washing" body tissues. Throughout the body, lymph is passed across capillary barriers to remove waste materials from healthy cell communities. The lymph is then returned to the bloodstream, where in a properly functioning body it is cleaned of waste material by the liver and kidneys. The waste then (hopefully) leaves the body via the usual urinary and digestive outlets.

Cleavers is used in virtually any condition that is characterized by general or localized swelling or in situations where lymphatic circulation has been impaired by the formation of scar tissue, ulceration, or infection. Although the activities of cleavers are subtle, the herb is believed to increase circulation of lymph in impaired areas of the body through dilation of small, almost cellular-level capillaries. This would explain the remarkable ability of cleavers in helping speed the healing of gastric ulcers and the herb's long-standing reputation for aiding drainage of lymph-engorged cysts, tumors, and inflamed tissues of the urinary tract. In addition to its lymphatic qualities, cleavers lends mild astringent activities to its job of relieving inflammations of the upper digestive and urinary tracts. In cats, these activities make cleavers a safe long-term aid in the treatment of feline lower urinary tract disease (FLUTD), also known as feline urinary syndrome (FUS), and the herb may also be useful for chronic low-grade kidney inflammation.

Because cleavers is thought to increase lymphatic flow throughout body tissues, it may be useful as an alterative therapy in the treatment of various skin disorders. From a holistic perspective, skin problems such as psoriasis and eczema are usually the result of poor elimination of systemic waste. Instead of being "washed" out by the lymph system, "filtered" by the liver and kidneys, and eliminated from the body, the waste materials build up in the body, resulting in diseases such as rheumatoid arthritis and conditions such as flaky, oily, or itchy skin. By improving lymphatic circulation, a critical level of systemic waste management is assisted.

Although relatively little scientific research has been done to validate these claims, its long history of use and safe track record make cleavers a worthwhile tonic for those who are willing to accept natural healing based on anecdotal evidence. A typical starting dose of the glycerin tincture for dogs, cats, birds, and other animals is 0.5–1.0 milliliter per 50 pounds of the animal's body weight, twice daily. Horses, rabbits, and other herbivores can be fed the fresh herb in their daily meals.

Availability: Cleavers is a common wild plant throughout most of the Northern Hemisphere. It is available in various forms at local herb retailers, but remember that the dried herb (or any preparation of the dried herb) is inferior medicine compared to the fresh plant. If you plan to purchase a commercial preparation of cleavers, check the label to make sure that it was produced from the fresh plant—otherwise, you might be buying an expensive but powerless herb. Fresh plant tinctures, in our opinion, is the best choice.

Propagation and Harvest: A few specialty seed catalogs offer cleavers (*G. aparine*) seed, and many nurseries sell starts of "sweet woodruff," a generic term for any variety of perennial *Galium* spp. sold as bedding plants. While these cultivars likely possess medicinal attributes, exactly how they measure up to the "herbalist-approved" *G. aparine* is unknown.

Alternatives and Adjuncts: For problems involving the lymphatic system, cleavers combines with calendula, echinacea, or astragalus. For skin and liver problems, cleavers is best if combined with alterative, diuretic, and liver-strengthening and stimulating herbs—dandelion, burdock, Oregon grape, milk thistle, and yellow dock should be considered. For treatment of tumors, cleavers is traditionally combined with red clover, licorice, violet, or aloe. For urinary tract problems, check out corn silk, marshmallow, and couch grass as alternatives or adjuncts.

Cautions and Comments: Cleavers is a safe herb. No contraindications have been noted with animal or human use, although allergic reaction is a possibility to consider before feeding.

COLTSFOOT

Petasites and
Tussilago species

Sunflower Family

Appearance: The common name of coltsfoot is shared by two distinctly different genera, *Tussilago* and *Petasites*. The classic Old World coltsfoot is *T. farfara*, a European native that produces light yellow, dandelion-like flowers and leaves proportionately large and heart shaped. The *Petasites* genus, on the other hand, produces its flowers on a leafless stem before the leaves fully develop. Five species of *Petasites* inhabit North America, while *T. farfara* is strictly a naturalized import here. Both genera of coltsfoot are equally valuable as medicines. For the purposes of identifying varieties native to North America, we focus on the *Petasites* clan of coltsfoot.

The flowers of *Petasites* are generally drab and featherlike, ranging in color from white to light purple, and are presented in a cluster at the top of the plant. Leaves vary in shape according to species, from triangular (*P. frigidus* and *P. nivalis*) or narrowly arrow shaped (*P. sagitta*), to broadly oval shaped with deep palmate (resembling a hand with the fingers spread) lobes (*P. palmatus*). The 3- to 10-inch-wide leaves are presented on long leaf stems that extend directly from thick, creeping rootstocks and are dark green on their upper surfaces and lighter green and feltlike on their undersides.

Habitat and Range: Coltsfoot requires consistent moisture at its feet and is usually found along streams, in wet meadows, and on shaded road margins, particularly where water seepage is continuous. Several species of *Petasites* range in forested areas from Alaska southward to California and eastward across the northern half of North America. The European variety of coltsfoot (*T. farfara*) has escaped

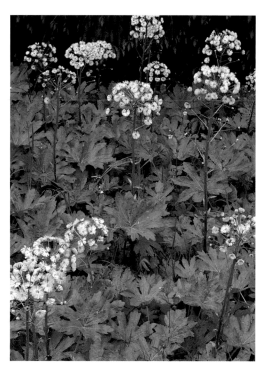

Petasites palmatus

cultivation in the northeastern portions of the U.S., where it enjoys similar habitat characteristics.

Cycle and Bloom Season: Late March to early June

Parts Used: Leaves and stems of the mature plant

Primary Medicinal Activities: Expectorant, eases cough spasms (antispasmodic), anti-inflammatory, antibacterial

Strongest Affinities: Lungs and upper respiratory tract

Preparation: Water infusion (tea), tincture, or syrup

Common Uses: People have been using coltsfoot for hundreds of years in the treatment of respiratory ailments ranging from chest colds to whooping cough, asthma, and viral pneumonia. Coltsfoot has long been regarded as a first choice for relieving the rawness and pain of unproductive spasmodic coughs. It is soothing because of its mucilage, and the ingredient petasin acts as an antispasmodic and nerve sedative for the bronchial rings and pulmonary receptors in the lungs.

Coltsfoot is useful in easing the discomforts of respiratory infections that are characterized by dry cough or seemingly immobile accumulations of thick phlegm in the bronchi. We find it particularly useful for tracheobronchitis in dogs (specifically kennel cough), especially when combined with anti-viral herbs such as licorice. Preparations of *T. farfara* have been shown to inhibit *Bordetella pertussis*, a bacterial component of the kennel cough malady, as well as various other strains of gram-negative bacteria such as *Staphylococcus aureus, Proteus hauseri, Pseudomonas aeruginosa,* and *Proteus vulgaris.* All of this makes coltsfoot useful as a respiratory disinfectant, expectorant, and cough suppressant in a wide variety of different animals—plus it acts in a holistic manner.

Many forms of cough suppressants (including wild cherry bark) simply suppress the body's efforts to heal itself by acting upon the brain to block the body's cough response mechanisms. Coltsfoot, on the other hand, gently assists the body in its efforts to clear invading microbes out of the upper respiratory tract.

Glycerin tinctures are the ideal form of administration of this herb. A good starting dosage for most animals is 0.5–1.5 milliliters (or about ⅓ teaspoon) per 20 pounds of an animal's body weight, two to three times a day.

Availability: Although coltsfoot is currently under FDA scrutiny and will likely be labeled as "unsafe for internal use," the tincture or dried herb remains widely available through herb retailers.

Propagation and Harvest: Coltsfoot (both Tussilago and Petasites) can be propagated in a garden if given ample shade and rich, consistently moist, slightly acidic soil. This winter-hardy plant does best in a cool climate.

Alternatives and Adjuncts: For deep coughs and bronchial congestion, coltsfoot may be combined with mullein, horehound, licorice, or elecampane. For respiratory infections that are believed to be bacterial or fungal in origin, coltsfoot can be boosted with echinacea, Oregon grape, bee balm, or thyme. For respiratory viruses, licorice and echinacea are good adjuncts.

Cautions and Comments: Coltsfoot contains PAs. The PA content of coltsfoot is about one-third of that contained in comfrey (*Symphytum* spp.), and most of this compound is contained in the plant's flowers, not the leaves and stems. What this means is that the PA content of coltsfoot is really quite low. Nevertheless, it can cause harm if it is used in absence of common sense. For more on pyrrolizidine alkaloids (PAs), see "Comfrey."

COMFREY

Symphytum officinale   Borage Family

Appearance: Comfrey is a robust plant with coarsely textured, broadly lance-shaped leaves that may exceed a foot in length at the base of the plant and become progressively smaller toward the top of the plant. The leaves and hollow stalk of the plant are covered with bristly hairs that tend to irritate human skin. The downy tubular flowers are presented among the small upper leaves in drooping clusters and are usually a shade of pink or purple but are sometimes white or pale yellow. Large plants may reach 3 or more feet in height and multiply vigorously by continuous root division, sometimes forming their own sort of hedgelike clump. *Symphytum uplandicum* (Russian comfrey) may grow in excess of 6 feet tall.

Habitat and Range: Over thirty-five species of Symphytum are in cultivation worldwide, most having originated from Europe and western Asia. In North America, common comfrey (*S. officinale*) and Russian comfrey (*S. uplandicum*) are the most common garden varieties.

Cycle and Bloom Season: A perennial that blooms from early spring to late fall

Parts Used: All aboveground parts

Primary Medicinal Activities: Heals wounds; anti-inflammatory; astringent; lubricates, soothes, and protects internal mucous membranes; expectorant

Strongest Affinities: Skin, digestive tract, respiratory tract

Preparation: Water or oil infusion, poultice, salve, fomentation

Common Uses: Where does one start with an herb that has had such a rich history as a healing device? Comfrey traditionally has been used for everything from mastitis in goats to cancer in humans. Virtual libraries of scientific research and anecdotal records have been compiled over the centuries to substantiate, deny, or otherwise argue comfrey's value and safety as an herbal

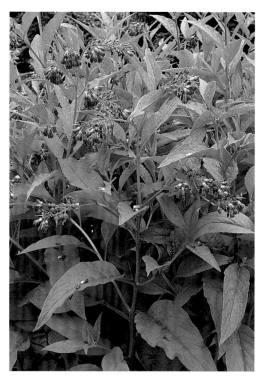

Symphytum officinale

medicine. Most of what you may have heard about this plant extends to animals (especially mammals), including toxicity issues, and almost everyone who has lived around horses, goats, sheep, llamas, and a comfrey patch knows how valuable this plant is.

Comfrey is among the first herbs to consider in the topical treatment of burns, skin ulcerations, abrasions, lacerations, flea and other insect bites, or just about any other irritation. Likewise, a poultice, salve, or infusion of the leaves can be applied directly to bruises, fractures, sprains, and other closed-tissue injuries. Most of the healing effects are attributable to allantoin, a compound that has been shown in several studies to speed cell reproduction, both inside and outside of the body. In fact, many herbalists have found that comfrey works so well at speed-healing injuries that it can actually seal bacteria into the site of an open wound. To prevent this from happening, a strong antibacterial herb such as Oregon grape, thyme, usnea, or Saint-John's-wort should be added to any comfrey preparation that is intended for open wounds, especially burns. In addition to its cell-proliferation activity, comfrey's mucilaginous nature provides a soothing, lubricating, and protective barrier to the skin and inflammations of the digestive tract. Comfrey also contains rosmarinic acid and several other compounds that have been shown to contribute anti-inflammatory, analgesic, and astringent qualities to its list of healing attributes.

For external treatment of closed injuries, skin ulcers, or mastitis, you can make a poultice or fomentation from the fresh or dried leaves and apply to the affected area. If you have access to fresh comfrey leaves, wrap a handful in a clean towel, then place the towel into a bowl of boiling water. Allow it to soak until the water just begins to turn green, then remove the towel and leaves and squeeze the excess water from the towel back into the bowl. After allowing the fomentation to cool slightly, apply the warm compress to the affected area. With horses and other large animals, this might require you to secure the compress onto a swollen limb with a strip of gauze or a clean piece of fabric torn from some old clothing. Leave the compress on for as long as possible—preferably eight hours or more. The extra "comfrey tea" that you squeezed back into the bowl can be applied to the compress from time to time and allowed to soak through to where it is needed. In cases of mastitis or other ailments where a fixed compress is not practical, an ointment or salve is a better option. If neither of these preparations is available, try making a strong tea of the leaves (fresh leaves are always superior to dried) and rinsing the entire area with the lukewarm liquid several times per day.

Internal use of comfrey has become a controversial issue and is strongly discouraged by the FDA, though millions of people have been using this herb safely and effectively in their animals (and themselves) for centuries. As is true for many other herbs, the safe use of comfrey is measured by moderation and common sense.

For treatment of colitis, stomach ulcers, or just about any other inflammation of the digestive tract, a handful of the fresh leaves or 2–3 ounces of the dried leaves can be fed directly to horses and other large herbivores on a daily basis for up to two weeks. For dogs and cats, ½–1 teaspoon of the dried herb for each pound of food fed should be of therapeutic benefit.

Comfrey is traditionally used for bronchitis and other respiratory ailments that are relieved by its soothing anti-inflammatory nature. A cooled tea serves this purpose well. Administer 1 tablespoon per 20 pounds of the animal's body weight, twice daily. In all cases of internal use, feeding of comfrey should be limited to occasional short-term therapies. By no means should comfrey be fed to an animal as a daily food supplement because the plant contains small cumulative amounts of potentially toxic PAs. For the same reason, highly concentrated preparations such as tinctures or strong decoctions should not be employed internally.

Availability: Any nursery that carries herb plants has access to comfrey. The dried herb and various salves, ointments, and other preparations containing comfrey are available through health food retailers and herb stores.

Propagation and Harvest: Comfrey can be easily started from root cuttings. It grows in just about any soil and is hardy as far north as central Canada. The biggest plants, though, are found in rich, deep, moist soil with a pH level in the range of 6 to 7.5. Once established, comfrey needs little attention. In fact, its rambunctious growth will amaze you. We live in an area of Montana that has a scant one hundred-day growing season and winter temperatures that may plunge to –40°F, yet our comfrey (which grows from beneath the foundation of the house) can be divided into multiple new starts at least twice per year!

Alternatives and Adjuncts: For external applications, comfrey combines especially well with calendula, chamomile, aloe, Saint-John's-wort, or bee balm. For gastric disorders, comfrey combines with cleavers, calendula, catnip, or chamomile.

Cautions and Comments: The issues of toxicity that have haunted comfrey in recent years have become a major subject of frustration for herbalists, a source of apprehension and political ammunition for opponents of herbal medicine, and a wealth of misinformation, confusion, and fear for the casual herb user. While the FDA and other protective agencies are doing their jobs as best they can during a major health care revolution—and it is not our intent to criticize them—most herbalists agree that comfrey has received an undeserved bad reputation. The FDA has banned the sale of comfrey for internal use, but in thousands of years of use by millions of people, only two reports of hepatotoxicity have been documented in humans.

Indeed, comfrey contains PAs, which are known to cause liver damage or cancer if ingested in large enough quantities. Most of the concern surrounding these alkaloids, however, comes from studies or cases where the alkaloids were isolated from the rest of the plant's chemistry and then fed or injected into test animals in quantities or concentrations hundreds of times greater than those that would occur in nature. Common sense dictates that anything ingested in overabundance is potentially toxic, but given the fact that the PA content in a fresh comfrey leaf amounts to only about 0.3 percent of its total chemistry, the average horse would need to eat several hundred pounds of the leaves each day before any toxic effects would be observed! Coffee contains over one dozen potentially toxic alkaloids—so does chocolate. However, the real threat from PAs comes from the fact that these alkaloids may accumulate in the body, perhaps to toxic levels, if used continually over a long period. Therefore, if you plan to use comfrey or any other herb that contains PAs in an internal application, do so with moderation and only for short periods. Don't use comfrey in pregnant or lactating animals or in animals with preexisting liver disease. Also, keep in mind that the PA content of the root is ten times greater than that of the fresh leaves; therefore, the root shouldn't be used internally. On the other hand, the PA content of the dried leaves, the form in which comfrey is most readily available in the marketplace, is practically nil.

CORN SILK

Zea mays   Grass Family

Appearance: We're sorry if you were expecting something other than the obvious here, but the corn silk we're referring to is simply the hairlike pollen-receiving portion of a corn stalk, the part most of us throw away first when we peel an ear of corn.

Habitat and Range: Farms and gardens throughout the world

Cycle and Bloom Season: An annual that blooms in early summer. The "silk" develops just as the plant is beginning to form cobs.

Parts Used: Silk

Primary Medicinal Activities: Diuretic; lubricates, soothes, and protects internal mucous membranes; anti-inflammatory, stimulates the liver (cholagogue), astringent

Strongest Affinities: Genitourinary tract, including the kidneys

Preparation: A low-alcohol (less than 25 percent alcohol) tincture or an infusion (tea) of the fresh silk is preferable. The dried silk may be used if it is fresh, but it is not as potent as silk that has been recently pulled from the plant.

Common Uses: First and foremost, corn silk is indicated wherever chronic inflammation exists in any portion of the urinary tract or kidneys. It is specifically indicated in FLUTD, where it serves to reduce inflammation without causing added irritation to the kidneys. Unlike many other diuretic and astringent herbs used to increase urine output by means of kidney irritation, corn silk does not contain harsh volatile oils that may compound the problems of inflammatory kidney disease. Therefore, it is useful for improving kidney function during early onset kidney failure or for helping with the reduction of pain and inflammation in the passing of kidney or bladder stones (especially when combined with marshmallow). The astringency factor of corn silk is enough to tighten and strengthen the lining of the bladder and the smooth-muscle

tissues of the urinary tract, making the herb useful in some cases of chronic urinary incontinence, but it is not strong enough to effectively stop acute cases of bleeding or inflammation. So, corn silk is best remembered as a long-term medicine for chronic urinary problems. Corn silk has been shown to lower blood pressure and blood sugar levels and to possess cholagogue and diuretic activities in laboratory animals. All of these activities serve as clues as to why corn silk is especially effective as a general kidney tonic.

The effectiveness of fresh silk over dried cannot be overstated, and the best methods of administration involve the direct feeding of the herb in a low-alcohol liquid base (a strong tea is ideal). Dosage is difficult to generalize because of the variable nature of genitourinary diseases. But a safe starting point is to use 1 milliliter (about 30 drops or so, or ¼ teaspoon) of the low-alcohol tincture per 20 pounds of the animal's body weight, twice daily. If the tincture is alcohol-free, it can be administered directly into the mouth. If not, it should be no more than 25 percent alcohol and should then be further diluted with at least an equal amount of water.

To make a tea of the fresh silk, chop it as finely as possible, then steep a heaping tablespoon of the herb in near-boiling water until the mixture cools. After the tea is strained, it can be fed to the animal—¼ cup (if possible) per 20 pounds of body weight, twice daily. Many herbivores enjoy eating corn silk. This is fine, but remember that if you want to get an optimum amount of the herb into your animal's urinary tract, it really needs to be administered as a liquid.

Availability: Finding dried corn silk is easy and several manufacturer's provide extracts of this herb, but if you want fresh corn silk, you might have to plant some corn in your herb garden. If you have access to organically raised fresh corn at your local health food store, you can use the silk from this. However, nonorganic sources of corn silk should be avoided because the silk has likely been sprayed with a pesticide. Corn silk should look fresh, juicy, and colorful. If it has turned brown, much of its medicinal activity has diminished.

Propagation and Harvest: Corn is easy to grow, and dozens of varieties are available to suit virtually any set of growing conditions. (We live at an elevation of 5,500 feet in Montana, and even we can grow corn.) Harvest your corn before the silk turns brown—usually in early summer. If you want to eat the corn, make sure that it has an opportunity to receive pollen from the tassels of the plants for at least a week before you harvest, otherwise your cobs will have no kernels. Plan to use your fresh silk immediately. Cooled corn silk tea can be stored in the refrigerator for about a week—a glycerin tincture keeps for at least a year if kept refrigerated.

Alternatives and Adjuncts: For chronic urinary tract inflammation, corn silk combines well with couch grass, calendula, or cleavers. If infection is evident, add echinacea, Oregon grape, yarrow, or thyme. For urinary incontinence, read about Saint-John's-wort, ginkgo, and uva ursi. To help pass kidney stones, try a half-and-half combination of corn silk and marshmallow. For use as a kidney tonic, corn silk combines with marshmallow, hawthorn, ginkgo, or goldenrod. For use in FLUTD, corn silk combines with couch grass, echinacea, marshmallow, and horsetail.

Cautions and Comments: Corn silk is known to be safe, but this herb is actually the

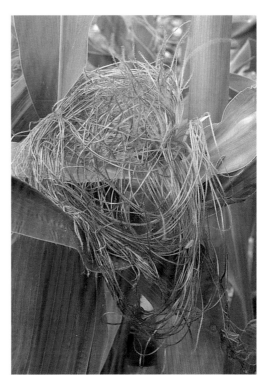

Zea mays

pollen-receiving part of the plant. It stands to reason that animals with pollen allergies may have adverse reactions to corn silk. Corn silk has been shown to stimulate uterine contractions in rabbits and therefore should be used with caution (if at all) in pregnant animals.

COUCH GRASS

Agropyron repens   Grass Family

Appearance: If you are a gardener, you probably already know, and hate, this plant by the name quack grass. Couch grass (pronounced "cooch grass" in much of Europe, its native birthplace and medicinal origin) is a profusely common weed in North America. To the untrained eye, *Agropyron repens* looks like every other waist-high wild grass—with perhaps the most distinctive exception displayed by its leaves. Each leaf, or blade, of couch grass looks as though somebody pinched a crimp in it 1 or 2 inches away from the tip. While this does not serve as a definitive means of identification, it provides a good point from which you can begin the process of ruling out look-alike grasses in your area, one species at a time. If you wish to gather this plant for medicinal use, find some samples of what you think might be couch grass, and then take them to your county extension agent, a botanist, or somebody else who can identify grasses. Unless you are experienced at using a botanical key (a scientific reference used to identify plants through recognition of their taxonomic features), identifying couch grass is hit or miss. Fortunately, the look-alike grasses are not toxic—but they're probably not medicinal.

Habitat and Range: Couch grass is native to the Mediterranean area. It now makes itself at home virtually everywhere on earth. In North America, expect to find it in areas where livestock grazing, farming, or other human-related activities have delivered the seeds.

Cycle and Bloom Season: An aggressive perennial that reproduces by seed or spreading rhizomes (horizontally creeping roots)

Parts Used: Rhizomes

Primary Medicinal Activities: Antimicrobial, astringent, anti-inflammatory, mild diuretic

Strongest Affinities: Urinary tract

Preparation: Tincture or decoction of the fresh or freshly dried rhizomes. Use fresh leaves as a dietary supplement.

Common Uses: Historically, many animal lovers have come to know A. repens as dog grass because dogs, cats, and other animals love eating the fresh spring leaves of the plant. Our dogs are no exception—we have clumps of dog grass growing in front of our house, and whenever an opportunity arises (one that doesn't interfere with a game of Frisbee), our dogs both actively graze on the plants. It's interesting to watch how they actually differentiate the couch grass from other grasses in their intuitive drive to eat the plants. But even more interesting is the way our dogs instinctively use this plant to fulfill special health care needs. Specifically, they eat couch grass to the point of vomiting, and while humans may find this somewhat disgusting, an inquisitive herbalist with a holistically oriented mind can clearly see what the animals are doing. They are either using the grass as a digestive cleansing agent or they are vomiting so they can reingest their stomach contents. The latter may be indicative of poor nutrient absorption—eating food twice, in effect, allows for more complete absorption of certain nutrients.

The point is this: if your animal eats grass, the grass is likely to fill a nutritional or medicinal need, and such activities should not be overlooked when assessing your animal's holistic health—even if you do wish to look away and forget about it.

As a food, a patch of couch grass provides grazing animals with a rich source of vitamins A and B, iron, rough fiber, and silica (for healthy bones, hooves, nails, and coat). But most of the medicinal value of couch grass is contained within the rhizomes of the plant.

Couch grass serves as an excellent tonic and disinfectant for the urinary tract. It is a soothing, anti-inflammatory demulcent and saponin-based diuretic with mild antimicrobial activity. Couch grass is considered a specific remedy for chronic or acute cases of cystitis and urethritis, where the root tea or tincture helps to reduce inflammation, inhibit bacterial reproduction, and lessen pain during urination. It should be noted that although couch grass has been shown to possess broad antibiotic activity, it may be too weak to be effective against infections that are already well established. In such cases, couch grass should be combined with stronger antimicrobial herbs such as echinacea, thyme, or Oregon grape (or certified organic goldenseal—don't buy wildcrafted goldenseal because the plant is at risk of becoming extinct).

As a diuretic, couch grass increases the volume of urine by stimulating sodium excretion, helping to wash away waste materials from the body via the kidneys. This makes couch grass an effective adjunct to a variety of liver-supporting, alterative herbs (such as dandelion or burdock), especially in the treatment of rheumatism or chronic skin problems.

The demulcent properties of couch grass soothe inflammation, so it can also be used for kidney stones and gravel. And because couch grass is gentle on the kidneys and seldom irritates the bladder or urethra during long-term use, it is a primary herb to consider when treating the symptoms of FLUTD in cats, a condition that is usually due to factors other than infection.

For use in urinary problems, the best way to administer this herb is in the form of a cooled decoction. Make the decoction by gently simmering a heaping teaspoon of the chopped dried root, or 2 heaping teaspoons of the chopped fresh root (rhizomes), in 8 ounces of water for about twenty minutes. The decoction can be squirted directly into the animal's mouth. A safe starting dose is

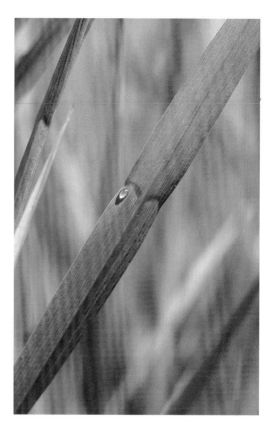

Agropyron repens

about a ½ teaspoon (2–3 milliliters) per 20 pounds of the animal's body weight, two to three times daily. If direct administration is too difficult, the dose can be added to the animal's drinking water. Try to figure out how much your animal drinks, then add enough couch grass to meet dosing requirements. Glycerin or alcohol tinctures can be used at half the above dosage and are best if diluted into water. Keep in mind that this is a subtle herbal medicine—the needs and systemic requirements of the animal you are helping may require several increases in dosage over several days or weeks of administration.

Availability: Couch grass is not a popular herb in the U.S. (although it is popular in Europe), and some of the dried rhizomes that you find in herb stores are on the verge of becoming useless dust. Fortunately, it grows everywhere. The only problem is identifying it among other weeds and finding the physical stamina to dig up the stubborn rhizomes. If you meet these criteria, you can easily become a garden hero in your neighborhood. (On the other hand, everyone may think you're nuts for actually *wanting* the weed.) The golden rule: Beware of pesticides. Finding "clean" couch grass is often difficult.

Propagation and Harvest: As far as propagating couch grass is concerned, go ahead if you don't mind sacrificing the engine on your tiller and if you don't care if the plant strangles the rest of your garden. The rhizomes can be harvested anytime throughout the growth season but are usually strongest when dug up in the fall. The best medicines are made from the fresh rhizomes, but dried roots are useful, too, if used within a year of digging.

Alternatives and Adjuncts: For urinary inflammations that are secondary to infection, combine with Oregon grape, organically raised goldenseal, thyme, or echinacea. For stones or any other cause of urinary tract inflammation, marshmallow, corn silk, and plantain are valuable adjuncts. If blood is present in the urine, see your holistic veterinarian—your pet needs stronger measures than couch grass.

Cautions and Comments: No toxicity has been noted for couch grass, although excessive amounts may lead to vomiting or diarrhea. Always be careful about verifying the cleanliness of the sources of this herb— it is on just about everybody's "noxious weed" list, and pesticide residues can remain with the plant for several years.

DANDELION

Taraxacum officinale   Sunflower Family

Appearance: It's time for all good herbalists to put their egos aside. Dandelion is actually confused with several other species of the sunflower family, and although we may hate to admit it, many of us have been fooled into using one of the look-alikes. The primary consideration to bear in mind when identifying *Taraxacum officinale* or any of its hundreds of variations is this: Dandelion has no branching characteristics but instead grows in a rosette fashion directly off of its taproot. And dandelion never has spines on its midrib as does *Lactuca serriola* (prickly lettuce), which otherwise looks similar to dandelion when young. Although dandelion impostors likely won't harm you, they won't offer you dandelion's benefits, either.

Habitat and Range: A native of Europe and Asia, dandelion has found its way onto every continent—except maybe Antarctica.

Cycle and Bloom Season: Dandelion is a perennial that may bloom several times throughout the year. In areas where there is severe winter climate, dandelion may appear only as a free-seeding annual.

Parts Used: All parts of the plant are useful for various applications.

Primary Medicinal Activities: Diuretic, stimulates the liver, stimulates salivation and improves digestion (bitter), nutritive, laxative, anti-inflammatory, tonic

Strongest Affinities: Liver, gallbladder, gastrointestinal tract

Preparation: Water infusion, decoction, tincture, fresh or dried leaves and flowers

Common Uses: To begin an accurate assessment of dandelion's deep-reaching medicinal attributes, we must first put healing into a whole-body perspective. All higher organisms (including dogs, cats, birds, mice, lizards, goats, and humans) maintain vital body functions within tightly knit parameters of systemic cooperation. A precise and balanced relationship between nutrition and elimination of waste is a critical part of this cooperation. If a systemic excess or deficiency occurs that the body cannot correct through elimination, supplementation, or immune system intervention, it will try to compensate by shutting down a system or storing waste materials wherever it can. In other words, a state of "dis-ease" results. Enter the dandelion.

Dandelion is one of the most complete plant foods on earth. A 1-cup serving of fresh dandelion greens provides as much as 2,000 international units (IU) of vitamin A (one and a half times the recommended daily allowance [RDA] for an adult human); 20 percent protein (by content, that's double what spinach provides); vitamins C, K, D, and B complex; iron, manganese, phosphorus, and many other trace minerals; and an especially rich supply of potassium. All of these vital nutrients are conveniently contained within a single source in quantities that the body can fully absorb. This means that dandelion can gently supplement a diet without overworking the liver and kidneys with excess vitamins and minerals (which is often signified by dark urine).

Supplementing your companion animal's diet with dandelion leaf is as simple as drying the greens and crumbling them onto

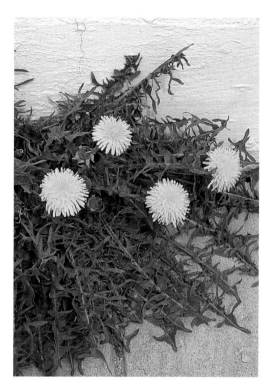

Taraxacum officinale

her food. If your animal doesn't like eating dandelion or if you need to get nutrients into her more quickly, try making a leaf tea using organic unsalted vegetable or meat broth in place of plain water. Plan on feeding about 1 teaspoon of the dried herb for each 20 pounds of body weight daily. Horses, llamas, sheep, goats, mules, and other large animals often eat the greens directly out of their pastures. If they don't, try hand feeding the greens to them or adding a little molasses. If your animal is sensitive to changes in diet, then start her off with a small amount of dandelion at a time.

In addition to providing your animal with many of the nutrients she needs, the leaves have what herbalists call a bitter tonic effect: the body's metabolism is "warmed up" before the digestive system is forced to go to work. When a small amount of a bitter herb is taken into the mouth, the recipient immediately experiences a sudden increase in salivation. As the bitter herb reaches the stomach, bile and other digestive agents are then triggered into production. The result is more efficient digestion, reduced indigestion, better absorption of nutrients, and increased appetite. Dandelion leaf is particularly useful in animals who have a chronic problem with indigestion. If your animal has frequent gas or passes food that does not appear digested, get her to chew a fresh dandelion leaf while you reconsider her diet, or apply a few drops of dandelion tincture (an herbal glycerite is most palatable) onto her tongue. It does not matter if the animal doesn't appear to swallow it; the bitter tonic action is triggered in the mouth.

Dandelion is well known among herbalists as a safe but powerful diuretic and liver stimulant. Congestive heart failure, pulmonary edema, arthritis, gallbladder disease, and kidney stones are all imbalances resulting from the body's inability to eliminate water or accumulated excesses. In mainstream practices, drugs such as furosemide are often used to drain off excess fluid from the body and thus promote the elimination of accumulated waste materials. Pharmaceutical diuretics are fast acting, easy to administer, and effective, but while they do a great job at expelling fluid, they tend not to discriminate between what the body needs to keep and what it needs to lose. As a result, the body often loses too much potassium, a crucial heart and brain nutrient, through urination. In this event, potassium must be supplemented throughout the therapy. Dandelion leaf, on the other hand, contains its own rich source of fully assimilable potassium, an attribute that helps to replace what would otherwise be lost through urination.

How effective is dandelion as a diuretic? Many contemporary herbalists claim that dandelion may be as effective as the aforementioned furosemide. The big trade-offs, though, are ease of administration, getting enough of the tea into the animal to bring about desired effects, and the time that it may take for dandelion to start working. While furosemide can be administered in a little pill, a dandelion therapy involves getting your animal to drink warm tea or take a tincture extract (the broth method works nicely). None of this is meant to encourage you to stop the diuretic therapy prescribed by your veterinarian. If you wish to seek the dandelion alternative, see a holistic veterinarian first.

While dandelion leaves are nutritive and diuretic, the root possesses its own usefulness as a safe, reliable liver tonic. The liver is the primary filtering organ of the body; it is responsible for removing toxins and excesses from the blood for elimination via the kidneys. The liver also plays critical roles in digestion through its production of bile, bilirubin, and various enzymes. If bile ducts in the liver or gallbladder become congested, blocked, or otherwise diseased to the point of dysfunction, the body invariably suffers one or more toxicity-related imbalances. Such imbalances may be characterized by symptoms such as jaundice, rheumatoid conditions, eczema, dandruff, or chronic constipation. And while dandelion leaf tea or tincture may do much toward relieving the symptoms of such conditions through a nutritive and diuretic action, the root will have more effect on the underlying causes.

Dandelion root has a well-validated ability to stimulate bile production and circulation throughout the liver. In one study involving dogs, researchers observed a three to four times increase in bile production after administration of dandelion root. The gallbladder, which stores bile from the liver, is also stimulated, causing this small, hollow organ to contract and release bile into the digestive tract, thus aiding in digestion and acting as a gentle laxative to promote the elimination of solid waste.

One of the best features about dandelion root as a liver and gallbladder stimulant is its gentle nature. Unlike many cholagogue herbs, dandelion does not further irritate an already inflamed condition. In fact, in clinical studies using an over-the-counter preparation of the root, dandelion was shown to be effective in treating inflammatory diseases of the liver and gallbladder, including gallstones.

The flowers of dandelion are known by herbalists to be high in lecithin and to have weak but useful analgesic qualities. Their usefulness as a pain reliever stems from the fact that they don't contain any salicylates, the alkaloid compounds found in aspirin that are toxic to cats and may be irritating to the stomach lining. To use the flowers, infuse a generous handful in a cup of near-boiling water. When the water has darkened as much as possible, it can be cooled and administered with a dropper: 30–40 drops per 20 pounds of body weight. If this proves to be too difficult for you and your animal, try drying the flowers and sprinkling them on her food. You shouldn't expect aspirin-like effectiveness, but this is a mild painkilling option worth considering.

Dandelion is perhaps the first herb to consider when optimized digestion and waste elimination is a necessary part of an herbal therapy. In holistic healing, the body, whether it be human or another kind of animal, should not be viewed as a collection of individual body systems but as an intricately balanced cooperation of relative components. From this perspective, it is easy to see how dandelion can serve a positive role in its effort to help the body at what it is designed to do—stay healthy. The body cannot achieve this goal unless it is able to effectively utilize nutrients and eliminate waste—and dandelion is here to help.

Availability: Everywhere!

Propagation and Harvest: If you wish to propagate dandelion (no, we're not insane), give the plants deep humus-rich soil and full sun. Gather dandelion greens for use in salads in early spring—they get bitter with age. Leaves intended for herbal teas and medicines can be gathered anytime in dry weather. Wet dandelion leaves tend to develop mold while they are drying, so don't wash them after picking. Shake them off and dry them on newspapers in a well-ventilated area, away from light. Then stir them often to prevent molding and store them in plastic bags only after they are completely crispy dry. Gather the roots as late in fall as possible; this is when they contain the greatest concentration of beneficial constituents. Chop them up (we use a food processor), then spread them onto newspaper and dry with the same consideration you gave to the leaves.

Alternatives and Adjuncts: For liver and digestive problems, consider milk thistle, burdock, yellow dock, marshmallow, chickweed, and Oregon grape as possible adjuncts or alternatives.

Cautions and Comments: The first and foremost consideration in using dandelion as food or medicine is the cleanliness of the plants you are using. Always make sure that the greens you are feeding have never been sprayed with herbicide. If they ever have, don't try washing them. Move on to another patch. You won't have trouble finding more.

DILL

Anethum graveolens   Parsley Family

Appearance: A healthy dill plant is an attractive addition to any herb garden. Plants may reach 6 feet in height. The dark green finely divided leaves have a delicate feathery appearance, and the yellow umbel (umbrella-like) flowers are attractive to bees. The entire plant is distinctively aromatic and delicious—just brushing past one can make your mouth water!

Habitat and Range: Originally a native of southeast Europe and southwest Asia, dill is a common resident in herb gardens worldwide.

Cycle and Bloom Season: An annual that blooms in early to midsummer, dill is successful at reproducing from the copious quantities of viable seed it produces shortly after blooming.

Parts Used: Foliage, flowers, and seeds

Primary Medicinal Activities: Expels intestinal gas, soothes the stomach (stomachic), stimulates milk production, antibacterial, diuretic

Strongest Affinities: Digestive tract

Preparation: Feeding of the fresh or dried herb, tea, tincture, poultice

Common Uses: Dill is good for relieving nausea and flatulence, especially when these maladies are secondary to a sudden change in diet—such as when your puppy decides to steal a tamale from your foolishly unattended dinner plate. The effectiveness of dill in this capacity is largely attributable to the plant's numerous volatile oil constituents, which combine to cause an antifoaming action in the stomach, like many over-the-counter antigas remedies. The highest concentrations of these oils are held within the seeds of the plant, but the dried leaves and stems (the herb you likely have in the kitchen) can be used too. If your dog is belching something that is suspiciously reminiscent of what was supposed to be your dinner and the problem appears to be getting progressively worse, try direct-feeding 2–8 ounces of cooled dill seed tea (1 teaspoon of dill seed to 8 ounces of water) to the animal. If your animal doesn't like the flavor, try adding the tea to her drinking water—or, if need be, disguise it as "yummy people food" by making the tea with some clear, unsalted broth instead of water. If belching, bloating, or other forms of indigestion are a problem after every feeding, call a holistic veterinarian and reassess your animal's diet. Think holistically—a sprinkling of ground dill seed on your pet's food may bring about symptomatic relief, but if the condition is ongoing, a deeper problem needs to be addressed.

In addition to providing relief from excess gas, dill also possesses antibacterial qualities that are strong enough to inhibit bacterial reproduction in the mouth but too weak to compromise beneficial microbes deeper in the digestive tract. This makes dill useful for treating halitosis and the early onset of gingivitis in dogs and cats. The herb or seeds can be infused and added to drinking water, or a poultice or glycerin tincture can be swabbed on the animal's gum line two or three times daily.

Dill is useful for treating mild to moderate cases of colic. If they will take it, horses and other large herbivores can be fed the seeds or even the entire fresh plant—as much as they need.

Dill seed contains carvone, anethofuran, and limonene, volatile oils that have been shown to increase the production of cancer-fighting enzymes (namely, glutathione s-transferase, or GST) in the body. These enzymes react with certain types of carcinogenic chemicals, eliminating them from the system. While this in itself represents only a small measure of cancer prevention, it makes dill another medicinal food to consider when custom-tailoring your animal's diet plan. While dill contains limonene, a substance known to repel fleas, its presence is not large enough to be of use by itself.

The carvone that dill contains, however, is believed to increase the effectiveness of various other natural insecticides (such as those contained in feverfew or oxeye daisy), making dill a useful adjunct in the never-ending battle against fleas. Dill has a folkloric reputation as a substance that stimulates the production of milk in nursing mothers.

Availability: The grocery store or your favorite nursery

Propagation and Harvest: Dill is easy to grow from seed or starts and can be seeded in fall for an early spring harvest in areas where winters are harsh. In areas where the growing season is long but not too hot, a continuous self-seeding crop of dill is not only possible but perhaps inevitable. Harvest the leaves and flowers when they are lush and aromatic, the seeds shortly after they have turned brown, before they begin to fall to the ground. This is best accomplished by clipping off the entire umbel, then shaking the seeds into a paper bag.

Alternatives and Adjuncts: For gas and other digestive problems, dill combines with fennel, parsley seed, or catnip. For infections of the mouth, Oregon grape, sage, and thyme are stronger options. For bad breath, a combination of parsley, dill, and peppermint makes an excellent formula. For

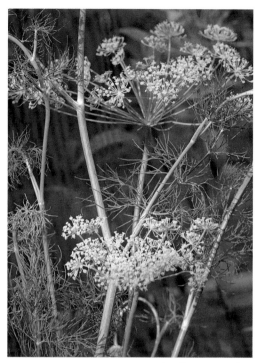

Anethum graveolens

fleas, try making a skin and coat rinse by combining dill, feverfew flowers, and yarrow into a tea.

Cautions and Comments: Dill is safe but because of its volatile oil constituents, dill should be used conservatively in pregnant or lactating animals.

ECHINACEA

Echinacea spp.   Sunflower Family

Appearance: Echinacea, also known as purple, pink, or white coneflower, is a taprooted perennial that may grow as high as 40 inches. Nine species of Echinacea are native to North America; all have flowers with distinctive conelike central disks, with the most common species ranging in color from pale to dark purple. The rays of most species droop away from the disk when mature. *Echinacea purpurea* (see photo on page 103) is by far the most widely distributed species in North America. For several decades, this species has been popular as a medicinal herb and garden flower. Dozens of varieties of *E. purpurea* have been developed, and it is estimated that the entire world market supply of this species comes from cultivated plants. Several other species, however, such as *E. angustifolia* and *E. pallida* are quickly succumbing to commercial and environmental pressures.

Habitat and Range: In the West, echinacea is largely an introduced plant. Partial to open plains and woodlands, its natural range once extended from eastern Canada southward into the Ozarks and westward throughout the corn belt states to the east slopes of the Rockies. Market pressures and continuing loss of habitat have eliminated most of the wild stands of echinacea. Its range continues to shrink, and today only small isolated populations of wild echinacea survive west of the Missouri River.

Cycle and Bloom Season: A perennial that blooms in early to late summer, depending on climate

Parts Used: Most often the root is used. The leaves, stems, and flowers are useful too, although they are much weaker medicine.

Primary Medicinal Activities: Immuno-stimulant, antimicrobial

Strongest Affinities: Immune system, lymph system, urinary tract

Preparation: Tincture, decoction, dried and powdered root, or direct feeding of the fresh leaves, stems, and flowers

Common Uses: First and foremost, echinacea is an immune-supporting herb—it serves to support intact immune functions through stimulatory and strengthening actions at various levels within the body. No single constituent contained in the root or flowering upper parts of echinacea can be attributed to the immune-tonifying functions of this plant. Instead, most herbalists agree that the complex structure of this plant should be viewed as a therapeutic synergy of dozens of biochemical influences. However, a few key elements stand out as strong clues to exactly how echinacea works.

A great deal of scientific research has identified echinacea's most influential immunostimulatory components as an extensive array of caffeic acids, volatile oils, polysaccharides, polyenes, polyines, and isobutylamides. In simpler terms, echinacea's immunostimulatory qualities are derived from a wide array of chemical compounds that allow the plant to be used in a variety of forms without sacrificing its effectiveness. For instance, while many of the acid constituents in echinacea are poorly water soluble and require a strong alcohol base to extract them into a tincture form, the plant's polysaccharide constituents are exactly the opposite—they are easily extracted into water—and, in fact, they are largely destroyed by alcohol. Since both of these chemical groups have been shown to possess very strong immunostimulatory qualities, it would appear that the plant is naturally designed to accommodate a wide variety of metabolic needs.

Echinacea serves to support disease resistance in several ways. At the blood level, it accelerates phagocytosis, the means by which macrophages and other antibodies attack and remove bacteria. At cellular levels, echinacea helps to reduce the production of an enzyme that breaks down hyaluronic acid, the compound that occurs between cells to bind them together. Eliminating this enzyme at the onset of an infection is believed to make body tissues less pervious to invading microbes and, in turn, the invaders more vulnerable to scavenging antibodies that have already been stimulated into action. Echinacea has also been shown to stimulate the lymph system, thus helping the body to eliminate waste materials from the tissues. And it possesses measurable antimicrobial qualities that assist the body's fight against infection by intervening with bacteria at the point of invasion.

Echinacea's multidirectional means of immune system support, its primary usefulness, depends on a healthy immune system. Without a healthy population of unencumbered antibodies to work with, echinacea's capacity to fight infection is limited to its simple, and less-than-impressive, antiseptic actions. This means that timing is critical to echinacea's effectiveness—this herb should be taken at the first onset of infectious symptoms, otherwise its activity will amount to a losing battle fought against microbial opponents that have already fortified their positions within the animal's body.

Learn to recognize minute variances in your animal's behavior and feeding habits. Take extra time to give your pet a cursory examination during your daily grooming session or playtimes, and look for anything that may point to the introduction of an infection—an inflamed gum, a swollen fleabite, or a slightly runny nose may be indicators for the proactive use of echinacea. If you are too late and an infection has set in, it's time to consider calling in some other troops from the herbal army. Don't despair. Try boosting echinacea with a small percentage of an antiseptic herb such as

Oregon grape, usnea, or organically grown goldenseal. By combining echinacea with about 10 percent by weight or volume of one of these other herbs, you will be offering a small measure of direct antiseptic intervention without compromising populations of the beneficial microbes the body needs in its fight. Applying antiseptics topically, directly onto the point of infection, also aids in the healing effort.

So how much echinacea should you give, for how long, and in what form? Many people think that the potency of an echinacea preparation can be determined by the intensity of the tingling sensation it causes when placed on the tongue. If this is your current method of judging echinacea preparations, please abandon it. A great deal of recent and continuing research has shown that the isobutylamides responsible for this sensation represent only a fragment of echinacea's active constituents and that their absence may not affect the overall effectiveness of echinacea. The more we learn about echinacea, the more complex and diverse its medicinal actions seem to be.

There is no best kind of echinacea preparation per se. As long as care and quality have gone into its propagation, its harvest, and the manufacture of the end product, all echinacea preparations contain adequate medicinal constituents. The question of what preparation to use internally in your animal hinges on how easy or difficult it is to get a therapeutic quantity into the animal. Echinacea is by no means a good-tasting herb, and its administration is complicated by the fact that dogs and cats have short digestive tracks and fast metabolic rates. In these animals, the problem isn't finding a preparation that contains high enough concentrations of active constituents but finding one that is both palatable and fully assimilable by their short digestive tracts. Cats in particular don't like alcohol and the sour tingle that alcohol extracts impart on the tongue. (They typically foam at the mouth and sometimes act as if you are force-feeding them a vile, poisonous fluid.) Dogs typically drink from toilets without complaint and are somewhat less picky, and since gel capsules often pass directly through them undigested, we prefer to use low-alcohol glycerin extracts for our carnivores. Glycerin-based preparations are low in tongue-tingling isobutylamides but rich in readily available polysaccharide constituents, and the sweet taste of the vegetable glycerin helps mask the unpleasant flavor of the herb.

Herbivores are naturally designed to efficiently metabolize plant materials; horses, goats, llamas, and other large animals can be fed the flowering plants, or dried root can be added to their feed.

Dosage and duration of use vary based upon the needs and individual nuances of the animal, but a conservative rule for dogs and cats is to give 12–25 drops of the tincture three times daily. Horses, cattle, sheep, and other large animals can be fed a couple of handfuls of the dried whole flowering herb per day. Several high-quality powdered echinacea preparations are now available for equines and other large animals as well. Use them as directed by your veterinarian or as suggested on the label.

In recent years, a rather heated controversy has arisen within the herbalist community concerning how long echinacea can be used before the body builds a tolerance to its immune-stimulating actions. In a German study conducted in 1989, a diminished response to echinacea was recorded in human subjects after five to ten days of normal dose administration. This result raised questions of whether echinacea is effective when used over the long term. Closer scrutiny of this study, however, has since led to the conclusion that while echinacea's activity does fall off sharply after about five days of use, its long-term use still maintains a level of immune system activity higher than that observed prior to its initial administration. Many herbalists believe that breaking the continuity of echinacea use every five to ten days allows for a greater immune boost each time the therapy is reestablished after a two- or three-day respite. We agree and believe that a break is necessary, in any case, to monitor the unassisted recovery of the animal. Five days on, two or three days off is a good guideline to follow.

Aside from its immune-stimulating qualities, echinacea is a good antimicrobial for the mouth and urinary tract. It is useful for treating bacterial or fungal infections of the bladder and urethra, especially when added to a demulcent and anti-inflammatory combination of herbs. Echinacea also has a long-standing reputation as a snakebite remedy. Used internally and externally simultaneously, the herb is said to antidote the venom. Although little scientific evidence exists to support such claims, hundreds of years' worth of use amounts to more than folkloric trivia. Knowing that about 85 percent of rattlesnake bites involve only a partial injection of venom (or no injection at all), it is likely that echinacea serves more to ward off infection and prevent tissue damage than to actually nullify the venom. Echinacea relieves the pain and swelling of most insect bites and stings, especially when applied as a clay poultice.

Echinacea is also used with some success for colic in horses, with free-feeding of the fresh leaves, stems, and flowers being the most popular method of administration.

Availability: Various preparations of echinacea are widely available through health product retailers. The seeds and plants are available through most nurseries. Because of continuing overharvest, wild stands of this plant are at risk of disappearing forever. Please make sure that the echinacea you are using is from cultivated sources.

Propagation and Harvest: Echinacea purpurea, the primary echinacea of commerce, is easy to grow and requires little care once the plants are established. Seeds require cold, damp stratification and light to break their dormancy. This means that the seeds must be sown on top of the soil or covered with just a trace of soil in order to germinate. Roots must be at least three years old to be of medicinal value. The plants are hardy and drought tolerant when mature. A well-established stand of echinacea reseeds itself, and mature plants can bear roots of up to 3 pounds each.

Varieties such as *E. pallida* and *E. angustifolia* are much more finicky. Before you choose to grow them, bear in mind that despite what herbalists once thought, the gardener-friendly *E. purpurea* provides medicine that is as potent as these other species.

Dig mature echinacea roots from the garden after the plant has gone dormant for the winter, following its third year of growth. The roots can be chopped and tinctured while fresh or dried and ground for use in teas. The dried roots can be tinctured as well.

Leaves, stems, and flowers can be selectively harvested when they are in full bloom in midsummer. If you opt to do this, bear in mind that a preponderance of leaves and flowers must remain on the plants to

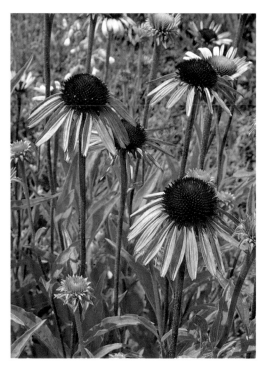

Echinacea purpurea

provide life support for the roots and to produce viable seeds.

Alternatives and Adjuncts: Virtually any of the alterative, diuretic, cholagogue, or expectorant herbs combine well with echinacea to support the body during microbial infections. To help fight infections of the mouth, digestive tract, or urinary tract, echinacea serves as an excellent adjunct to Oregon grape or couch grass. As a lymphatic, echinacea combines well with cleavers.

Cautions and Comments: Echinacea is a very safe herb. But remember, echinacea can only be expected to support a healthy immune system. If the animal is malnourished or immune-compromised by preexisting disease or by other factors, you should consider dietary changes and/or other measures that feed and support the immune system before jumping into Echinacea therapy. Before using echinacea, it is a good idea to consult a holistic veterinarian—especially if you are uncertain of your animal's level of disease resistance.

ELECAMPANE

Inula helenium   Sunflower Family

Appearance: Elecampane is a stout, impressive plant. Healthy specimens may grow in excess of 6 feet high. We have seen these plants in tightly clustered hedgelike stands so thick that one cannot see daylight through them. The narrowly lance-shaped leaves may exceed 16 inches in length and 4 inches in width. The daisylike flowers may reach 4 inches in diameter, are burnt orange, and have narrow rays that contrast with the robust overall appearance of the plant—a splendid addition to any herb or flower garden!

Habitat and Range: Probably a native of southeastern Europe, elecampane has become naturalized throughout much of Europe and the eastern portions of the U.S. It has been cultivated throughout much of the world.

Cycle and Bloom Season: A perennial that generally blooms in early to midsummer

Parts Used: Rhizomes (roots)

Primary Medicinal Activities: Expectorant; sedative; respiratory stimulant; lubricates, soothes, and protects internal mucous membranes; antibacterial, fungicide, expels worms

Strongest Affinities: Lungs

Preparation: Decoction or tincture

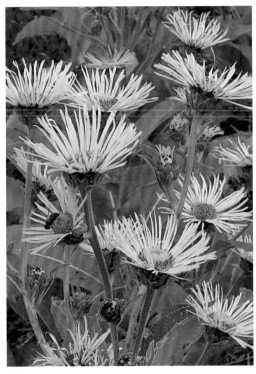

Inula helenium

Common Uses: Elecampane has long been regarded as a valuable medicine for a wide variety of lung disorders. Among herbalists, it is regarded as an expectorant that also lends antibacterial support, mild cough-suppressive qualities, and relief to mucous membranes by virtue of its slippery, oily, soothing mucilage. In other words, elecampane helps make coughing more productive by stimulating excretion of mucus, acts to protect and lubricate inflamed mucous membranes in the respiratory tract while inhibiting bacterial infection, and serves to suppress the cough response just enough so that the body is relieved of unnecessary stress. Unfortunately, relatively little scientific study has been performed to support all of these claims. Science has uncovered evidence to suggest that elecampane may have sedative qualities in mice, and we know that it contains a volatile oil constituent called alantolactone, which is active against roundworms, whipworms, threadworms, and hookworms in humans. Regardless of a lack of scientific study, this plant has been used for thousands of years as a treatment for bronchitis, pneumonia, and tuberculosis—and it is regarded by herbalists as safe enough for use in children with a dry, irritating cough. In animals, we find it useful for soothing a raspy hack that is the result of too much trail dust or perhaps even for kennel cough. Proper dose and duration of therapy must be determined through recognition of specific symptoms and should be based on the special needs of the individual animal. Most of what we know about this herb is centered on the hands-on experience of those who are familiar with it. Therefore, if elecampane seems to be a viable option for your animal, seek the advice of a holistic practitioner before you proceed with its use.

Availability: The dried rhizome or tincture is available through herb retailers. Plants, root cuttings, and seeds are available through specialty nurseries.

Propagation and Harvest: Elecampane likes full sun and a moist clay loam with an acid pH of 4.5 to 6. Aside from these requirements, you can grow it just about anywhere. Roots are dug in the fall of their second year. They can then be processed into tincture while fresh or dried in a warm location for future use.

Alternatives and Adjuncts: For respiratory disorders associated with heavy congestion, elecampane combines well with mullein or grindelia. For kennel cough, it can be combined with coltsfoot.

Cautions and Comments: Elecampane has been shown to be highly allergenic in animals and humans with sensitivity to plants in the sunflower (Asteraceae) family.

FENNEL

Foeniculum vulgare   Parsley Family

Appearance: Fennel looks very much like dill—delicate finely divided leaves, yellow umbel flowers, and hollow stems. The most obvious difference between fennel and dill is the aromatic nature of the plants—fennel smells somewhat like anise (or licorice), whereas dill smells like, well, dill pickles. Fennel also has sturdier stems and a proportionately large bulb, which is considered a gourmet delicacy by salad and sautéed vegetable connoisseurs. The entire plant may grow in excess of 6 feet tall.

Habitat and Range: Native to Eurasia, fennel has become a full-time, naturalized resident in the southern half of California, where it is frequently found on the edges of waste areas.

Cycle and Bloom Season: There are many subspecies of *Foeniculum vulgare*—many are perennials, others are annuals or biennials. In northern climes, fennel usually grows as an annual.

Parts Used: Seeds, leaves, roots

Primary Medicinal Activities: Expels intestinal gas, relieves stomach cramps, stimulates milk production, stimulates digestion, nutritive, and antibacterial

Strongest Affinities: Digestive tract

Preparation: Fresh or dried leaves, seeds, or roots; or a tincture of the seeds or roots

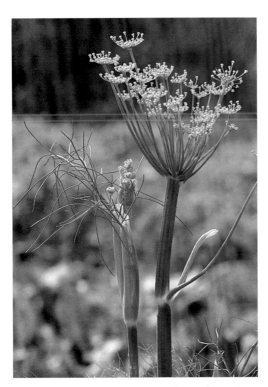

Foeniculum vulgare

Common Uses: Fennel seed is among the first herbs to reach for in cases of flatulence or colic. Its activity in the digestive tract is similar to that of catnip. Fennel tastes different from any mint, however, and its flavor is often favored by dogs and cats who dislike "minty" herbs. About 20 percent of cats won't go near a flake of catnip, making fennel the herb of choice for gastric upset and irritability. In chronic cases, it serves as a gentle antigas and antispasmodic agent that can be added directly to the animal's food to bring symptomatic relief while the caretaker looks for the deeper cause of the problem. In acute cases, such as when your horse finds an open bag of molasses and oats that you forgot to put away (or when she grazes on too much fresh alfalfa because you left a gate open), fennel may help to reduce

the subsequent bloating that is caused by intestinal gas buildup. For flatulence or colic, horses can be free-fed fresh fennel greens—as much as they want—until they find relief. For dogs and cats, fennel seed works to relieve gastric discomfort from the "no-no's" that are inevitably consumed as a result of human weakness such as tidbits fed from the Thanksgiving dinner table or from the dishes that "can wait until morning." A cooled tea works well for this purpose—1 teaspoon of the fresh or dried seeds (fresh are better) in 8 ounces of boiling water, steeped until cool. The tea can be fed at a rate of 2–4 tablespoons for each 20 pounds of the animal's body weight, or it can be added to drinking water as generously as the animal will allow. A glycerin tincture also works well, especially for finicky animals, because it allows for the convenience of a small dosage of 10–20 drops (or more precisely, up to 0.75 milliliters) per 20 pounds of the animal's weight, as needed. Fennel is high in vitamin C, vitamin A, calcium, iron, and potassium and has varying amounts of linoleic acid. It is an especially good nutritional adjunct for dogs and cats with chronic indigestion that cannot be attributed to a specific disease entity. Fennel also helps increase appetite and reduce bad breath by minimizing belching and by acting as an antibacterial in the mouth. The leaf tea is said to be an effective skin and coat rinse for repelling fleas. Traditionally, fennel is fed to increase milk flow in nursing mothers.

Availability: Fennel seed, root, and sometimes the greens can be found in food stores that stock specialty vegetables. Fennel tinctures are available through herb retailers.

Propagation and Harvest: Fennel is easy to grow from seed or nursery starts. It does best in areas with a cool climate and likes light, dry, slightly alkaline soil. The seeds should be harvested in the fall, just as they begin to dry and turn to a light brown color. The leaves and flowers can be harvested and used anytime. For food use, the 1-inch-wide bulbs are "blanched" throughout the remainder of their growth by covering them with hills of soil. This makes the bulbs white and tender with a mild flavor.

Alternatives and Adjuncts: Catnip serves as an excellent alternative, as does anise seed, celery seed, or dill seed. For chronic flatulence, try using a bitter herb such as dandelion leaf or Oregon grape a few minutes before each feeding. Fennel can then be used after meals if flatulence persists.

Cautions and Comments: The volatile oils in fennel are thought to cause or contribute to photosensitive dermatitis in some animals, but such occurrences are rare. In general, this herb is safe.

FEVERFEW

Tanacetum parthenium   Sunflower Family

Appearance: Feverfew is a stout, fast-growing plant with sturdy ridged stems, deeply divided alternate leaves, and yellow-centered white flowers that look like miniature (1-inch-wide) white daisies. The entire plant is aromatic.

Habitat and Range: Feverfew is native to the Balkan region of Europe and has since been naturalized throughout North America.

Cycle and Bloom Season: A perennial or biennial that usually blooms from June through August

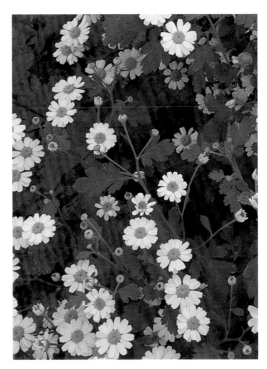

Tanacetum parthenium

Parts Used: All aerial parts

Primary Medicinal Activities: Anti-inflammatory, helps reduce arthritic inflammation (antirheumatic), dilates blood vessels, insecticidal, promotes menstruation

Strongest Affinities: Vascular, gastrointestinal, and reproductive systems

Preparation: Dried herb, tincture, and tea

Common Uses: Feverfew has become a well-known remedy for migraine sufferers. Several studies have shown that part of its effectiveness in treating migraines is attributable to a group of chemicals known as sesquiterpene lactones (especially parthenolide) that are contained in the plants' leaves and flowers. These compounds act to inhibit platelet aggregation in the bloodstream, thus preventing blockage of small capillaries and helping to relieve the pounding, high-pressure pain of a migraine headache. In animals, this activity helps relieve posttrauma or postsurgical discomfort, especially where capillary circulation is diminished or impaired. Feverfew has been shown to block or inhibit the release of histamine, serotonin, thromboxane, and prostaglandins, while inhibiting proliferation of certain types of mononuclear cells in the synovia of injured or arthritic joints. This means that feverfew might be useful in the proactive reduction of inflammation associated with arthritis, joint injuries, and various other diseases.

Feverfew is especially useful in cats as an alternative to aspirin, which can be toxic to felines. And many of the classic anti-inflammatory herbs, including willow, poplar, and meadowsweet, contain salicylic acids, the natural precursors to aspirin. Feverfew may not address pain as directly as aspirin, but it does not contain any salicylate compounds and can therefore be used with a greater margin of safety. A glycerin-based tincture works well for this purpose, as does a cooled tea. A safe starting dosage is 12–20 drops of the tincture or ½ teaspoon of a strong tea for each 20 pounds of the animal's body weight, twice daily.

The upper parts of feverfew (especially the flowers) contain pyrethrins, compounds that are known to paralyze fleas. To make a flea rinse for your pet, pour boiling water over some fresh herbs. Cover the container, and let the mixture stand until it is completely cooled. Strain the herb from the liquid, and pour the liquid onto your animal's coat, making sure that it soaks down to the skin. Do not towel dry your pet. Let the rinse dry naturally and be sure to use all of the rinse as the pyrethrin will not remain active for more than a few hours.

Availability: Feverfew is readily available wherever herbal remedies are sold. The plants are available through most nurseries. For use against fleas, however, you really need a fresh plant—so plant one in your garden.

Propagation and Harvest: Feverfew is easy to grow from seed or nursery starts. The plants are extremely winter hardy, drought resistant, and tolerant of poor soil. Tuck a plant into the corner of your garden, give it a little water, and watch it grow. (In fact, it will reseed its way right out of the garden!) Harvest the leaves and flowers as you need them.

Alternatives and Adjuncts: For relief from pain and inflammation, feverfew combines well with skullcap, valerian, and licorice. For fighting fleas, combine with yarrow and celery or dill seed.

Cautions and Comments: I (Greg) have heard that feverfew should never be fed fresh, because it may cause mouth ulcers. But throughout two decades of using and recommending this herb, I have yet to witness an adverse side effect. Nevertheless, caution dictates that we should take care in assuring that the herb is entirely dried first.

FLAX

Linum spp.   Flax Family

Appearance: Almost three hundred species of flax are distributed worldwide. The most common species have bright blue, five-petaled, ½- to 1-inch-wide flowers, narrow single-veined leaves, small five-chambered fruits, and wirelike stems that sway in the slightest breeze and seem to have a hard time supporting their own weight. Plants range in height from 6 to 32 inches.

Habitat and Range: Common blue flax (*Linum perenne*) and several other blue-flowered species are found in prairies, in open meadows, and along roadways throughout North America.

Cycle and Bloom Season: An annual or perennial (depending on species) that blooms from June to August and reseeds itself readily

Parts Used: Seeds (called flaxseed)

Primary Medicinal Activities: Nutritive, soothes the digestive tract, laxative, antioxidant, tonic

Strongest Affinities: Skin, nervous system, digestive system

Preparation: Ground seeds, seed oil, stabilized seeds

Common Uses: Flaxseed contains alpha-linolenic acid and linoleic acid, as well as omega-3 fatty acids. Essential fatty acids are important in the development and maintenance of a healthy brain, liver, heart, and immune system—in fact, these acids are so important, animals cannot survive without them. Several studies have confirmed that omega-3 fatty acids are essential factors in the brain development of young animals and may even help protect the brain against certain types of neurotoxins. Numerous studies also have shown that daily supplementation with EFAs may dramatically improve the skin, coat, and nails in animals who receive it as a supplement to a good diet. Essential fatty acids have been linked to retinal development and antioxidant activities. The point is this: All animals require EFAs in order to enjoy healthy lives. The problem is that many animals do not receive enough to adequately support

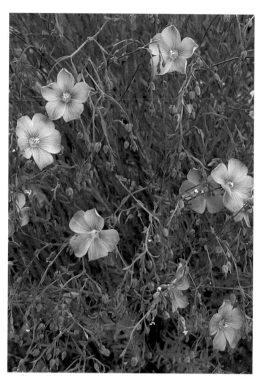

Linum sp.

their bodies' needs and, as a result, suffer from chronic diseases that could have been easily prevented. Flaxseed oil is one of the richest plant source of omega-3 fatty acids known to humanity—but it is not the "totally complete," stand-alone source of omega-3 fatty acids we once thought. A piece of the complex puzzle is missing, namely, gamma linolenic acid (GLA)—a fatty acid that is needed to support the body's inflammatory responses to allergens and other inflammatory stimuli. The problem is due to the lack of a critical enzyme, called delta-6 desaturase (or D6D), that is needed to convert the linoleic acid constituents in flax into GLA. Although most mammals, including humans, should be able to produce D6D, most cannot. This is due to environmental factors, such as various pollutants, and perhaps even emotional stress factors, which have been shown to inhibit the body's production of this important enzyme. So if you are searching for a more complete omega-3 supplement, you should turn to fish oil, borage seed oil, or chia seed. All of these sources already contain gamma linoleic acids, and no metabolic conversion (or D6D) is required for the body fully utilize it.

There are various ways to feed flaxseed to an animal. One option is to buy a nutritional supplement that includes flaxseed as part of a balanced herbal formula. Other options are to buy the seeds in their whole form and grind them immediately before adding them to your companion's food. You can also use flaxseed oil. When deciding which form of flaxseed is best for you and your companion, you should consider several factors. First, it's important to know that flaxseed oil (the fraction of the plant that contains the highest concentration of EFAs) becomes rancid very quickly. While flaxseed oil offers omega-3 EFAs in a form that can be fed in relatively small quantities and that is quickly and completely absorbed into the body, it requires constant refrigeration and its shelf life is variable and unpredictable. On the other hand, its flavor is relatively easy to mask in an animal's food. If you wish to use flax for digestive problems, you will need the seeds. Whole seeds keep for several months if refrigerated but must be ground into powder each time they are used. If you grind them ahead of time, they will quickly spoil. The freshly ground seeds can be used as an EFA supplement, but it's difficult to gauge the amount of EFAs your animal receives with each feeding because as the seeds age, their EFA content deteriorates. Another problem with the seed option is palatability—many animals don't like the flavor of ground flaxseeds, and getting an appreciable amount of the powder into a finicky animal can be challenging. The solution: buy a

natural pet product that contains stabilized flaxseed.

Stabilized flaxseed is treated with zinc and vitamin B6, which makes the seed taste better and helps to prevent the EFA-containing oil from becoming rancid. If you buy a stabilized flaxseed product that is designed especially for animals, follow the manufacturer's feeding instructions. You can also buy stabilized flaxseed that is intended for humans and prorate the recommended dose up or down to your animal's body weight. Human doses are generally based on the needs of a 150-pound person; therefore, if you have a 50-pound dog, you need to feed the dog one-third of the recommended dose for humans. It's also a good idea to consult your veterinarian for the correct dosage for your pet's weight.

If you don't wish to use a stabilized flaxseed product and have access to a source of fresh flaxseed, buy weekly supplies and grind a ½ teaspoon of the seed into a fine powder for each 20 pounds of your animal's body weight. Sprinkle the powder onto your companion's food each day, and be sure that she has plenty of water to drink with her meal because flaxseed absorbs water and gains mass while in the stomach. This swelling action is due to the combined fiber, mucilage, and oil content of the seed, which make flaxseed an excellent herb for colic, constipation, and other digestive problems. The oily mucilage of the seed helps lubricate the digestive tract while the swollen fibers serve as a safe but efficient intestinal cleanser (it works the same way as psyllium husks do). For cases of constipation, 1 teaspoon of ground flaxseed can be thoroughly mixed with 4 ounces of cool water. Allow the mixture to stand for an hour, or until it thickens—you should be able to rub a drop between your thumb and forefinger and feel its oily nature. If the mixture doesn't feel slippery, add more powder and let it stand again. The idea is to activate the flaxseed before putting it into your companion's body and thus alleviate any possibility of expansion-related discomfort. Once you get a slippery consistency, 2 teaspoons of the mixture can be fed for each 30 pounds of the animal's body weight (start with ½ teaspoon in cats). If possible, the slurry should be fed on an empty stomach so the mixture can work its way throughout the digestive tract.

Propagation and Harvest: Flax is easy to grow from seed. Simply scatter the seeds as thinly as possible, rake them into the top ⅛ inch of soil, and water thoroughly. Sprouts will usually emerge within seven days. Flax is a pretty border plant, but it really isn't a practical herb to grow for medicinal purposes. It takes several plants to yield a useful quantity of seed, which must be thrashed and separated from the stems, leaves, and seed capsules. Without special equipment, this is a tedious task that yields only a handful of seeds that could have been purchased for a few cents at a health food store.

Alternatives and Adjuncts: Borage seed oil, evening primrose oil, and black currant seed oil are also excellent sources of EFAs. Flaxseed oil can be combined with cod liver oil or other fish oils to make a rounded supplement of omega-3 and omega-6 fatty acids. For digestive problems, psyllium husks, plantain, and marshmallow serve as good alternatives.

Cautions and Comments: Dry flaxseeds should be fed with plenty of water, otherwise digestive upset and discomfort may result from rapid expansion of the seed fibers in the digestive tract. The best

way to avoid this possibility is to premix flaxseed with water prior to feeding or to use a balanced flaxseed formula that is specially designed to be used in powder form.

GARLIC

Allium sativum   Lily Family

Appearance: Need we describe garlic? It's what makes Italian dishes worthwhile. It is the aromatic bulb that repels vampires yet attracts hungry people with its nose-tantalizing, mouthwatering scent. While most of us can readily identify a head of garlic in the supermarket, relatively few of us are familiar with the living green plant. Garlic is a member of the *Allium* genus, a branch of the lily family that also includes hundreds of varieties of onions, leeks, chives, and shallots. In terms of appearance, the numerous varieties of garlic are differentiated from what we know as onions by the nature of their bulbs (commonly known as heads) and their leaves. Commercial varieties of garlic produce heads that are divided into segments (cloves), whereas onion bulbs are comprised of singular, multilayered globes. Garlic leaves are characteristically flat and almost grasslike, whereas most onions' leaves tend to be hollow and erect. Shallot leaves fall somewhere in between. For the purposes of holistic healing, it's important to know that all of the *Allium* species come from the same source—nature. All of the various colors and shapes of onions, garlic, and their relatives have originated from wild *Allium* species that range throughout the world. On the slopes surrounding our Montana home, several species of wild *Allium* are among the first greens to emerge from the receding snows of early spring. With their emergence come winter-weary bears, grouse, deer, elk, and moose, all of whom wish to indulge, if only briefly, in a snack of garliclike wild onions. As one watches these animals while they browse, it soon becomes apparent that they eat wild onions and garlic to fill some instinctive need other than hunger—they pick and choose only a few select plants, then move on to others. Could it be they know something we don't? Certainly! It is obvious that nature put the *Allium* genus here for reasons far deeper than epicurean delight. Fortunately for those who cannot forage the wilds of North America on behalf of their pets, the "supermarket varieties" of garlic are of optimum medicinal potency.

Habitat and Range: It has been theorized that garlic's wild ancestors originated from west-central Asia. Garlic's use as a medicine dates back at least five thousand years, and since then hundreds of cultivars have been propagated worldwide. In North America, dozens of varieties can be found in open forest clearings and grasslands at foothill to subalpine elevations. Most are montane residents.

Cycle and Bloom Season: Although commercial varieties are typically harvested during their first year of growth when the bulbs are prime, most *Allium* species are self-seeding perennials that bloom in midsummer.

Parts Used: Bulb (the segments of which are called cloves)

Primary Medicinal Activities: Antibacterial, stimulates the immune system, anticancer, nutritive, antioxidant, expectorant, lowers blood pressure, antitumor, antiviral, antifungal, tonic

Strongest Affinities: Liver, blood, cardiovascular system, immune system

Preparation: Fresh, dried, tincture, or oil infusion

Common Uses: Garlic contains considerable amounts of protein, fiber, potassium, phosphorus, calcium, sodium, vitamin A, thiamine, niacin, taurine, zinc, riboflavin, and dozens of other nutritive compounds. A single clove of fresh garlic may contain as much as one hundred sulfur compounds, all of which have been shown to possess medicinal qualities.

Most of us who read the ads and labels for garlic preparations or supplements at health food stores are continually reminded of allicin—a volatile oil constituent of garlic. Once believed to be the definitive factor in garlic's healing abilities, allicin represents only a segment of garlic's complex, medicinally versatile chemistry. This is not to say that allicin is not useful; actually it is one of the most impressive broad-spectrum antimicrobial substances available in nature, with dozens of scientific studies to back up this claim. Researchers have found that allicin may be more effective against harmful microbes than tetracycline, a frequently prescribed antibiotic drug. And unlike conventional antibiotics, garlic works against many forms of virus and won't compromise populations of beneficial flora in the digestive tract when ingested in the appropriate amounts.

Despite its clear value as a healing agent, allicin is not the only healing agent in garlic worth considering. In fact, the presence of allicin in garlic preparations is not required at all in many situations where garlic may prove beneficial. At least thirty other compounds that are contained in garlic have been shown to be useful for conditions that range from skin disorders to cancer.

Allicin is an unstable compound that dissipates quickly when exposed to air, moisture, or heat. Unless special measures are taken to preserve it, the allicin content in many garlic preparations are nil by the time they reach someone who needs them. To confront this dilemma, several garlic preparations that have been "standardized to allicin" are available on the market. These extracts, powders, capsules, and tablets have had a certain percentage of allicin added in the laboratory to "guarantee their potency." Such formulas are safe and effective when used properly for specific antimicrobial purposes but are generally unnecessary and expensive for use in most other instances where garlic is indicated. And, despite the claims of many manufacturers, consumers can't tell if the allicin content in a standardized preparation still exists at the time of use. Unless a laboratory analysis is performed after the product has reached store shelves, there's no way of knowing whether the allicin's potency has vanished from the formula.

Before you use a standardized formula, try to find out how the manufacturer can guarantee the allicin content in the product after it leaves the lab. If the company's answer is satisfactory, then bear in mind that many of garlic's other medicinal constituents may be absent or overpowered by an unnatural abundance of allicin and that you will be using garlic in a manner beyond nature's design. Regardless of what the manufacturer might say, nature endows garlic with a specific amount of allicin as well as hundreds of other compounds that serve unified purposes.

When we isolate a single constituent from the whole plant, we are no longer

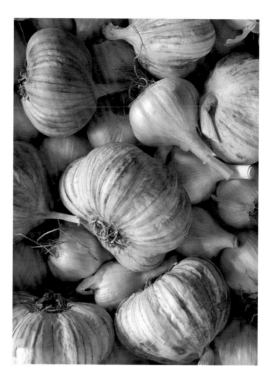

Allium sativum

working within a natural context, and we limit the healing potential of that plant to the confines of what we know, as opposed to what might be possible. While scientists are beginning to understand how single chemical elements and compounds work in or on the body, we still know very little about how they work in a synergistic capacity. In this realm, just beyond our understanding, a great many healing secrets are waiting to be discovered. Any good herbalist will tell you that the whole is always greater than the sum of its parts.

The chemical complexity of garlic is good news for the self-reliant herbalist because in addition to allicin, garlic contains a multitude of compounds that are stable and easy to use. Despite its widespread recognition as a healthy food for humans, garlic demands some added respect, caution, and therapeutic consideration if it is to be used effectively in the care of animals. Here are three general rules of proper use:

- Allicin is essential in applications where garlic is to be used as a natural form of antibiotic but may not be necessary if you are using garlic for general health maintenance or other purposes.
- If you wish to employ garlic as an antibiotic, you need to use raw garlic or raw garlic juice within three hours of chopping or pressing the fresh cloves, or you need a good garlic extract from a reputable source. A properly dried garlic powder may be useful for internal antibiotic applications as well, though only a residual trace of allicin remains in the powder until it is used. In this case, two compounds, alliin and allinase, meet with enzymes to form allicin as they enter the mouth. The allicin then does its work within the body—from the inside out.

If you use garlic as a topical antibiotic, bear in mind that raw garlic juice is strong and may cause acute reddening and irritation of skin and mucous membranes if applied undiluted. Cut the juice with olive oil, vegetable glycerin, or water at a starting rate of one part pure garlic juice to two parts inert liquid (oil, water, etc.). If irritation persists, further dilute the juice. Such problems can be avoided by infusing fresh cloves of garlic directly into olive oil.

- If you wish to use garlic as a cancer-inhibiting antioxidant agent, immune-system enhancer, blood-thinning agent, cardiovascular tonic, or nutritional supplement, any form of garlic will probably have the desired results. Perhaps the only exceptions are preparations of garlic that have been subjected to heat such as pickled, sautéed, boiled, roasted, or otherwise hyperheated cloves that have

likely been depleted of their medicinal potential and a considerable percentage of their nutrients.

Used properly and in the correct form, garlic is valuable for treatment of virtually any form of internal or external bacterial, viral, or fungal infection, including parasites (such as tapeworms) and protozoan organisms (such as *Giardia*). Fresh garlic or properly dried powder (from a reputable market source) can be fed as part of your animal's diet to fight infections of the mouth, throat, respiratory tract, stomach, or intestines. In sheep, goats, and cows, it is said to help alleviate mastitis. Freshly crushed garlic or fresh garlic juice can be infused or diluted into olive oil for use as a topical antiseptic for minor injuries, ear infections, or mites. The rule here is to be sure the garlic is diluted sufficiently—the volatile oils are strong and can cause burning irritation if applied to the skin in concentrated form. Never apply essential oil of garlic to any part of the body; it's too concentrated. And never use garlic preparations in the eyes.

To use in topical applications, you don't need much garlic—just enough to impart a mild garlic odor to the oil. To make a garlic oil, crush two or three cloves of garlic, wet them with vodka to help release the oils, and cover them with 4 ounces of olive oil. Shake the mixture vigorously and let it stand in the refrigerator for an hour before using. The oil should have an obvious, but not overpowering, garlic odor. Within three to twenty-four hours, the allicin will begin dissipating from your oil, and its usefulness for killing microbes will be diminished. But don't discard it. It still possesses immune-supporting and disease-preventing qualities, and it can be added to your pet's meals. Use ½ to 1 level teaspoon per pound of food per feeding, depending on the oil's strength. Keep your garlic oil in the refrigerator in a glass jar with a tight-fitting lid. Expect it to keep for no more than a month. Contrary to what many believe, garlic will not act as its own preservative, and old garlic oil may develop botulism—a bacteria that can be deadly to animals and people. The added alcohol (vodka) is not enough to prevent botulism either, but adding ¼ teaspoon of vitamin E oil to the garlic oil before it goes into the refrigerator will help extend its shelf life while adding a new element of nutritional support. As you can see, this justifies the task of making your own oil. Many commercially prepared oils produced from raw garlic offer no information on how long they will remain fresh and effective.

Scientific studies have shown that various compounds in garlic stimulate immune functions in the bloodstream at levels of activity that are unparalleled by any other herb (yes, even by echinacea). Perhaps most intriguing is garlic's effect on the body's natural killer cells—those cells that seek out and destroy cancer cells and invading microbes. In a study conducted with human subjects who have AIDS, garlic was found to increase killer cell activity threefold. Similar animal studies have been conducted with similar results. Given the fact that these studies were done on subjects with depressed immune functions, it stands to reason that companion animals with healthy immune functions may benefit from the added measure of immune support supplied through moderate garlic supplementation in their diets.

A 1988 study found that diallyl sulfide, a garlic constituent, prevented tumor formation in rats, and several other studies have shown that garlic inhibits various forms of cancerous growths in the body. This effect may be attributable to the liver-strengthening actions of at least six garlic components. In this capacity, garlic gently enhances overall liver function and triggers enzyme responses to help break down waste materials before they go into the bloodstream. In other words, garlic helps the liver cleanse the body and thus helps prevent toxic accumulations that may lead to cancerous growths. Garlic also helps to lower blood cholesterol and triglyceride levels, making it useful for miniature schnauzers, beagles, and other breeds that may be predisposed to hyperlipidemia—a condition that may lead to chronic seizures. Any form of uncooked garlic performs these functions, and its use is as simple as sprinkling it onto an animal's food. A once-a-day dosage of ⅛–¼ teaspoon (powdered or freshly chopped) per pound of food fed is usually sufficient for most animals.

We have seen very good results from the use of garlic against tapeworms. Used in powdered, fresh, or extract forms, garlic might not kill these persistent parasites, but it will make their living quarters much less desirable. Intestinal parasites don't seem to like volatile oils or sulfur compounds, and if fed to an animal in correct dosages over a period of one to two months, garlic helps to drive these pests out. In our experiences with dogs, an increase in visible tapeworm segments in an animal's stool is likely to occur after two to three weeks of daily garlic ingestion. After about two months, populations of these parasites are usually back to acceptable levels, or they may disappear completely.

Garlic works in a similar fashion against protozoan infestations such as *giardiasis*, but in these cases a strong presence of allicin is needed to be effective. Use fresh garlic and add Oregon grape root to your animal's diet. This adds an antimicrobial "double punch" against these tough organisms.

Garlic is one of the best all-around cardiovascular tonics in the plant world. In studies conducted in collaboration with the New York Department of Health, a component called ajoene found in both fresh and dried forms of garlic was found to be effective at preventing the formation of blood clots in the vascular system. In some provinces of France, racehorses suffering from blood clots are routinely fed garlic in their grain feed, and, as a result, the clots sometimes disappear in a matter of days. In fact, many researchers believe that garlic may be as useful as aspirin in this capacity, which makes it especially promising for use in cats since they cannot tolerate the salicylate constituents of aspirin. Garlic has also been shown to reduce cholesterol levels and the occurrence of atherosclerosis (fat buildup in the arteries) in both animals and humans, thus reducing the possibility of stroke or heart attack. All of these attributes, combined with the immune-supportive, liver-strengthening capabilities of garlic, make this herb an excellent multisystem tonic for older animals—especially dogs, who tolerate regular feeding of garlic better than cats do.

Garlic's effectiveness as a systemic flea or mosquito repellent is the subject of a great deal of debate among those who have tried it. Some people claim good results; others believe that the usefulness of garlic in this capacity is largely unfounded.

Availability: Supermarkets and health food retailers

Propagation and Harvest: Garlic is easy to grow. When sown in the fall, the plants thrive in even the harshest of winter climates, usually producing bulbs by late summer. A sandy loam with a slightly alkaline pH level is the best growing medium. In areas where winters are mild, the cloves can be pressed about 1 inch into the soil in late fall for an early summer crop. In northern climes, plant your cloves 4 inches deep as late as you can still work the soil in fall. Cover your planting with at least 6 inches of mulch. Expect to see sprouts shortly after the last hard frost. Garlic should be harvested in midsummer to late summer, after the tops of the plants have died back. Dig up the bulbs, then allow them to dry in the sun for two or three days before you store them in a cool, dry place indoors.

Alternatives and Adjuncts: For topical treatment of bacterial infections, consider Oregon grape, Saint-John's-wort, bee balm, thyme, and chamomile as alternatives. For immune system and antioxidant support, investigate echinacea, astragalus, licorice, alfalfa, red clover, and burdock as adjuncts or alternatives. For treating *giardiasis* and *E. coli* infections, garlic combines well with Oregon grape or organically raised goldenseal.

Cautions and Comments: Toxic side effects from the consumption of garlic are rare in animals and humans alike, but the possibility of harming your dog, your cat, or your herbivore with garlic does exist, and there is a growing controversy about how much garlic is enough and how much is too much. At the root of this controversy is a dangerous misconception: the notion that more garlic is always better. Despite all of the grand attributes we have just described, moderation—the cardinal rule of all herb use—applies strictly to garlic, particularly when it is used in cats.

When misused (used excessively or over an extended period), garlic may cause Heinz-body anemia, a potentially life-threatening blood disease. Scientists theorize that two chemical compounds contained in garlic may be related to this disorder: s-methyl cysteine sulfoxide, or n-propyl disuldhide. These compounds are believed to deplete a naturally occurring glucose enzyme called Glucose-6-phosphate dehydrogenase (G6PD). This enzyme has a special function of protecting the walls of red blood cells. Depletion of G6PD causes oxidative damage to the cells, thus forming Heinz bodies and triggering the body to reject them from the bloodstream (usually via dark-colored urine). If left unchecked, this process continues until the numbers of red blood cells are lowered to the point that the animal becomes anemic and eventually dies. Fortunately, this nightmare is easily prevented with some common sense and a few precautions.

Other side effects of garlic are more predictable and less threatening: digestive upset and gas when ingested (in which case, reduce the dose and relieve the gas with chamomile) or redness and irritation when applied to the skin (usually indicative of a preparation that is too concentrated).

First, it stands to reason that animals with preexisting anemic conditions should not receive garlic internally in any quantity. Puppies don't begin reproducing new red blood cells until after six to eight weeks of age. Until then, they need every red blood cell they are born with, so a diet that includes garlic is not appropriate for young puppies.

It's important to know that the possibility of Heinz-body anemia is dose dependent, meaning the more garlic fed, the greater the chances of a problem developing. While we still don't know exactly how much is too much, most recorded instances of Heinz-body anemia in animals involve the ingestion of large quantities of onions and other garlic relatives, many of which are likely to contain much larger percentages of enzyme-depleting constituents than a typical dose of garlic. Recorded cases of allium poisoning typically involve onion doses exceeding 0.5 percent of the subject animals' body weight—this means that a healthy 60-pound dog would have to eat a whole 5-ounce onion, or several cloves of garlic, just to start the Heinz-body process. And since red blood cells are regenerated quickly from the bone marrow, this grotesque overdose would probably have to be repeated several times on a frequent basis to cause permanent harm. In further defense of garlic, several other foods can cause Heinz-body anemia as well—large amounts of turnips, kale, rape, or anything rich in vitamin K may lead to the disorder, especially in herbivores.

Small doses of garlic added to your companion animal's food three or four days per week, perhaps ⅛ teaspoon of garlic powder per pound of food fed, are probably going to be of great benefit to the overall health of your pet. Just don't overdo it.

Cats are much more sensitive to the side effects of garlic than dogs are, so they require more caution and attention with its use. Watch for digestive upset and behavioral changes. And if your cat simply doesn't want any garlic, don't force the issue. Your cat's behavior may be more than just a finicky attitude—animals know their needs better than we do.

Remember to use common sense and moderation and to have respect for garlic as more than just a table condiment. No two animals are alike; one person's miracle cure is another one's poison. If you wish to use garlic in a therapeutic capacity, get to know your animal first, then consult a professional (or carefully read the label on your garlic product) before you proceed.

GINKGO

Ginkgo biloba   Ginkgo Family

Appearance: Characterized by its unique fan-shaped leaves, ginkgo is a slow-growing tree that may reach 100 feet in height. A healthy tree can live to be one thousand years old. Ginkgo is one of the oldest plant medicines on earth. In fact, it is one of the oldest species of trees still in existence.

Habitat and Range: It is estimated that the *Ginkgo* genus once included several hundred varieties that spanned the globe for over two million years. Today, however, there is only one species, *G. biloba*, a native of China that has been introduced into North America and most of Europe and Asia for ornamental and medicinal purposes.

Cycle and Bloom Season: Ginkgo is a deciduous tree that blooms in early spring, just as the leaves are beginning to develop into their fanlike shapes. Fruits (known as ginkgo nuts) develop and ripen by midsummer. The leaves turn yellow and begin falling in early to late fall.

Parts Used: Although ginkgo nuts were used almost exclusively for thousands of years, the fall-harvested leaves are of primary interest to contemporary herbalists.

Primary Medicinal Activities: Dilates blood vessels, anticoagulant, antioxidant, tonic

Strongest Affinities: Brain, circulatory system, eyes

Preparation: Tincture, tea, capsule

Common Uses: Over four hundred scientific studies have been conducted to validate ginkgo's effectiveness in both animals and humans. In fact, in Germany and other European countries, *G. biloba* extract (commonly known as GBE) is among the most frequently prescribed drugs of commerce.

For a long time it was thought that almost all of ginkgo's medicinal activity could be attributed to two groups of chemical constituents: flavone glycosides and terpene lactones. Dozens of human and animal studies have shown that these two groups of constituents act to improve blood circulation in small capillaries, a trait that makes gingko especially useful in the treatment of various forms of vascular deficiency—including the effects of old age. But current research indicates that these compounds represent only a small part of a complex array of interactive components. Specifically, ginkgo inhibits the platelet aggregation factor (PAF), the mechanism that causes slow-moving or obstructed blood to become "sticky" and begin forming into clots. Ginkgo does this especially well in small capillaries that are particularly susceptible to blockage and that serve tissues that are not reached by larger vessels such as areas of the brain, ears, and extremities. Ginkgo also helps regulate the tone and elasticity of blood vessels, making them stronger and less susceptible to degenerative disease. These actions make ginkgo a first choice cerebrovascular tonic for older animals. Increased blood flow in capillary-rich tissues of the brain means that the brain is better fed and oxygenated, which in turn can reduce the likelihood of stroke and may equate to a longer, higher-quality life for your pet. In fact, several studies have shown that the cerebrovascular activities of ginkgo may be beneficial in treating degenerative age-related cases of chronic depression or abnormal behavior. If the brain is not getting the blood it needs, mood and behavior will likely be affected—and Rover might start getting rather snippy in his old age.

Most of the current hoopla surrounding ginkgo is focused on its use in the treatment of Alzheimer's disease and other forms of dementia, but its effectiveness as a vascular tonic in other parts of the body deserves equal consideration. Ginkgo works as an effective vascular tonic throughout the body, especially in smaller, peripheral capillaries of the legs, ears, and rectum. This makes it useful in a wide variety of circumstances where circulation has been impaired by trauma, chronic or degenerative disease, or surgical intervention. By opening up and strengthening the structural integrity of small capillaries in impaired areas, gingko improves circulation and enables the body to heal itself more effectively, which is the primary goal of using herbal tonics.

Ginkgo also has been used for hundreds of years as a tonic for weak kidney function. While relatively little research has been conducted to validate such use, ginkgo's effectiveness in this capacity is likely attributable to the same vascular tonic activities since the kidney is a blood-dependent organ. In fact, its vulnerability and demise in the event of diminished blood supply is second only to the brain. In recent months, we have heard from veterinarians and pet owners who have been using an herbal combination that includes ginkgo and hawthorn in the treatment of early-stage renal failure. The anecdotal reports claim a general improvement in kidney function. This makes sense because hawthorn acts to reduce blood pressure as it increases circulation within the larger arteries, while ginkgo serves to open and tonify the smaller vessels.

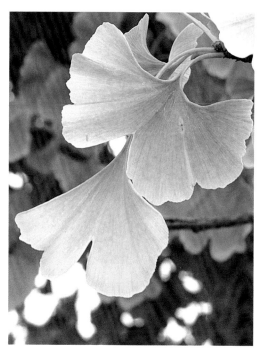

Ginkgo biloba

In addition to its vascular actions, ginkgo also works as a nervous system tonic in the brain. Although the mechanisms of its neurological activity are complex and still hold many mysteries, studies indicate that ginkgo somehow increases energy levels in the brain and stimulates the release of various neurotransmitters, many of which regulate constriction of important smooth-muscle tissues throughout the body—such as those of the heart, bladder, and uterus. The fact that ginkgo works to influence brain function in ways that are exclusive of its circulatory activities makes for a broad scope of therapeutic usefulness. In many cases, urinary incontinence, seizures, various forms of neuralgia, skin problems, chronic digestive upset, cardiac arrhythmia, and behavioral disorders (to name just a few) may be the result of cerebrovascular or neurological dysfunction that might be relieved with the proper use of ginkgo.

Many studies suggest that GBEs have been standardized to contain at least 24 percent ginkgolides. In our opinion, however, excellent results can be obtained from any high-quality extract of the leaves. A typical dose for elderly animals or for those who exhibit early signs of cerebrovascular deficiency, kidney failure, or impaired circulation in the extremities is anywhere between 0.25 milliliters and 0.75 milliliters of the liquid extract, two or three times daily for each 50 pounds of the animal's body weight. Exact dosage varies according to the specific circumstances of disease, size of the animal, potency of the extract, and duration of use. In other words, you are advised to seek a qualified holistic practitioner for a complete workup of your animal before proceeding with ginkgo therapy.

Availability: Widely available through health food stores and herb retailers. Ginkgo trees are available through landscape nurseries.

Propagation and Harvest: Ginkgo trees are not difficult to grow—all they need is room to spread their roots, a moderate climate (hardy in the southern two-thirds of North America), and some water from time to time. The problem is that they are slow growers, with yearly growth often measured in fractions of an inch. If you are lucky enough to have access to a mature ginkgo tree, however, take advantage of the fresh leaves, which are far superior to the dried leaves that are available at herb stores. Analysis of ginkgo leaves indicates that the broadest diversity of medicinal constituents is found when the leaves are just beginning to turn yellow (in the fall). Gather the leaves just as they are turning yellow, before they fall from the tree and in advance of any evidence of mold on the leaf surfaces. The leaves can then be used

fresh to make tincture, or they can be dried for future use. The dried leaves keep for about one year.

Alternatives and Adjuncts: Gingko combines well with hawthorn for cardiovascular or kidney disorders. For use as a general vascular tonic, ginkgo can be combined with garlic, cayenne, or yarrow.

Cautions and Comments: By most standards, ginkgo is safe. But because of its ability to inhibit platelet aggregation in the blood, its use may be contraindicated in the presence of blood-thinning drugs or in animals with blood-clotting disorders. While ginkgo improves the body's ability to heal after surgery, its use should be delayed until all risk of postoperative hemorrhage has passed.

GOLDENROD

Solidago spp.   Sunflower Family

Appearance: Goldenrod is a common wayside weed that is easy to identify by its spire-shaped or triangular clusters of tiny bright goldenrod-yellow flowers. The leaves of the most common species are narrowly lance-shaped and may or may not have serrated edges. Plants are erect and range from 2 inches (*Solidago multiradiata*— mountain goldenrod) to 70 inches (*S. canadensis; S. occidentalis; S. gigantea*) in height. Most species share similar appearances. This is especially true of the larger species, which may differ only in leaf texture or the presence of stem hairs.

Habitat and Range: The *Solidago* genus can be divided into two categories: those that grow in moist soils and those that prefer drier habitats. Generally speaking, most of the smaller mountain varieties are found in dry soils, often at the edges of forest roads or in open meadows. The larger varieties are common to river and lake habitats, irrigated fields, drainage ditches, and so on, from below sea level to about 4,000 feet in elevation. Several species are widespread throughout North America, with *S. canadensis* (Canada goldenrod) being perhaps the most common.

Cycle and Bloom Season: Perennial, sometimes annual. Blooms throughout the summer months

Parts Used: Entire flowering plant—roots and all

Primary Medicinal Activities: Astringent, tonic, diuretic, reduces inflammation of respiratory mucosa (anticatarrhal), strengthens kidney functions (nephritic), anti-inflammatory, helps prevent or eliminate urinary stones (antilithic), antibacterial, antifungal, stops bleeding

Strongest Affinities: Respiratory tract, urinary tract, and kidneys

Preparation: Dried herb, tincture, tea

Common Uses: As with many common wayside weeds, goldenrod's usefulness is usually overshadowed by that of other herbs that have greater mass-market appeal. This is unfortunate because while many people spend their hard-earned money on the latest herb sensation, a better alternative may be growing in profuse abundance just behind the house. Goldenrod is one such herb. It is extremely useful but far less marketable than many others simply because it is too abundant to give notice to.

Goldenrod is an excellent anticatarrhal, an herb that helps to reduce the production

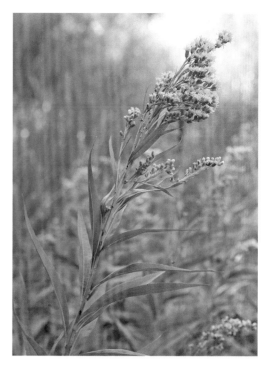

Solidago canadensis

of mucus in the bronchi by decreasing inflammation of the mucous membranes. While the production of mucus is essential in the body's holistic efforts to eliminate pathogens and waste products from the respiratory tract during bacterial, viral, or fungal infections, reducing the irritation of swollen membranes helps to comfort the sufferer while making the overall healing effort more productive. For dogs and cats, a teaspoon or two of a flower or leaf tea (made with a teaspoon of the dried herb in 8 ounces of water, cooled to lukewarm) often brings quick relief for a persistent wet cough. Horses and other large herbivores can be fed a handful or two of the fresh herb for the same purpose.

Although relatively little scientific research has been conducted into goldenrod's effectiveness as a kidney tonic, it has been used successfully in this capacity for hundreds of years. Specifically, goldenrod is said to boost renal function quickly, making it especially helpful for acute cases of nephritis, especially where anuresis (an inability to pass urine from the kidneys) is a prevalent symptom. Goldenrod can also be useful in preventing or assisting in the elimination of kidney stones. However, the activities of goldenrod may be contraindicated in advanced chronic cases of kidney disease, where stimulation of renal function may cause added stress to overworked kidneys. The various mechanisms and pathologies of kidney disease are difficult to assess accurately, and finding the correct approach should be left to your holistic veterinarian.

In topical applications, goldenrod has remarkable hemostatic qualities, especially when the dried and powdered flowers are used. The powder can be applied liberally to stop bleeding and inhibit bacterial infection of minor cuts and abrasions.

Goldenrod may moderate allergic reactions to airborne pollen and other allergens if taken for several weeks prior to the start of hay fever season.

When a measured amount of golden-rod—a potentially allergenic plant—is introduced into the body just before hay fever season, the body begins building its antiallergen defenses before the real onslaught.

Availability: Available through herb retailers; profusely abundant in vacant lots and forests throughout North America, Europe, and Asia.

Propagation and Harvest: Harvest the entire plant when it is in full bloom. The entire plant can then be chopped and made into a tincture, or it can be dried for later use in teas.

Alternatives and Adjuncts: For upper respiratory infections, goldenrod combines especially well with echinacea and Oregon grape. Consider mullein, coltsfoot, wild cherry, marshmallow, slippery elm, and grindelia as adjuncts or alternatives for coughs. Dandelion, couch grass, corn silk, ginkgo, uva ursi, marshmallow, echinacea, and hawthorn should be investigated for treating urinary and kidney disorders.

Cautions and Comments: Goldenrod has no known toxicity but may be contraindicated in animals with certain forms of kidney disease. Although goldenrod is not as allergenic as once thought (often it is blamed for allergies caused by ragweed and other plants), it should be used with caution in animals who are predisposed to pollen allergies.

GOLDENSEAL

Hydrastis canadensis   Buttercup Family

Appearance: Goldenseal is a perennial that may grow to 12 inches in height. The main stem of the plant is typically forked to produce two nearly circular 2-inch to 6-inch-wide leaves, one of which is usually larger than the other. The leaves are deeply lobed, five to seven times, with toothed margins. The plant may require three or more years of growth before it blooms, then it produces a single whitish green flower that has no petals. In midsummer, the flower develops into a single raspberry-like red fruit that contains ten to thirty small seeds. Stems are hairy. The horizontally creeping root is thick and woody. All parts of the root have deep goldenrod-yellow inner tissues.

Habitat and Range: The range and population of this North American native are rapidly diminishing. The original range of goldenseal once included most of eastern North America—from Minnesota and Vermont south into Georgia. Today, most remaining stands of wild goldenseal are isolated in the central and northern reaches of the Appalachians and, to a lesser extent, the Ozark Mountains.

Cycle and Bloom Season: A long-lived perennial that blooms in early spring

Parts Used: Primarily the root; to a lesser extent the leaves

Primary Medicinal Activities: Antimicrobial, reduces inflammation of respiratory mucosa, tonic, astringent, stimulates the liver, antiparasitic

Strongest Affinities: Mucous membranes of the respiratory tract, lower urinary tract, gastrointestinal tract, mouth, and eyes.

Preparation: Tincture, tea, or poultice

Common Uses: Wild goldenseal is vanishing because of greed, sensationalism, and misinformed use. The greatest misconception about goldenseal is that it acts as an herbal antibiotic in the body, coursing its way through the body systems via the bloodstream to attack any pathogenic microbes in its path. This is untrue. Goldenseal does not act as an antibiotic. In fact, the antimicrobial alkaloids of this plant (namely berberine and hydrastine) act only to inhibit bacteria, fungi, parasites, and protozoan bodies that they come in direct contact with in the mouth, gastrointestinal tract, and urinary tract. These infection-fighting compounds are not absorbed into the bloodstream; they simply act as contact disinfectants. With this in mind, goldenseal can be used against a broad spectrum of

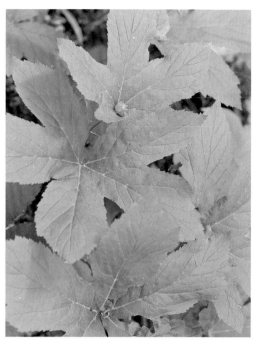

Hydrastis candadensis

pathogens, including *Streptococcus* sp., *Staphylococcus* sp., *Shigella dysenteriae*, *Salmonella*, and several others.

As an anti-inflammatory, goldenseal is effective for ulcers and irritations of the mouth, upper respiratory tract, eyes, and, to a lesser degree, the digestive and urinary tracts. A poultice made from the powdered root can be applied directly to infections or ulcers in the mouth. Results are often seen within hours of application.

For conjunctivitis that is secondary to bacterial or fungal infection in dogs, cats, birds, ferrets, rodents, horses, or reptiles, a goldenseal eyewash serves as a strong antimicrobial agent and also quickly reduces inflammation and redness. To use goldenseal in this capacity, make a strong tea from the chopped dry root, then add 12–20 drops of the dark golden-yellow fluid into 1 ounce of sterile saline solution—the liquid marketed for people with contact lenses. A few drops in each eye (or a fraction of a drop for small birds, rodents, and such) two or three times daily usually brings relief quickly. Internally, we like to use goldenseal in conjunction with garlic for ridding our dogs and cats of tapeworms, and we have received good reports from veterinarians we work with who find this combination useful for treating *giardiasis* or *E. coli* infections in dogs, cats, and larger animals. Studies of the active component berberine substantiate these claims.

Wild goldenseal is one of the most endangered wild medicinal plants in North America, and it is still being exploited by the "bad apples" of the herb industry. Fortunately, goldenseal can be replaced (in most cases) with Oregon grape root (*Mahonia aquifolium*), a naturally abundant member of the barberry family that also contains an impressive amount of the active constituent berberine. The continued survival of wild goldenseal is totally dependent on human conscience and responsibility—if you think you need goldenseal, give Oregon grape a try first. Chances are you will be pleased with the results. If you still see a need for goldenseal, spend the extra money to buy goldenseal roots or goldenseal preparations that have come from certified organic (cultivated) sources. If you use wildcrafted goldenseal, you are contributing to the rapid demise of a great healing treasure that can never be replaced.

Availability: Herb retailers. Please buy goldenseal harvested from a cultivated source only.

Propagation and Harvest: If you have a piece of ground that can support goldenseal, grow some. The future success of this plant may depend on people like you. The best place to plant goldenseal is in the shade of a dense,

hardwood canopy of a north-facing hillside. The plant requires deep compost-rich, well-drained soil with a pH level between 5.5 and 6.5. With enough shade and the right soil amendments, goldenseal can be propagated in a garden as well.

Goldenseal can be propagated from stratified seeds or from rhizomes spaced 4 inches apart in rows that are 12 inches apart. Planting should occur in fall. Goldenseal requires at least four to five years (preferably seven) to reach maturity.

Alternatives and Adjuncts: In many applications where an antimicrobial or anticatarrhal is indicated, any number of plants that contain the yellow alkaloid berberine can be employed in place of goldenseal. Choices include Oregon grape (*Mahonia* sp.), twinleaf (*Jeffersonia diphylla*), or yerba mansa (*Anemiopsis californica*). Before any of these herbs are employed, however, a fundamental question of holistic responsibility should be addressed in the minds of all earth-conscious herb users: Does substituting a wildcrafted herb for an overharvested one benefit the future of wild medicinal plants, or does it simply defer impact onto another species? The fact that Oregon grape is an abundant wild substitute is beside the point. Humanity is efficient at disturbing or depleting virtually anything on earth, and when we elect to abandon one natural resource for another in the absence of proactive holistic thinking, we are only contributing to a continuum of human impact. With this in mind, we should elect to use wild substitutes only when cultivated goldenseal is not available. *Coptis sinensis*, a species of goldthread that is widely cultivated in China, may also serve as an excellent substitute for goldenseal. A small portion of goldthread or goldenseal added to echinacea serves as a direct-intervention "double-punch" for infections of the mouth, urinary tract, and gastrointestinal tract, while the echinacea does its job at boosting the immune system.

Cautions and Comments: Some animal studies have shown that berberine calms the uterus, but other studies show that it stimulates uterine contractions, so it is inadvisable to use goldenseal, Oregon grape, or other berberine-containing plant medicines in pregnant animals. Goldenseal lowers blood sugar, so don't use it in animals who are hypoglycemic. Goldenseal also may alter the metabolism and may have the potential to cause hypertension. Long-term internal use of goldenseal may overstimulate the liver and trigger excessive production of bile—a situation that is likely to result in vomiting. Cats are especially prone to this side effect. In light of this, goldenseal should not be used continuously, in excess of seven days, without a break. For proper dose and duration of therapy, and to ascertain if internal use of goldenseal is indicated for your animal, consult a holistic veterinarian.

An unpleasant but not really threatening side effect may occur in cats that are fed goldenseal or any other plant that contains berberine: excessive salivation. Since first writing this book we have heard from several cat owners and veterinarians who report a "foaming at the mouth." If this occurs, simply discontinue use—it simply means that this may not be the best herbal choice for your particular kitty.

GOTU KOLA

Centella asiatica   Parsley Family

Appearance: Gotu kola produces dark green, nearly circular, 1- to 3-inch leaves and purple flowers that are atypical of the parsley family. The leaves have long petioles (stems) and

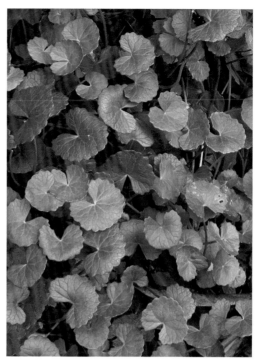
Centella asiatica

leathery smooth surfaces that give the plant an appearance similar to what lily pads would look like if they grew on land instead of in water.

Habitat and Range: Gotu kola is a native of India, south Asia, eastern Europe, and the Philippines. It inhabits drainage ditches, streambeds, and moist waste areas, often in ground-covering abundance.

Cycle and Bloom Season: A perennial that blooms in summer

Parts Used: Leaves

Primary Medicinal Activities: Active against various skin problems (antidermatitic), peripheral vasodilator, helps reduce arthritic inflammation, antioxidant, wound healing, diuretic

Strongest Affinities: Skin, nervous system, circulatory system

Preparation: Tea or tincture or any variety of topical preparation such as salves, lotions, and poultices

Common Uses: Gotu kola is especially useful for burns, skin injuries, or dermatitis that involve vascular insufficiency or accumulation of subcutaneous swelling. When taken internally it increases peripheral blood circulation and serves as a mild diuretic, thus assisting with the body's natural ability to cleanse and heal the epidermis. When applied externally, it serves as an antioxidant and speeds the healing process by stimulating regeneration of skin cells. It has also been shown to accelerate the production of healthy scar tissue after surgery. It is known to promote hair and nail growth.

Gotu kola is useful in treating leprosy (mycobacteriosis), an ulcerous bacterial infection of the skin that can occur in dogs, cats, and other animals. In these cases, it is believed that a terpene compound called asiaticoside breaks down the protective waxy coating of the disease-causing bacteria, leaving the invading microbes vulnerable to the body's immune system. Recent studies also suggest that the betulinic acid content of gotu kola is active against melanoma, a life-threatening form of skin cancer.

Gotu kola is said to improve mental clarity and to act as a mild sedative and nervine (moderates nerve transmissions) in animals. In a study where rats were trained to do simple tasks, gotu kola was shown to improve learning and memory. Researchers correlated this finding to a deceleration of neurotransmitter reproduction in the brain—in other words, memory was retained

because the process of neurotransmission remained less interrupted. This makes gotu kola a potential candidate for treating senility in aging animals. Gotu kola may also be useful in the treatment of epilepsy.

For animals with arthritis, gotu kola improves circulation in the legs and helps to reduce inflammation. It has also been shown to promote healing and reconstruction of connective tissue in the joints.

For external applications, gotu kola can be used as a skin rinse, poultice, or fomentation. Salves and oil infusions work well too, especially when vitamin E oil is added. For internal uses in a dog or cat, a tea from the dried leaves (1 teaspoon of herb to 8 ounces of near-boiling water) can be fed directly or put in the animal's food. Feed 1 tablespoon of the cooled tea per 30 pounds of the animal's body weight, once daily. Alternatively, a tablespoon of the fresh leaves can be finely chopped and added to each pound of an animal's food (the young light-green leaves are delicious in salads). Horses can be fed a handful of the leaves each day as a dietary adjunct. A low-alcohol tincture is yet another option. For each 30 pounds of a dog's body weight, add 0.5–1 milliliter of tincture to food daily. Add 0.5 milliliters of tincture to your cat's food daily.

Availability: Herb retailers and a few specialty seed and plant suppliers

Propagation and Harvest: Although gotu kola is seldom grown in North America, its cultivation is certainly possible. The plants must be kept warm—at tropical temperatures—throughout their lives, meaning that they will need a greenhouse or a consistently warm, sunlit place indoors in order to flourish in most of North America. The plants like nitrogen-rich soil, a mix of shade and sunlight, and room to spread.

Alternatives and Adjuncts: For external treatment of skin problems, consider calendula, chaparral, aloe, comfrey, and chamomile as alternatives or adjuncts. For internal treatment of skin problems or arthritis, gotu kola combines with alternatives such as burdock, red clover, or yellow dock. Diuretic, nutritive, and cholagogue herbs such as dandelion leaf and root, Oregon grape, cleavers, and nettle should be considered as well. Licorice, devil's claw, or yucca root serves as anti-inflammatory adjuncts. For vascular problems, gotu kola combines with ginger, cayenne, peppermint, ginkgo, yarrow, or hawthorn. To improve mental clarity and circulation in the brain, add ginkgo to your gotu kola.

Cautions and Comments: Although never witnessed by the authors or anyone we consult with, there is some scientific literature that presents the theory that excessive doses of gotu kola may have narcotic effects in animals, may cause photosensitivity, and may interfere with hypoglycemic therapies. Large doses may also present abortifacient activities and therefore should not be used in pregnant animals.

GRAVELROOT

Eupatorium purpureum   Sunflower Family

Appearance: Gravelroot is a large perennial, sometimes reaching 12 feet tall. The lance-shaped leaves have short petioles and grow directly off of the main stem in whorls of four or more. Leaves are distinctively textured and have coarsely serrated edges. Stems are smooth, succulent, and covered with purple spots, especially at the leaf axils. Flowers are small and pink, presented in showy slightly globe-shaped clusters at the top of the plant. Spotted gravelroot

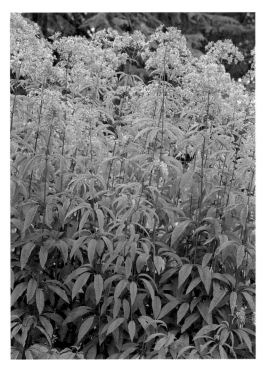

Eupatorium purpureum

(*Eupatorium maculatum*) shares the habitat of and looks similar to *E. purpureum*, except the mature plants tend to be much smaller. Both are equally useful.

Boneset (*E. perfoliatum*), a close relative of gravelroot, is a proportionately smaller plant that offers a different range of therapeutic usefulness.

Habitat and Range: Gravelroot is common at the edges of moist forest clearings, where it often forms dense thickets. Its range includes most of the eastern United States from Minnesota and Nebraska eastward to the Atlantic Ocean and south to Florida. In the West, *E. maculatum* is sporadically distributed from South British Columbia to New Mexico.

Cycle and Bloom Season: A perennial that blooms in midsummer

Parts Used: Roots

Primary Medicinal Activities: Diuretic, anti-inflammatory, tonic, helps reduce arthritic inflammation, helps prevent or eliminate urinary stress

Strongest Affinities: Urinary tract

Preparation: Decoction or tincture of the root

Common Uses: Gravelroot is traditionally used for expelling small kidney and bladder stones (gravel) from the urinary tract. It is effective for reducing the pain and inflammation of cystitis, and is sometimes used to treat swollen prostates. The diuretic activities of gravelroot may help in the elimination of excess uric acid from the body, making it potentially useful in the treatment of gout and other forms of rheumatism. Although little scientific validation exists for the medicinal uses of this plant, its abundance and long-standing reputation among herbalists as a safe and effective urinary tract remedy warrants attention. While this herb has been safely used in dogs and cats, we cannot recommend gravelroot as a first-choice herb simply because we don't know it as well as its alternatives. However, gravelroot is a profusely abundant plant in many areas of North America, and it is a valuable resource when other urinary tract herbs may not be available. It is also a plant that is likely to gain market popularity in coming years, and chances are it will someday enter the market in some kind of pet formula. In any case, gravelroot is a good herb to remember as an emergency standby resource.

Availability: Despite its long history as an herbal medicine, commercial sources of gravelroot are difficult to find in many parts of North America, especially in the West. The solution to this problem is simple—grow your own! Seeds are available through specialty catalogs.

Propagation and Harvest: This perennial is easy to grow. It sends up shoots from its rhizomes shortly after it is planted and forms a self-sufficient thicket. All it really needs is plenty of sun, rich soil, and frequent watering. Plants do best if sheltered from wind because the stems tend to break easily.

Alternatives and Adjuncts: For removal of gravel from the urinary tract, gravelroot is often combined with demulcent herbs such as marshmallow root, plantain, and corn silk. In urinary disorders that also involve inflammation or bleeding, gravelroot can be combined with stronger astringents or other anti-inflammatory herbs such as uva ursi, cleavers, and corn silk. As an alternative, consider couch grass.

Cautions and Comments: Only the root of this plant should be used because the leaves, stems, and flowers contain echinatine, a pyrrolizidine alkaloid that may be harmful to the liver if consumed in large enough quantities. Although direct side effects appear to be rare in animals who eat this plant, raw milk taken from animals who have grazed on gravelroot and then fed to humans and other animals may have toxic effects. The symptoms of overdose may include weakness, nausea, vomiting, liver damage, tremors, collapse, difficult breathing, convulsions, coma, or death. It is highly advisable to contact a veterinarian familiar with gravelroot before administering it to your dog or cat.

GRINDELIA

Grindelia squarrosa   Sunflower Family

Appearance: When grindelia is first encountered in the field, two thoughts often come to mind: This is a weed, and this is obviously a member of the sunflower family. Grindelia has strong but flexible 1- to 3-foot-tall stems, saw-toothed leaves, and bright yellow flowers that grow one per stem. Beneath the yellow rays, the flowers have distinctive curved bracts. The flower heads have a sticky gumlike substance that has earned the plant the common name of "gumweed."

Habitat and Range: Several species of Grindelia range throughout the western two-thirds of North America. All share similar appearances and most are inhabitants of wide-open plains or dry, sunny forest clearings.

Cycle and Bloom Season: A biennial or short-lived perennial that reproduces by seed

Parts Used: Flowers and leaves

Primary Medicinal Activities: Expectorant, sedative, cough suppressant, anti-inflammatory, lowers blood pressure, relieves poison ivy–induced contact dermatitis

Strongest Affinities: Respiratory tract and skin

Preparation: For internal uses: tincture or tea. For contact dermatitis: tea (skin rinse), salve, lotion, ointment, or liniment (an externally applied tincture).

Common Uses: Very little scientific attention has been directed toward grindelia, but its effectiveness and usefulness as a respiratory herb is well known among Western herbalists. Native Americans, who passed their herbal wisdom to us, used grindelia to treat everything from tuberculosis and

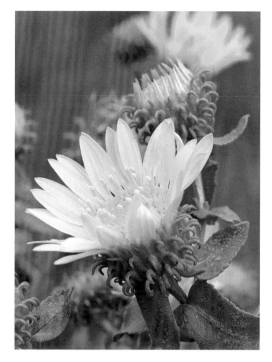

Grindelia squarrosa

pneumonia to gonorrhea and postpartum pain. From a scientific perspective, we know that the gummy substance secreted from the flower heads contains at least 20 percent resins, which are composed of substances that stimulate mucus secretion and reduce inflammation in the upper respiratory tract, making a dry, hacking cough more productive. Adding to grindelia's expectorant qualities are sedative and antispasmodic activities that calm a spastic cough by relaxing the smooth muscles of the upper respiratory tract while dilating the bronchioles. This makes grindelia useful for relieving the symptoms of asthma in dogs and cats, especially when it is administered at the early onset of an attack. We also find it useful for easing the symptoms of bordetella (kennel cough). To evaluate whether grindelia is appropriate for your pet and to determine a proper dosage, talk to a holistic practitioner.

Many North American Indian tribes used decoctions or simple teas of grindelia leaves and flowers as a soothing skin rinse for poison ivy–induced dermatitis, and in recent years, grindelia lotions have started to appear in European markets for the same purpose. A simple homemade decoction or tincture serves this purpose—apply as needed to the affected areas once or twice daily.

Availability: Grindelia herb or herbal preparations are available through herb retailers. The seed is available through specialty seed catalogs.

Propagation and Harvest: Grindelia tolerates poor soil and can be propagated easily from seed. Harvest the flowers and leaves when the plants are in full bloom.

Alternatives and Adjuncts: For asthma, a small amount of grindelia can be combined with nettle. Look at lobelia as a possible adjunct or alternative. For kennel cough and other respiratory infections and irritations, check out horehound, coltsfoot, comfrey, mullein, and wild cherry as possible alternatives or adjuncts.

Cautions and Comments: Internal use of grindelia may have a relaxing effect on the heart muscle and may cause a decrease in blood pressure. As a result, grindelia may be contraindicated in animals with heart or other circulatory problems. Excessive doses of grindelia are believed to cause renal irritation; therefore grindelia may be contraindicated in animals with renal failure or other forms of kidney disease. Although it is generally regarded as nontoxic but unpalatable to livestock and other animals, little research has been done on the effects of grindelia. Its use should be limited to

what the holistic pet care community has learned through clinical experience. See your holistic veterinarian before administering this herb internally. Barring allergic sensitivity, external applications are generally safe for home treatment of poison ivy dermatitis on most animals.

HAWTHORN

Crataegus sp.   Rose Family

Appearance: Hawthorn is a small deciduous tree or large shrub (up to 16 feet tall) that is easily recognized and quickly remembered by its nasty 1- to 3-inch curved thorns that are strategically spaced along the branches, often at eye level. The leaves of most species are narrowly fan-shaped or oval. The margins of the 1- to 2-inch-long leaves are toothed with all leaf tips pointing distinctly forward. The white ¼-inch flowers are presented in flat clusters, each blossom having five petals and numerous stamens (the pollen-bearing structures). When in full bloom, the blossoms often have an unpleasant "dead" odor. In late summer, the flowers are replaced with clusters of red to black berries that contain two to five seeds each.

Habitat and Range: The *Crataegus* genus is large and varied with hundreds of species (all of which readily hybridize) in North America. Most species are found in riparian thickets or moist meadows, where they serve as important forage and nesting habitats for birds and other wildlife. They are found in Alaska and British Columbia southward into California and are widely distributed eastward throughout the western interior states at valley and foothill elevations. *C. douglasii* (black hawthorn, see photo) is one of the most common and widespread species.

Cycle and Bloom Season: Deciduous perennial; blooms sometime between April and June

Parts Used: Fruits (berries) or flowers and leaf buds

Primary Medicinal Activities: Tonic (strengthens cardiovascular structures and functions), lowers blood pressure, dilates blood vessels, nutritive, antioxidant

Strongest Affinities: Cardiovascular system

Preparation: Fresh or dried berries, tincture, tea, and decoction

Common Uses: Hawthorn berries have been considered one of nature's best and safest heart and vascular tonics for millennia. A great deal of scientific study has validated hawthorn's usefulness in this capacity, and herbalists and researchers agree that hawthorn benefits the heart and arteries in at least three ways:

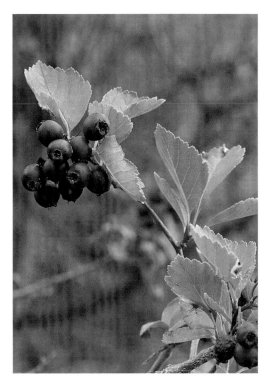

Crataegus douglassi

• Hawthorn dilates both coronary vessels and vessels of the brain, helping to increase circulation and the transport of nutrients and oxygen throughout the body. It accomplishes this in an effective and unique fashion: while it dilates major vessels, it also increases blood flow from the heart to compensate for any reduction of arterial blood volume. In other words, it helps the body push more blood around by increasing cardiac output and decreasing blood flow resistance in the arteries so there is more blood flow at lower pressure. This effect has been shown in studies performed with dogs, especially when used in small doses over an extended period.

• Hawthorn possesses antioxidant properties. It scavenges free-radical molecules that are known to rob the blood of oxygen and may lead to various forms of vascular disease.

• Hawthorn acts to steady and strengthen a weak or erratic heartbeat. In fact, it has been shown to be a possible alternative to the drug digitalis and may actually serve as a potentiating adjunct to this cardiac drug.

All of these activities are largely attributable to the vast array of flavonoid constituents held in hawthorn. Flavonoids are typified as red pigments found in many kinds of fruits and vegetables, and hundreds of studies have indicated that these compounds are essential in maintaining disease resistance and the integrity of smooth-muscle tissues throughout the body. It so happens that hawthorn may be the richest natural source of these vital nutrients. In a recent study using unfortunate rats, the flavonoid constituents held in hawthorn were shown to help prevent myocardial damage in situations where the heart muscle was subjected to physiological stress. This means that animals such as racehorses and working dogs, who are constantly under cardiovascular stress, are likely to find preventative benefits from daily supplements of hawthorn berries in their diets. It stands to reason that this cardiovascular tonic is useful in the daily care of older animals, especially those who suffer from chronic heart problems such as congestive heart failure, postsurgical dysfunction, or cardiac anomalies that have resulted from heartworm, bacterial or viral infections, or protracted chemotherapy. When combined with herbs that strengthen kidney function, hawthorn may also serve as a good adjunct therapy in the early treatment of kidney failure. Hawthorn's vasodilator and hypotensive actions may help to improve blood circulation through the renal arteries and smaller vessels of the kidneys without the added stress of increased blood pressure.

One of the nicest things about using hawthorn in treating animals is the fact that it tastes pretty good and is one of the easiest herbs to feed to your pet. If you are lucky enough to have a hawthorn tree near your home and an animal who likes red fruit, you can pick the ripe berries and feed them as tonic treats. As an alternative, the fully ripe berries can be picked, dried on a clean sheet of paper, and ground by hand with a mortar and pestle (be forewarned: the dried berries burn out small coffee grinders) into a coarse powder. The powder can then be added to your pet's diet—1 teaspoon per pound of food fed each day.

If your animal won't eat the berries either way, try making a tea and pouring it over the food. If that doesn't work, you can use hawthorn gel capsules wrapped with a little cheese, or, better yet, you can use a low-alcohol hawthorn extract.

The berries are the commonly used and marketed part of the hawthorn plant, probably because they make such a pretty and palatable medicine. But in early spring, before the berries are available, the flowering branch ends (leaves, flower buds, twigs, and thorns) can be clipped into small pieces and made into a decoction. Good luck getting it into your animal though— unlike the berries, the "twig tea" tastes awful!

Availability: Hawthorn berries and the dried leaves and flowers are available through herb retailers. Various hawthorn preparations are available at health food stores.

Propagation and Harvest: A few species of hawthorn are available through nurseries, particularly those specializing in native plants. Hawthorn is not difficult to grow— all it really requires is plenty of water. But it tends to be a slow grower. Gather the berries when they are completely ripe, usually in midsummer. Depending on the species, the berries are red or blue-red (almost black in the case of *C. douglasii*). The berries can then be used fresh, or they can be dried for future use. When properly stored, they should keep for at least a year. The flowering end-twigs should be harvested and used as soon as the blossoms open in early spring.

Alternatives and Adjuncts: When combined with a good natural diet and other tonic herbs, hawthorn acts exactly as an herbal heart tonic should, filling the special cardiac needs in the golden years of an animal's life. Other tonic herbs can be used in combination with hawthorn to round out the supplemental needs of older animals. These might include ginkgo or yarrow (for strengthening capillary walls), garlic (for added antioxidant and immune system support), alfalfa and red clover (to nourish the blood, increase appetite, and raise energy levels), dandelion leaf (to assist in the removal of excess water and lend tonic support to the kidneys), and oatstraw (as a nervous system tonic).

Cautions and Comments: Hawthorn is safe. In fact, in the hundreds of animal studies that have been conducted with this herb since 1900, hawthorn has shown extremely low toxicity in every animal tested. We place the toxicity potential of hawthorn berries on the same level as that of rose hips, raspberries, or blueberries—in other words, hawthorn is a medicinal food.

HOP

Humulus lupulus   Mulberry Family

Appearance: Hop is a beautiful trailing vine with deeply lobed leaves reminiscent of those of grapevines.

Habitat and Range: Originally a Eurasian plant, several varieties of hop are grown throughout the world. Many have escaped cultivation and now adorn waste areas, railway easements, and ravines throughout North America.

Cycle and Bloom Season: A perennial that blooms in mid– to late summer.

Parts Used: Strobiles (strobili), commonly known as hops

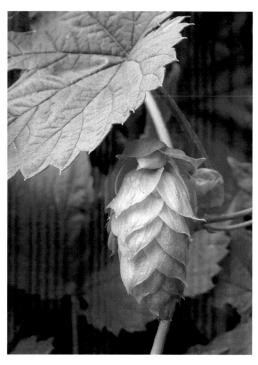

Humulus lupulus

Primary Medicinal Activities: Sedative, diuretic, stimulates digestion

Strongest Affinities: Nervous system, urinary tract, digestive tract

Preparation: Tea, tincture, fresh strobiles

Common Uses: Unlike many of the calming herbs we refer to as herbal sedatives, hop is truly sedative in nature. It works as a mild but reliable nervous system depressant and hypnotic, whereas most other calming herbs work more as muscle relaxants. Provided it is used with prudence and respect, hop serves as an excellent general-purpose calming agent in cases of acute anxiety such as the dreaded trip to the groomer or a long horse-trailer ride on the interstate. Provided the animals accept the bitter flavor, a handful or two of the fresh or dried strobiles can be fed to horses, llamas, mules, or other herbivores just before or during an emotional crisis. A few drops of the tea or tincture can be fed to dogs and cats.

Hop is also good for separation anxiety and for episodes of hyperexcitability that occur subsequent to traumatic events such as intermittent episodes of insomnia, whining, and restlessness that haunt an adopted pet who is recovering from physical or emotional abuse. Giving 10–20 drops added to each quart of the animal's drinking water usually serves this purpose well. Hop is also good for helping an animal to relax in the presence of physical pain, especially when hop is combined with valerian. While hop does not lend appreciable painkilling activities, it does assist the animal in dealing with pain naturally. (Animals are much better at this than we are.) Giving ⅛ teaspoon for each 20 pounds of the animal's weight, no more than three times daily, usually suffices for pain or acute anxiety problems.

While hop may help to relieve the severity of pain or an emotional crisis, it is important to remember that it cannot treat the underlying causes of behavioral disorders. Hyperactivity and excitability may be symptoms of a nutritional deficiency, a metabolic imbalance, an infection, or hyperthyroidism. Look deep into your animal's crisis from as many perspectives as you can. Even if hop seems to be solving the problem, it may be only masking the symptoms of a serious disease.

Animal studies have confirmed that the humulone and lupulone constituents in hop are active against many forms of gram-positive bacteria as well as some of the troublesome fungi, including *Candida* spp. Human studies have also shown promising results from the use of hop in treating gallbladder inflammation and urinary

incontinence. In the incontinence study, 772 of 915 human patients who received a formula containing hop, uva ursi, and vitamin E experienced excellent results.

Availability: Dried hop is available through herb retailers or wherever beer-making supplies are sold. Avoid the compressed pellets or strobiles and the concentrated hop syrups used for brewing. What you want is the whole dried strobiles. The compressed pellets and syrups are concentrated and may cause a serious toxic reaction in your animal. Ideally, of course, you should grow your own hop.

Propagation and Harvest: Hop vines are easy to grow, cold hardy, and attractive when trained to climb a trellis or garden archway. The plants need moist, rich soil and full sun in order to thrive and bloom. Plants and root cuttings are available through nurseries.

Alternatives and Adjuncts: For pain and posttraumatic irritability, hop combines especially well with valerian. If the pain is attributable to nerve trauma or dysfunction, consider skullcap, oatstraw, or Saint-John's-wort as possible adjuncts or alternatives. For anxiety and restlessness characterized by trembling or hyperexcitability to touch or a sudden sound (the animal jumps when surprised), hop can be combined with skullcap or passionflower.

Cautions and Comments: In 1998, the National Animal Poison Control Center had recorded eight instances of dogs dying after eating hops that had been used and discarded during the process of brewing beer. All of these dogs succumbed to malignant hyperthermia—an acute, uncontrollable fever the first symptom of which is heavy panting, followed by rapid heartbeat and a rapid and continued rise in body temperature. Seven of the dogs were greyhounds, and it appears that this breed is especially susceptible to hyperthermia from eating discarded hops. It also should be noted that the deaths of these dogs were from the ingestion of the spent (postbrewing) hops used in making beer, not from the medicinal-quality hops used in making tinctures. The problem appears to stem from three common denominators:

- The chemistry of spent hops or the manner by which they are metabolized by greyhounds may be quite different from the manner in which fresh or dried strobiles are processed by the same animals. It is evident that the chemical and biochemical relationships among hops, malt syrup, various sugars, and other elements of beer-making may be responsible for the ultimate results and should be investigated. Heat raises yet another question—the process of boiling the herb is likely to change the chemistry of hop and the entire beer-making combination.
- The hops used may have been compressed and therefore would have been concentrated.
- Although we still do not know why, it appears that greyhounds are especially predisposed to this problem, and therefore they should never be fed hops.

In light of this problem, a subsequent study was conducted and published in *The Journal of the American Veterinary Medical Association*. The study found that all of the greyhounds examined in an emergency clinic for the disorder had ingested approximately 250 milliliters of spent hops each—that's about one cup.

Spent brewing hops are sweet and tasty, making them a target for gluttony and toxic excess. Despite the fact that there have been no additional reports of hops-related hyperthermia in dogs ten years later, caution dictates that it is best to limit your dogs' access to spent home-brew hops, especially if your pet is a greyhound. Limit your use of hops to small quantities of a high-quality formulation designed for animals, or use unadulterated fresh or dried hops with moderation.

HORSETAIL

Equisetum arvense   Horsetail Family

Appearance: The horsetail family is generally divided into three groups: (1) annual varieties that produce separate and distinctly different fertile and sterile stems, (2) annuals that produce sterile and fertile stems that are similar in appearance, and (3) evergreen perennials that produce fertile and sterile stems that are alike. Despite these variances, the entire family shares fundamentally similar characteristics: hollow, distinctively grooved and jointed stems and dark, scalelike leaves that appear as sheaths surrounding the stems at the joints. In early spring, *Equisetum arvense* produces a small 3- to 12-inch fertile stem that lacks chlorophyll (the constituent that makes plants green). This stem dies back as its larger green, sterile counterpart matures. The subsequent, 6-inch to 2-foot-tall sterile stems have whorled branches that resemble green bottlebrushes. *Equisetum hyemale* is much larger (up to 5 feet tall) and lacks any branching characteristics. It looks like a prehistoric cross between miniature bamboo and an asparagus spear. Both species are often seen growing side by side.

Habitat and Range: Lakeshores, stream banks, and other wet areas, up into alpine elevations throughout North America. Horsetails often represent the primary ground cover in shady wet thickets.

Cycle and Bloom Season: The green sterile plants emerge in spring. Perennial varieties remain green and usable throughout the year; annual varieties die back in late fall.

Parts Used: All aerial parts

Primary Medicinal Activities: Diuretic, astringent, stops bleeding, tonic

Strongest Affinities: Musculoskeletal system, skin, and hair

Preparation: Tincture or decoction for internal uses; a poultice for external compresses

Common Uses: Horsetail contains a vast array of synergistic chemical compounds that all contribute to myriad medicinal uses, but most notable is its usefulness in healing bone and connective tissue injuries.

Most of horsetail's regenerative actions in the musculoskeletal system can be attributed to its remarkable content of bioactive silicon. In the body, silicon is a fundamental starting point, or matrix, for the formation of bone, cartilage, skin, and other connective tissues, including those of the aorta and trachea. Silicon is perhaps the most common element on earth. In fact, most of the sand on our planet is composed largely of silicon but not in a form that can be absorbed and used by the body. The silicon contained in horsetail is unique in that it is in a form that can be metabolized for tissue repair and development.

For you and your companion, horsetail can help speed recovery from joint and bone injuries, including postsurgical trauma. For internal use, a decoction or tincture preparation is needed. Horsetail is poorly water soluble and is abrasive, so unless it is put into a form that the body can easily absorb, it may cause irritation to the urinary tract and kidneys.

To make a decoction, take a large handful of the dried herb and place it into a nonmetallic cooking vessel (to avoid picking up metallic residues). Add a ½ teaspoon of sugar and enough water to barely cover the herb. The sugar helps to extract the silicon constituents and makes a more palatable finished product. Simmer the mixture over low heat for about twenty minutes or until the water has turned dark green. Strain through a fine cloth and allow to cool. The clarified decoction can be added directly to your companion's food—1 tablespoon per 20 pounds of the animal's body weight daily, five days a week. Horsetail tincture can be used the same way but at a smaller dosage of ¼ teaspoon (1 milliliter) per 20 pounds of body weight.

Horsetail is also useful for a variety of urinary tract problems, particularly those that involve bleeding or an accumulation of superfluous tissue in the urinary tract. The hemolytic and antimicrobial properties of horsetail make it beneficial for urinary tract infections that involve minor bleeding from the bladder or urethra. To help avoid urinary tract irritation during long-term use (more than ten days), it's a good idea to use horsetail in conjunction with soothing, protecting, and lubricating herbs such as marshmallow, plantain, or chickweed. Marshmallow is our first choice because it adds excellent antimicrobial properties to the therapeutic effort.

There is evidence to support claims that horsetail may help prevent bone degeneration, skin and coat disorders, and even senility in older animals. Scientific studies have concluded that as a body ages, silicon levels in the circulatory system and skin decrease, which in turn leads to tissue degeneration and a diminished capacity to form new tissue. Other studies suggest that horsetail may be useful in preventing certain forms of senility and degenerative bone disease, namely those directly related to the balance between silicon and aluminum in the body. In theory, these ailments may result from a toxic excess of aluminum, a condition normally counteracted by the presence of silicic acid, silicon, and other vital compounds that are contained in horsetail. In other words, dietary supplementation with horsetail may help maintain a healthful balance of silicon in the bodies of aging animals. See your holistic veterinarian to ascertain if and how much horsetail is suitable for your companion.

Availability: A common plant throughout most of the world. The dried herb and tincture are available through herb retailers.

Propagation and Harvest: For medicine of optimum quality, harvest E. arvense in mid– to late spring while the leaves of the bottlebrush-like plant still point skyward. Later, as the leaves spread horizontally, they become less water soluble and therefore do not make as good a medicine. Clip the plants just above ground level, and spread them out on a piece of newspaper to dry thoroughly before use.

Alternatives and Adjuncts: Combines well with marshmallow, cleavers, plantain, chickweed, corn silk, or couch grass for urinary tract problems. To help in the healing of bone and connective tissue injuries, horsetail tincture combines well with comfrey

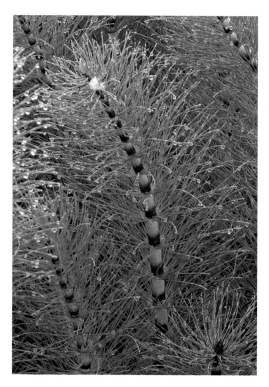

Equisetum arvense

or nettle and serves as an excellent adjunct to glucosamine and chondroiton sulfate supplements. For nervous system support in older animals, horsetail serves as an excellent adjunct to hawthorn and ginkgo.

Cautions and Comments: Do not use horsetail in cases of hypertension or cardiac disease. Horsetail may cause breast milk to change flavor during lactation. If there is a history of silicate stones of the urinary system, caution should be used. Do not gather this plant from areas that are downstream of commercial farming activities as it may contain inorganic nitrates that are metabolized into abnormal nicotine-like alkaloids. Livestock have reportedly been poisoned by eating large quantities of horsetail, possibly due to alkaloid interfering with either the production or use of vitamin B_1.

JUNIPER

Juniperus spp.   Cypress Family

Appearance: There are over 130 species of juniper worldwide; about 26 of these species are native to North America. The berries of all are useful, but *Juniperus communis* (common juniper) has a reputation among herbalists and wild food epicureans as having the berries with the strongest medicine.

Species of this large genus of evergreens are differentiated by their size (trees or low-growing shrubs) and the specific characteristics of their leaves (needlelike or scalelike). All junipers can be easily identified by their foliage and cones (commonly called juniper berries), which have a strong and distinctive ginlike aroma.

Habitat and Range: Common juniper is generally a mountain shrub that can be found on rocky hillsides and forest clearings up to about 10,000 feet in elevation. Juniper is widespread from Alaska to California and throughout much of temperate North America. The aforementioned tree varieties are high-desert dwellers of eastern California, Nevada, Utah, Colorado, Wyoming, Arizona, and New Mexico.

Cycle and Bloom Season: Evergreen, producing fruits that take two to three years to ripen

Parts Used: Fruits (berries) and leaves (often called needles)

Primary Medicinal Activities: Astringent, diuretic, antimicrobial, strengthens kidney function, lowers blood sugar, tonic

Strongest Affinities: Genitourinary system (including the kidneys), skin

Preparation: Decoction of the leaves or berries, tincture (berries), or whole (dried or fresh) berries can be fed directly or as a food additive.

Common Uses: Recent scientific studies conducted at the College of Medicine at Taiwan National University and the Universidad de Granada in Spain have shown that juniper offers new hope in the treatment of diabetes and cardiovascular disease. In the study conducted in Spain, a decoction of ripe juniper berries was administered to both diabetic and healthy rats. In both test groups, the decoction was found to lower blood glucose levels by increasing glucose uptake in the diaphragm, while at the same time increasing the amount of insulin released from the pancreas. The result was a lower mortality rate in animals with insulin-dependent diabetes and new hope for those with other forms of diabetes. In the study conducted in Taiwan, a compound derivative of the berries called 14 acetoxycedrol was found to have anticoagulant effects in the blood and a relaxing action on vascular tissues, actions that should prove useful in reducing the risk of cardiovascular disease in humans and other animals. In the minds of modern herbalists, these wonderful new discoveries only add to juniper's long history as a healing ally.

During the black plague, many European physicians carried three or four juniper berries in their mouth at all times to prevent infection. Medical instruments were soaked in a disinfecting decoction of the berries. Native Americans used every part of the shrub for a variety of ailments ranging from sore throats to dandruff, sometimes bathing their horses in a root tea to improve their coats. In fact, juniper has been used as a food and medicine for thousands of years by cultures the world over and remains an ingredient in several mainstream over-the-counter diuretic and laxative remedies today. The berries are a valuable culinary commodity as well, being used as the primary flavoring agent in gin and as a rather expensive seasoning for gourmet dishes. (We like to use them in place of bay leaves in chili and wild-food dishes.)

Modern-day herbalists use juniper to treat edema and arthritis as well as acute and severe cystitis and other infections of the urinary tract. Juniper is also known to stimulate kidney function by increasing the rate of glomerulus filtration, the process by which the kidneys filter out impurities and cleanse the blood. In lay terms, juniper increases urine production and waste elimination. This effect is due to an irritant action attributable to juniper's generous content of volatile oils, especially one called terpineol. Because of these irritating effects, juniper should never be used in animals with preexisting kidney problems, nor should it be used over long periods of time. Also, juniper is known to have a vasodilating action in the uterus and was once used to promote menstrual flow; therefore, it should never be used in pregnant animals. Fortunately, all of this sounds more ominous than it really is since many stimulatory herbs work because of their abilities to selectively irritate the body. When used over a very short period in the correct dosages, and in nonpregnant animals with healthy kidneys, juniper can safely increase renal circulation and boost overall kidney function.

The antiseptic and astringent properties of the berries or leaves may be useful in relieving itchiness and infections of the skin when applied topically in the form of a cooled dilute rinse. Because the plant is not water soluble, you will first need to make a simple decoction (see chapter 1). After the

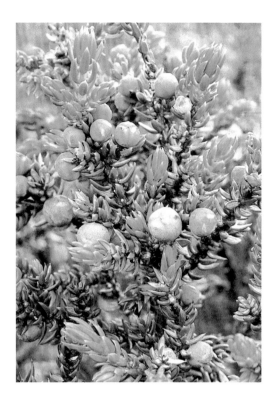

Juniperis communis

decoction has cooled, dilute it with enough cold water to give it the appearance of a weak tea (you should be able to see through a clear 8-ounce glass of the liquid. Now you can pour the liquid over your dog (and as long as you don't mind a few claw scratches, your cat) until the animal is thoroughly soaked. Avoid getting any into your animal's eyes.

Before using juniper in a rinse, be sure that the decoction is well diluted. While problems seldom occur when using juniper as a skin rinse, the volatile oils in the plant can be irritating if the solution is too strong, especially if your animal has sensitive skin to start with. (By the way, this applies to peppermint, pennyroyal, and eucalyptus rinses as well.)

After you rinse your pet, she will smell like a conifer forest on a warm spring day!

Materia Medica

Availability: Juniper berries are available at the supermarket, but they are much too expensive considering how common the shrubs are. Juniper leaf and berry extracts are available through herb retailers. Several shrub and small tree varieties are available from nurseries.

Propagation and Harvest: Several species of juniper have been domesticated and are available at your local nursery. *Juniperus communis* is frequently used as a low-growing landscaping shrub and is an excellent choice for walkway borders and flower beds. Junipers are easy to grow but tend to grow slowly. Once established, they are cold hardy (especially *J. communis*), drought tolerant, and they require minimal maintenance. Soil quality is of little concern to these plants, but they do appreciate at least a slightly acidic pH level, so if necessary, amend your soil with some redwood compost. When you visit the nursery, remember that only the female plants bear the sought-after berries and that you will need at least two plants (a male and a female) to produce fruit.

Alternatives and Adjuncts: For inflammations of the urinary tract, consider couch grass, gravelroot, corn silk, plantain, and uva ursi before using juniper. Marshmallow adds soothing and lubricating protection when added to juniper. For urinary tract infections, look at echinacea, sage, thyme, and Oregon grape as alternatives or adjuncts. For treating fleabites and other skin irritations, juniper combines well in a skin rinse with calendula, chamomile, or peppermint (or for that matter, any kind of mint).

Cautions and Comments: Do not use juniper internally in animals with preexisting kidney disease or in pregnant or lactating animals. The key rule with juniper is one that applies to all herbal remedies: Use with caution and always in moderation. And remember, what may be deemed excessive for one animal may be inadequate for another. Proper use of juniper is entirely dependent upon an accurate assessment of your companion's specific needs and medical condition. Please see your holistic veterinarian first.

LAVENDER

Lavandula angustifolia   Mint Family

Appearance: With its delicate spikelike flowers, narrow silvery leaves, and sweet fragrance, lavender is a beautiful adornment to any garden. There are several cultivars of *Lavandula*; the one most commonly found in nurseries is English lavender (*L. angustifolia*).

Habitat and Range: A Mediterranean native that is in cultivation throughout much of the world

Cycle and Bloom Season: A perennial that blooms in early to midsummer

Parts Used: Flowers, leaves, and stems

Primary Medicinal Activities: Elevates mood (antidepressive), antibacterial, astringent, analgesic, antispasmodic, tonic

Strongest Affinities: Skin, nervous system, respiratory tract, joints

Preparation: Diluted essential oil, tea, dried flower bunches, sachets

Common Uses: The essential oil of lavender works wonders to calm a nervous or excited animal. In depressed or aggressive animals, lavender can be used to lift spirits and adjust attitudes. In these applications, the oil is not applied to the animal itself but is used in aromatherapy. An open bottle of the oil is waved under the animal's nostrils, or a few drops are put on a piece of cardboard that is placed near the animal's bedding, under a car seat, or on the outside of a travel carrier. The sweet aroma helps the animal (and her human guardian) to relax during an otherwise restless experience. Oftentimes the effects are instantaneous. A small sachet bag can be filled with lavender flowers and placed near the animal for the same (but less reliable) effect.

A few drops of the essential oil can be added to some water and placed in a vaporizer (or a potpourri simmering pot) and used to treat coughs and respiratory infections. When emitted near the animal in a closed room, the vapor helps to open respiratory passages and inhibit bacterial reproduction in the lungs.

For joint inflammation, stiffness, or pain, 10 drops of the essential oil can be added to 1 ounce of apricot kernel or almond oil (these absorb into skin more readily than olive oil). The mixture then can be liberally massaged into the affected area to bring relief. The oil mixture is also useful for insect bites and stings and is an excellent addition to first aid salves.

A good tick repellent oil for dogs can be made from 300 milliliters of olive oil or other oil, 500 milliliters of essential oil of terebinth, 100 milliliters of Saint-John's-wort–infused oil, and 100 milliliters of essential oil of lavender. This recipe makes about a liter of the oil. It can be massaged on affected areas to help ticks drop off. As a preventative, it can be massaged on areas of the dog that are most likely to come into contact with ticks. Avoid using essential oils on or around cats.

A tea of the fresh or dried flowers, leaves, and stems can be used as an external skin rinse for relief from pain and itching caused

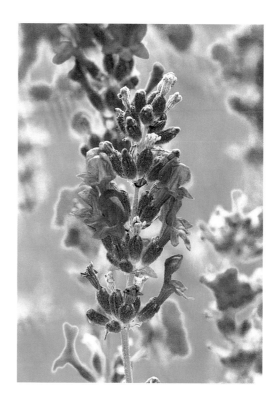

Lavandula angustifolia

by seborrhea, contact dermatitis, or fleabites. The rinse helps to fight bacterial infection as well. Be sure the rinse is well diluted— the water should be slightly tinted but still fragrant.

Availability: The essential oil can be purchased through natural product retailers, as can the dried flowers. Plants are available through most nurseries.

Propagation and Harvest: Lavender is winter hardy, drought resistant, and easy to grow from transplants. Plants prefer well-drained, sandy soil with a pH between 6.4 and 8.3 (acidic soil should be amended with hydrated lime or soft rock phosphate).

Alternatives and Adjuncts: For joint problems, lavender combines with yarrow, arnica, Saint-John's-wort, or cayenne. For respiratory infections, try adding yarrow to a vaporizer. For calming effects, lavender aromatherapy used in conjunction with an internal dose of passionflower, skullcap, valerian, or hop can be effective.

Cautions and Comments: Although all parts of the dried or above-ground parts of this plant are generally safe when used in raw form or in simple teas, the highly concentrated essential oil of lavender can be very hard on the liver and kidneys. Therefore, it should not be ingested. Nor should the oil be used on the skin in undiluted form because it may cause irritation. Avoid using essential oils on or around cats.

LICORICE

Glycyrrhiza glabra   Pea Family
and *G. lepidota*

Appearance: Licorice is a member of the pea family and can be characterized by its greenish white, pealike axillary flowers; pinnately divided pealike leaves (divided into pairs of lance-shaped leaflets); and inclination to climb and tangle among other plants. At first glance, licorice looks like any one of thousands of wild legumes. Fortunately, our wild American licorice (*Glycyrrhiza lepidota*) has characteristics that make it unique and easy to identify. It is a large legume (3–7 feet tall when mature) with an exceptionally stout reddish main stem. But even more distinguishing are its ½-inch-long, tightly clustered seed pods, which are covered with conspicuous hooked spines. No other legume in North America presents this characteristic.

Habitat and Range: The vast majority of licorice root sold in North America is

G. glabra, a native of southeast Europe that probably came over with the first Anglo settlers. Of the twenty-five or so species that can be found worldwide, we have only one native species in North America: *G. lepidota*. All other species have been naturalized from Europe or Asia. American licorice occurs sporadically across North America, and like its alien relatives that in many areas have escaped cultivation, it is generally to be found in moist ravines, in roadside ditches, in waste areas, and along the banks of irrigation canals where soils are rich and deep.

Cycle and Bloom Season: A biennial or short-lived perennial that reproduces by seed. Blooms in midsummer.

Parts Used: Roots

Primary Medicinal Activities: Expectorant; helps with blood cleansing; lubricates, soothes, and protects mucous membranes; anti-inflammatory; antiviral; adrenal stimulant; mild laxative; immunostimulant.

Strongest Affinities: Respiratory, digestive, and endocrine systems

Preparation: Fresh or dried chopped root, tea, tincture

Common Uses: Numerous studies have confirmed that licorice is an effective and fast-acting anti-inflammatory agent. In fact, many herbalists regard it as nature's answer to hydrocortisone and claim that it potentiates the effectiveness of other herbs when added to compound formulas. All of this is primarily attributable to licorice's content of glycyrrhizin, a compound with a chemical structure similar to that of the corticosteroids that are naturally released by the body's adrenal glands. Glycyrrhizin effectively stimulates the adrenals into action and is especially useful for treating Addison's disease.

Licorice provides anti-inflammatory, antimicrobial, immunostimulant, and corticosteroid-like actions—thus helping to relieve pain, itching, and inflammation without completely bypassing the body's normal anti-inflammatory functions and without seriously compromising the immune system. This makes licorice useful for a wide variety of inflammatory diseases. In a study where arthritis was induced in rats through injections of formaldehyde, a by-product of glycyrrhizin called glycyrrhetinic acid was produced in the body and was shown to have obvious antiarthritic actions that were comparable to those of hydrocortisone. Glycyrrhizin has also been shown to potentiate the effects of cortisone-like drugs in the body, which makes licorice a useful adjunct in hydrocortisone therapies. The theory here is that the potentiating effect of licorice allows for lower drug dosages without compromising therapeutic effectiveness. Used in this capacity, licorice should help reduce the debilitating side effects of steroid drugs in long-term therapies and may also assure safe withdrawal when the patient is weaned off of the steroids.

The anti-inflammatory properties of licorice root are also apparent when the herb is topically applied. Licorice tea, salve, or oil infusion can be used to relieve the uncomfortable symptoms of various skin disorders such as psoriasis, eczema, contact dermatitis, and flea allergies. Used in this capacity, licorice provides a degree of relief during long-term holistic therapies, including a detoxification and allergy therapy consisting of internal doses of burdock, dandelion, alfalfa, or other alterative herbs. In this example, the animal receives

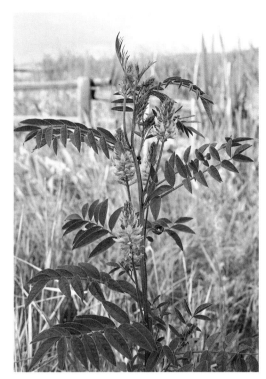

Glycyrrhiza lepidota

relief from suffering, but the underlying metabolic causes are also addressed through tonification of the involved body systems.

To make a simple oil infusion, all you need is some chopped dried licorice root (available at any good herb retailer) and some olive oil. Put the root into a glass jar and cover it with enough oil to leave a ½-inch layer of liquid above the herb. Cover the jar tightly, put it in a warm (55–75° F) place, away from sunlight, and let it sit for one month. After a month, strain the oil through a sieve, then squeeze what you can from the herb by wrapping it in unbleached muslin or cheesecloth. You'll have a sweet-tasting licorice oil that keeps for several months if refrigerated. Use it topically as needed, but expect your companion to lick it off—it tastes like candy.

In addition to its powerful anti-inflammatory actions, licorice root is beneficial in the treatment and prevention of many forms of liver disease. Over the past two decades, medical researchers in China and Japan have found (through animal studies) that extracts of licorice root are useful in the treatment of chronic and chemically induced hepatitis and that the herb has liver-protectant qualities similar to those offered by the popular liver herb milk thistle (*Silybum marianum*). However, the mechanisms by which licorice root works in the liver are quite different from those of milk thistle. While milk thistle has been shown to resist liver cell destruction largely through protection of the cell walls and by antioxidant actions, licorice works through a broader set of effects. In addition to a protectant action that glycyrrhizin has upon the liver cells, licorice also enhances interferon and T cell production, two natural actions that are critical to liver repair and general resistance to disease. In Chinese medicine, licorice is commonly used as a liver detoxifier in the treatment of obstructive jaundice. And in several studies, licorice has been shown to benefit animals suffering from liver damage due to absorbed or ingested toxins such as carbon tetrachloride.

In a recent study, the root of *G. uralensis* (an Asian species of licorice) was found to have a potentiating effect on the reticuloendothelial system, the body's first line of defense against infection. In essence, the reticuloendothelial system is composed of specialized cells whose jobs are to seek out and eliminate invading microbes and dead blood cells, and licorice helps to stimulate these little bloodstream warriors into action.

Licorice is also an excellent demulcent, anti-inflammatory, and expectorant for the gastrointestinal and upper respiratory tracts. It is especially good for healing ulceration

of the stomach and reducing the gastric acid secretions that often contribute to the severity of ulcers. For bronchitis, licorice works well at reducing inflammation while adding antiviral, antibacterial, and soothing demulcent actions to any variety of other respiratory herbs that may be employed such as mullein, coltsfoot, and grindelia.

When giving licorice to your animal, you are likely to find the best results when using liquid extracts (tinctures). Feeding dried chopped roots to herbivores is fine if tolerated, but dogs and cats have short digestive tracts that may not absorb the active constituents quickly and completely. Herb tinctures are free-form medicines: their active components are readily available and quickly assimilated early in the digestive process. This means that less of the active material is lost during digestion and more ends up in your cat instead of in her litter box. Dosage is entirely dependent upon individual needs and circumstances and should be determined by a trained practitioner, but 12–20 drops per 20 pounds of body weight, two times daily, of low-alcohol licorice extract is a conservative starting point for dogs, cats, and other small animals. Horses can be fed the equivalent of up to 1 ounce (10–30 grams) of the dried root, or about ¼ ounce of the tincture daily. You can triple the liquid dosages if you are using a cooled tea (1 teaspoon of the root to 1 cup of water).

Availability: Licorice can be planted from root cuttings or seed, both of which are available from nursery catalogs that specialize in herbs.

Propagation and Harvest: To grow licorice in your garden, plant it in moist, deep, well-drained, nutrient-rich sandy loam with a neutral to slightly alkaline pH. Although it is adaptable to various climates, licorice does best in areas with long, warm growing seasons. (If you can't meet these demands, don't worry. This plant survives just about anywhere.)

Dig the perennial roots during the fall of their third or fourth year of growth— younger roots won't be as potent. After digging, cut the roots into small pieces and dry them on newspaper, away from sunlight. The completely dried roots keep for one to two years if properly stored in plastic bags in a cool, dry, dark place.

Alternatives and Adjuncts: For stomach ulcers and other gastric disorders that are secondary to bacterial or parasitic infection, licorice combines with Oregon grape. To provide secondary anti-inflammatory relief in the gastrointestinal or urinary tract, consider corn silk, couch grass, or uva ursi as adjuncts. For respiratory problems, consider elecampane, coltsfoot, grindelia, mullein, slippery elm, plantain, marshmallow, and wild cherry bark as possible substitutes or adjuncts. For liver problems, look toward milk thistle, dandelion root, Oregon grape, red clover, and burdock as possible adjuncts.

Cautions and Comments: As for all herbal medicines, the primary rule is moderation and insight when using licorice. Throughout its long history as a medicine, licorice has been the subject of controversies. When used in large, highly concentrated doses, especially over long periods, several hydrocortisone-like side effects may occur: water retention, hypertension, loss of potassium, sodium retention, and other symptoms of adrenal hyperactivity. In human studies, the large majority of these side effects have been observed following the excessive consumption of European

licorice candy, which is made from a concentrated pressed extract of the root. (American-produced licorice candy contains ab-solutely no real licorice but instead an artificial flavoring or the extracts of other plants that taste similar.) Most herbalists and practitioners agree that the risks of adverse side effects from licorice are limited to those who abuse it. We, however, have never seen a case of licorice-induced toxicity. Nevertheless, licorice should not be used with reckless abandon or in normal doses for periods exceeding two weeks without the in-struction of a qualified practitioner. If a licorice therapy does exceed two weeks, then the treated animal's diet should be adjusted to accommodate increased needs for potassium and to eliminate excess sodium. Dandelion leaf is well indicated here because it works as an effective diuretic to prevent water retention while providing an excellent source of supplemental potassium. Animals with preexisting cardiovascular conditions should not be given licorice without professional guidance.

Licorice may temporarily elevate blood sugar levels and should be used with caution in diabetic animals. It has also been shown to have estrogenic properties that may affect uterine functions. Therefore, licorice should be used with caution in pregnant or nursing animals.

MARSHMALLOW
Althea officinalis   Mallow Family

Appearance: Marshmallow is a stout plant that may grow as high as 7 feet. It has alternate 3- to 5-lobed leaves and showy 2- to 3-inch flowers that range in color from white to pale pink. The entire plant is covered with fine, soft hairs, a trait that gives the foliage a dusty appearance.

Habitat and Range: A native of western and central Europe, marshmallow has become naturalized in the U.S., where it grows in marshes and moist meadows throughout the New England states. It has become a popular garden herb throughout the world and is easy to grow.

Cycle and Bloom Season: A perennial that blooms from late June through September

Parts Used: Primarily the root. The foliage is useful, too, but does not make as good a medicine.

Primary Medicinal Activities: Soothes and lubricates internal tissues, soothes skin, antimicrobial, lowers blood sugar, immunostimulant.

Strongest Affinities: Skin and respiratory, digestive, and urinary tracts

Preparation: Tea, low-alcohol tincture, fresh or dried chopped root

Common Uses: Marshmallow has a long history as a medicine. The word *Althea* is derived from the ancient Greek word *altheo*, meaning "to cure." With few exceptions, marshmallow is among the safest and most versatile herbs for animals. The root of the mature plant contains up to 35 percent mucilage. This makes marshmallow useful in situations that involve surface irritation of the skin or internal mucous membranes. It is particularly helpful for urinary tract inflammations compounded by the presence of gravel in the urine (urinary calculus) and in digestive disorders where ulceration or infection is further aggravated by the presence of food or other solids. In these cases, marshmallow provides a soothing, lubricating, protective barrier between mucous membranes and substances that contribute to the irritation. Marshmallow also soothes upper respiratory irritations that are secondary to a dry, raspy cough. Used on the surface of the body, marshmallow brings relief to insect bites, stings, abscesses, and inflammations that are secondary to injury or infection. In addition to the soothing nature of mucilage, marshmallow has antimicrobial and immune-stimulating properties. In animal studies, it has been shown to be active against *Pseudomonas aeruginosa*, *Proteus vulgaris*, and *Staphylococcus aureus*, bacterial infections that are commonly seen in the digestive tract, urinary tract, skin, and ears of dogs, cats, horses, ferrets, and other animals. A dab of marshmallow tincture also serves as an excellent antimicrobial lubricant for a rectal thermometer.

For internal use of marshmallow root, a tea or low-alcohol tincture is usually the best choice. The dried or fresh root may be a better option for problems such as colitis that are deep within the digestive system. This is because marshmallow's mucilage is highly water soluble and may not reach the lower end of the digestive tract unless it is carried there in a solid container, namely the chopped or ground root.

If you opt to use a tincture of this herb, make sure that it doesn't contain more than 20 percent alcohol (actually, none is needed). The mucilage constituents aren't taken up well in alcohol, and if too much is used in the tincture-making process, the end product will cause nausea when ingested. We like glycerin tinctures of this herb, not only for this reason but because the glycerin itself adds soothing, protective qualities to the medicine. Marshmallow glycerite can be squirted directly into an animal's mouth—about ¼ teaspoon (1 milliliter) per 20 pounds of the animal's body weight, three times daily or as needed. Alternatively, a tea can be made by steeping a teaspoon of the dried chopped root (or 2 teaspoons of fresh root) in 8 ounces of very hot water. Stir the tea frequently until it has cooled to lukewarm. You should be able to feel the slippery, oily nature of the mucilage when you rub a few drops of the tea between your thumb and index finger. If not, add more marshmallow root. One teaspoon of the tea is a good starting dose for dogs. Cats usually benefit from a ½ teaspoon. It's also good for lubricating and expelling fur balls. For lower gastrointestinal problems or to help relieve constipation (in a manner similar to that of psyllium husks), the dried powdered root can be added to an animal's food at a rate of a ½ teaspoon for each pound of food fed (¼ teaspoon for cats and other small animals), once or twice daily. For horses, 1 ounce of the powdered root can be added to feed each day to aid in cases of cystitis, colitis, or chronic spasmodic colic.

For problems that are close to the rectum such as a swollen anal gland irritated by bowel movements, a small gel capsule might be necessary to carry the root powder through the digestive tract to the problem area. Another option is to administer a small amount of the cooled tea or glycerite as a rectal suppository using a soft plastic pipette or ear syringe.

Marshmallow has been shown to cause hypoglycemic activity in animals. Although more research is warranted, marshmallow might be useful in treating certain forms of diabetes. See your holistic veterinarian before trying it in this capacity.

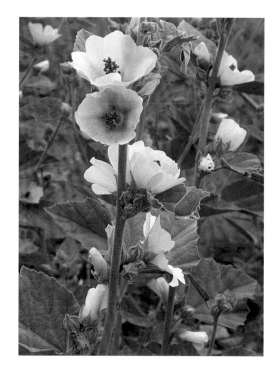

Althea officinalis

Availability: Marshmallow plants are available through most nurseries. Marshmallow root and various preparations are available through herb retailers.

Propagation and Harvest: Marshmallow is easy to grow. It can be propagated by seed, root cuttings, or transplants. Although it requires ample water, it's not picky about soil and is hardy and drought tolerant once established. Planting should occur in early spring. The roots are ready for harvest anytime during their third year of growth and every year thereafter. You do not have to kill your plant to dig up some of the root—simply divide what you need from the existing root system, and give the plant extra water until the roots regenerate.

Alternatives and Adjuncts: For urinary problems, marshmallow combines well

M

with couch grass, horsetail, uva ursi, corn silk, echinacea, ginkgo, or any of the diuretic herbs. For coughs and upper respiratory irritations, marshmallow combines with mullein, coltsfoot, elecampane, or grindelia. For digestive problems, consider combining licorice, chamomile, calendula, cleavers, fennel, dill, or any variety of mint with marshmallow. In horses, a combination of marshmallow, valerian, slippery elm, and licorice is good for a spastic colon. For infections or irritations of the skin of most animals, calendula, mullein flower, garlic, comfrey, and aloe are all complemented by marshmallow.

Cautions and Comments: Marshmallow has long been used as a food plant, and its safety is substantiated by many years of use in both humans and animals. It is known to lower blood sugar levels, however, and therefore should be used with caution in hypoglycemic animals. It may also retard the intestinal absorption of some drugs— at least for short periods, until the thick, viscous mucilage can be broken down in the digestive tract.

MILK THISTLE

Silybum marianum   Sunflower Family

Appearance: From a distance, milk thistle looks very much like any other thistle: deeply lobed, often spiny leaves; stout, often spiny stems; and large, up to 2 inches wide, white to purple disk flowers, each resembling a miniature artichoke (another thistle). Closer inspection of milk thistle reveals a weblike pattern on the surfaces of the leaves, a characteristic that sets it apart from its many cousins. Milk thistle may grow to 7 feet tall.

Habitat and Range: A native of the Mediterranean region of Europe, milk thistle

has become naturalized in many portions of North America. In many areas it has earned the reputation of being an invasive weed. Milk thistle is cultivated throughout much of the world for its medicinal seeds.

Cycle and Bloom Season: An annual or biennial that blooms June through July

Parts Used: Ripe seeds

Primary Medicinal Activities: Protects and strengthens the liver

Strongest Affinities: Liver

Preparation: Alcohol tincture or a standardized powder extract (usually contained in gel capsules). A high concentration of alcohol is required to extract the active constituents from the ground seeds. Be skeptical of milk thistle tincture products whose labels claim low or no alcohol.

Common Uses: Milk thistle has a long ethno-botanical history that gives it stature as much more than a liver herb. It has been used to treat everything from cancer to poor milk production in nursing mothers, but it is most effective in protecting and regenerating the liver.

Most of milk thistle's usefulness can be attributed to its silymarin constituent. Dozens of studies have confirmed that silymarin and its related compounds support and protect the liver during crisis by accelerating the rate of protein synthesis and stimulating production of new cells to replace damaged ones. These compounds work as powerful antioxidants and strengthen liver cell resistance to toxic compounds, while at the same time stimulating cellular reproduction. Much of what we know about these activities stems from the discovery that silymarin can be used to antidote amanita (death cap) mushroom poisoning. When intravenous silymarin is administered within twenty-four to forty-eight hours of ingestion, toxic compounds that would normally destroy liver cells are prevented from penetrating the cell walls, and liver damage is greatly minimized.

Scientific research has also confirmed that milk thistle protects the liver from the harmful effects of various other toxins. Specifically, milk thistle protects an animal's liver during a toxicity-related crisis (such as exposure to toxic chemicals or potentially harmful drug therapies) and helps the animal through a liver damage or disease crisis. It can be used in dogs, cats, horses, goats, ferrets, and rodents to aid in liver or kidney damage, hepatitis, jaundice, leptospirosis, and parvovirus recovery. Milk thistle may prove helpful for treating liver tumors, cancers, and skin problems that are secondary to liver disease. Animals who have been on allopathic drugs, heartworm medication, dewormers, vaccinations, anticonvulsive drugs, or chemotherapy might benefit from this herb as well. Milk thistle can also help block the potential liver-damaging effects of anesthesia and is often used both before and after surgery in Germany. Medical and biological studies support its use in reducing the toxic effect of heavy metals if administered soon enough.

Despite much of the publicity that has been generated about this "wonder herb," milk thistle should not be used as a daily food supplement. Milk thistle is a medicine that is best reserved for situations in which the liver is already under abnormal stress. When used in absence of preexisting stress, milk thistle probably won't do any harm,

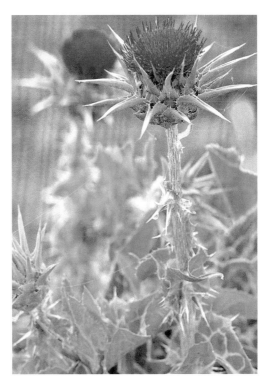

Silybum marianum

but on the other hand it might cause digestive disorders or it might impair other body-cleansing functions of the liver. Many herbalists believe that it can actually slow the metabolic functions of a healthy liver. In any case, milk thistle is unnecessary unless there is a real and present need, and its use as a dietary supplement constitutes waste.

Alcohol tinctures are the best for administering milk thistle because they allow quick and complete absorption of silymarin into the body. But in cases in which severe liver damage might be compounded by alcohol, or in animals with alcohol hypersensitivity, a standardized powder extract (formulated to contain 60–80 percent silymarin) might be a better choice. In cases in which stress on the liver is suspected but not yet serious, the alcohol extract can be administered at a starting dose of ¼ teaspoon (1 milliliter) per 20 pounds of the animal's body weight. Before feeding it to your animal, dilute each dose with an equal amount or more of water to make the tincture more palatable and to minimize the astringency and burning sensation of the alcohol. The tincture can then be added to the animal's food. In any suspected case of liver disease, a holistic veterinarian should be consulted before proceeding with the use of milk thistle or any other herb.

Availability: Available in various formulations through herb retailers

Propagation and Harvest: Milk thistle is easy to grow, but the small yield of seeds per plant makes cultivation a pointless endeavor unless you own a farm rather than just a garden. Harvesting must be done when the seeds are completely ripe and dry but before they leave the plant with a gust of wind. In other words, leave the task to the people who farm it.

Alternatives and Adjuncts: Licorice is another excellent liver-repairing herb that possesses a broader spectrum of medicinal activities than milk thistle. For mild to moderate liver disorders that are believed to be toxicity related and that are signified by chronic constipation, indigestion, or skin problems, milk thistle can be combined with dandelion, burdock, yellow dock, red clover, Oregon grape, or turmeric.

Cautions and Comments: Milk thistle is a very safe herb. In studies that involve giving laboratory animals high doses of silymarin over long periods, the animals display no toxicity.

MULLEIN

Verbascum thapsus Figwort Family

Appearance: This conspicuous plant is recognized during its first year of growth as a ground-hugging rosette of large, up to 12 inches long, broadly lance-shaped, profusely fuzzy leaves. During its second and final year of growth, mullein heads skyward with a stout central stalk that may exceed 6 feet in height. Numerous yellow flowers are then presented in a coblike cluster. There are several species of mullein to be found in North America. *Verbascum thapsus* is the most common and widespread.

Habitat and Range: Mullein is a Eurasian import that has made itself at home in any variety of disturbed sites throughout North America. It is common to clear-cuts, burned areas, and partially developed lands in the West, where it often serves as an important earth regenerator, helping to regain biological balances and prevent erosion.

Cycle and Bloom Season: A biennial that blooms throughout the summer

Parts Used: Leaves, flower heads, roots (each part represents different medicines)

Primary Medicinal Activities: Expectorant; antimicrobial; antiviral; cough suppressant; lubricates, soothes, and protects mucous membranes; astringent

Strongest Affinities: Respiratory and urinary tracts, skin, and ears

Preparation: Tea, tincture, oil infusion, compress, poultice

Common Uses: This wayside weed is extremely useful, providing safe and effective medicine for a wide variety of ailments. The leaves are well known for their ability to ease spasmodic coughs while reducing inflammation and increasing mucus production in the bronchi, making coughs more productive and allowing sufferers to rest easier. These qualities combine with antimicrobial and antiviral properties, making mullein an herb of choice in the treatment of canine tracheobronchitis (kennel cough) and various other forms of respiratory distress in animals.

Scientific studies have shown that a synergy of compounds contained in mullein leaf actively inhibits reproduction of herpes simplex virus (HSV). This activity, combined with the antitussive and expectorant qualities of the plant, might prove useful in treating canine herpes virus (CHV) and feline viral rhinotracheitis (FVR). Although more study is needed to ascertain the effectiveness of mullein against HSV infections in animals, the safety of this plant and its demonstrated ability to relieve many of the discomforts of these diseases justifies giving it a try. A strong leaf tea can be used (10 milliliters per 30 pounds of a dog's body weight, twice daily; 5 milliliters twice daily for cats), or a glycerin tincture can be given directly into the mouth (1–2 milliliters per 20 pounds of an animal's weight, twice daily). Mullein leaf is also practical in the treatment of asthma, especially when it is combined with elecampane, grindelia, or lobelia. (Please see the Lobelia section in the "Supplemental Herb List" for cautions about this herb.)

The large leaves of mullein also make an excellent antimicrobial and astringent poultice for minor wounds and insect bites. Just mash up a few fresh or dried leaves with some water and apply the poultice directly

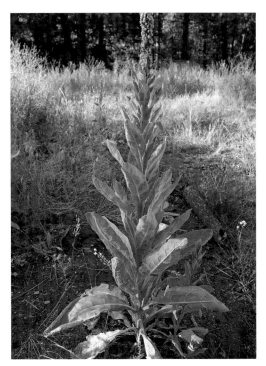

Verbascum thapsus

to the affected area. Mullein leaf is said to lower the acidity of urine, as well, making the herb useful in the treatment of various urinary disorders where urine pH levels are too low.

The flowering tops of mullein have antimicrobial properties with a special affinity toward infections of the ears, including those caused by ear mites. (Note: Ear problems are a sign of chronic disease in an animal who is on a commercial diet.) The best way to use the flowers is in the form of an oil infusion. The flowers also contain rotenone and a synergy of other insecticidal compounds, making mullein effective in the fight against fleas and mange.

Some herbalists maintain that a tincture of the root can be used to treat urinary incontinence. Urinary incontinence can be due to estrogen or testosterone deficiencies, neurogenic dysfunction, anatomical abnormalities, or paradoxical obstruction from urethral calculi or neoplasia, so contact your holistic vet to find the cause before proceeding with the use of mullein root.

Availability: An abundant weed in much of North America. The seeds are available through specialty seed catalogs.

Propagation and Harvest: The leaves of mullein can be harvested anytime, provided they look healthy. The flowers do not appear until the plants' second year and should be plucked from the flower heads when they are wide open (we prefer to use them fresh). The first-year roots should be dug in fall, whereas the second-year roots should be dug in the spring, before the biennial plant begins to die.

Alternatives and Adjuncts: For kennel cough and other respiratory problems, mullein leaf combines well with elecampane, grindelia, or horehound. For use in the ears, nothing compares to a combination of garlic and mullein flower oil. Saint-John's-wort oil and vitamin are also great adjuncts here. Other herbs to consider for urinary incontinence (alone or as adjuncts) include corn silk, uva ursi, couch grass, Saint-John's-wort, and horsetail.

Cautions and Comments: Keep mullein away from fish and amphibians. The rotenone contained in mullein is toxic to aquatic life.

NETTLE

Urtica dioica   Nettle Family

Appearance: Stinging nettle is an erect plant that may grow as high as 7 feet where conditions permit. It reproduces largely from its shallow horizontally creeping root system and is often found in dense patches. Its leaves are broadly lance-shaped with coarsely toothed margins. Flowers are presented in inconspicuous drooping clusters. Stems are covered with fine stinging hairs. Young plants often emerge a reddish color, later turning green as they mature.

Habitat and Range: Several species of nettle inhabit drainage ditches, stream banks, and other moist soils throughout North America and much of the Northern Hemisphere.

Cycle and Bloom Season: A perennial, annual, or biennial (depending on species and climate) that blooms in early summer

Parts Used: Leaves and stems of the preflowering plant and, to a lesser extent, the root

Primary Medicinal Activities: Nutritive, antihistamine, astringent, tonic, helps with blood cleansing

Strongest Affinities: Genitourinary tract, blood, skin, and eyes

Preparation: Dried herb (directly fed), tea, poultice, tincture

Common Uses: All species of *Urtica* cause an instantaneous contact dermatitis that is characterized by tiny blisters and a burning sting. Fortunately, nettle's unpleasant, self-initiated introduction is usually short lived, and those who can learn to accept nettle's characteristics are bound to realize the precious gifts this somewhat obnoxious plant has to offer. Despite its downside, we recognize this plant as one of nature's best nutraceuticals. Ironically, nettle is actually quite delicious, nutritious, and rich with healing opportunities.

Although gloves and a long-sleeved shirt must be worn when gathering the greens, complete drying or cooking neutralizes the plant's antigenic proteins and formic acid compounds—the constituents responsible for the plant's sting. These compounds break down quickly when exposed to air or heat, and when correctly prepared, the leafy greens of young nettle plants are delicious and contain a vast array of vitamins, minerals, and nutrients. In fact, 100 grams of dried preflowering nettle plant contains up to 30.4 grams (30 percent by weight) of crude protein, 2,970 milligrams of calcium, 680 milligrams of phosphorus, 32.2 milligrams of iron, 650 milligrams of magnesium, 20.2 milligrams of beta-carotene, and 3,450 milligrams of potassium, along with vitamins A, C, D, and B complex—all in a highly palatable form that can be effectively assimilated into the body without adding excess stress upon the liver, kidneys, or digestive tract. Nettle therefore makes an excellent addition to food for animals who need extra trace minerals and vitamins in their diet but not necessarily in huge, multivitamin doses. This applies to animals who are already on a natural diet or those who are sensitive to excessive vitamin or mineral supplementation because of chronic digestive disorders, existing systemic toxicity, or urinary tract problems. The completely dried herb can be sprinkled directly onto the animals' food—½ teaspoon for each pound of food fed to dogs, or ⅓ teaspoon per meal for cats. Herbivores can be fed the dried greens in their usual diet, and many will relish nettle as a special treat. In Sweden and Russia, where the problem of producing nutrient-rich feeds is compounded by a short growing season, winter-hardy nettles are sometimes cultivated as fodder crops and then dried.

For finicky pets who despise anything but what their humans are eating, try cooking the fresh young plants with enough water

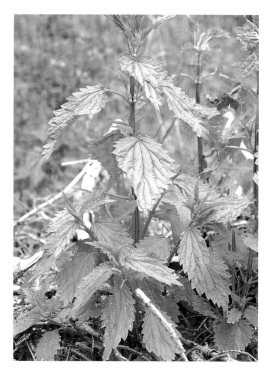

Urtica dioica

to cover them until they are soft and tender. The cooked greens are excellent with butter, and after your furry friend has watched you relish them for a while, you can stir some into her food.

Although many herbal preparations for the eyes typically use a plant called eyebright (*Euphrasia* sp.) as a primary anti-inflammatory agent, many herbalists are becoming concerned about the increasing scarcity of this wild-harvested herb. Fortunately, nature always provides us with a diversity of herbal options—all that is required is for us to ignore market sensationalism and embrace the use of our less compromised plant allies. Nettle, a much more abundant plant, is a good alternative to eyebright.

Nettle leaf tea is an excellent skin and coat rinse that nourishes animals' fur and provides symptomatic relief for itchy skin and flea bites.

Many herbalists who suffer from seasonal allergies have found that nettle leaf tincture or tea helps lessen their symptoms if taken on a regular basis. In a recent study involving sixty-nine patients who suffer from allergic rhinitis, 58 percent found relief after taking a freeze-dried preparation of the leaf.

Although the theories behind the medicinal actions of nettle are varied, we believe that part of the basis for nettle's antiallergenic usefulness may lie in the plant's histamine content, which may work in a like-versus-like manner similar to the concepts of homeopathy. What we mean is that by introducing a substance into the body that acts mildly as an allergenic antagonist, the body is triggered into protecting itself from what it believes to be an inevitable, all-out attack of allergens. In short, nettle may prompt the body into preparing itself. For animals with predictable seasonal occurrences of allergies, dietary supplementation with dried nettle leaf may help.

Nettle root may be useful in the treatment of prostate enlargement, especially at early onset of the disorder. Although a swollen prostate is not as common in animals as in humans, this disorder is sometimes secondary to a chronic or acute infection, poor diet, inflammatory disease, or injuries of the urinary tract, especially in older animals. In a study conducted on human subjects who had mild cases or early onset of prostatic adenoma (a degenerative enlargement of the glandular part of the prostate that typically results in frequent urination during the night), the fluid extract (tincture) of nettle root was found to reduce the duration and volume of urine retention and thus the need to urinate throughout the night. The active constituent in this case is believed to be Beta-sitosterol, a phytosterol known to possess mild anti-inflammatory activity. Although this action is not likely to reduce the formation of scar tissue within the urinary tract and prostate, it is believed to relieve symptoms through reduction of swelling in surrounding tissues. Given the safety of this herb and the functional similarities between the prostates of animals and humans, nettle is certainly worth a try. Keep in mind that large doses of nettle can be irritating to the kidneys if given over an extended period of time, particularly if an animal has preexisting kidney disease or if the herb was gathered too late in its growth cycle.

Availability: Available wherever bulk herbs are sold

Propagation and Harvest: Nettle can be transplanted from root cuttings, but the plant tends to be somewhat choosy about where it grows. Although we know exactly where the plant should thrive, our efforts to introduce nettle to such an area have met with a less than 50 percent success rate. In other words, you are probably better off finding a healthy patch of wild plants to collect your herb. Gather the plants before they bloom—the younger the better. Mature plants begin to develop cystoliths, tiny crystalline particles in the leaf tissues that can irritate the urinary tract and kidneys when ingested in large enough quantities. After gathering, you can boil the greens and serve them as you would spinach, or you can spread them onto clean newspapers and allow them to dry in a well-ventilated, sunlight-free location until they are crispy.

For obvious reasons, gloves and a long-sleeved shirt should be worn when handling nettle plants. If a leaf or stem manages to sneak under your shirtsleeve, try this trick: grasp a piece of the stem and squeeze some of the nettle juice onto the affected area. The stem juice is rich in lecithin, which is believed to antidote the sting. We manage to get stung by this plant several times each spring, and we find relief by using this method in many of our adverse encounters.

Alternatives and Adjuncts: For anti-inflammatory eye and skin washes, alternatives include raspberry leaf, chamomile, dandelion, calendula, or oxeye daisy. For conjunctivitis that is secondary to bacterial or fungal infection, nettle combines well with Oregon grape. Nutritive adjuncts include spirulina, flaxseed, red clover, and alfalfa. For allergies, nettle combines well with elecampane, coltsfoot, goldenrod, lobelia, or licorice as lesser adjuncts. For urinary incontinence and inflammations of the urinary tract, consider couch grass, corn silk, cleavers, uva ursi, goldenrod, and marshmallow as adjuncts.

Cautions and Comments: Touching the live plant results in a painful, blistering sting. Thorough drying or cooking neutralizes the toxic constituents. Some herbalists believe that this plant should be used before it flowers—mature plants contain gritty particles that can irritate the kidneys. Animals who are predisposed to plant allergies may be sensitive to nettle—proceed with care.

OAT

Avena sativa   Grass Family

Appearance: Oats look very much like any other tall grass, and positive identification can be difficult if you're not familiar with the fine details specific to the various cultivars of the Avena genus. Wild oat (*A. fatua*), a common and often hated weed, has the same medicinal attributes as its cultivated relatives. The leaves of the seedlings and

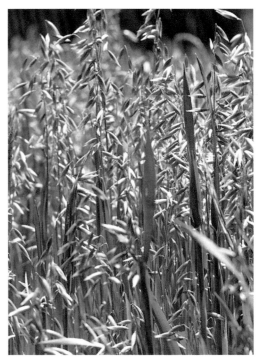

Avena sativa

seeds of this 1- to 4-foot-tall plant have two unique features that differentiate it from its cultivated cousins and most other wild grasses. The first feature is the leaves. Early in growth, they have a counterclockwise twist in them; as the plant matures, the leaves progressively straighten out. The second unique characteristic is the plant's seeds, which at maturity are presented in loosely arranged drooping spikelets. Each spikelet contains two or three foxtail-like seeds that have proportionately long hairlike awns, each of which has a right angle kink in it, giving the appearance of a crimped cockroach feeler.

Habitat and Range: Several cultivars of *A. sativa* are commercially grown throughout the world. Wild oat (*A. fatua*) is a native of Europe that has been introduced into meadows, pastures, and waste areas throughout much of North America.

Cycle and Bloom Season: An annual that blooms from June to August. The seeds of wild oat can remain dormant in the soil for more than eight years, making it difficult to eradicate from areas where it isn't wanted.

Parts Used: Post-flowering tops are used before the seeds fully mature. This is called the plant's milk stage. Herbalists refer to these parts as oatstraw.

Primary Medicinal Activities: Improves nerve functions, nutritive, anti-inflammatory

Strongest Affinities: Nervous system

Preparation: Tea, tincture, fresh or dried herb

Common Uses: Oatstraw is perhaps the best nervous system tonic for aging or debilitated animals. Not only does the herb contain considerable amounts of protein (gluten), vitamins, and minerals (especially calcium, manganese, iron, copper, and zinc) that are essential to the maintenance of health, but it contains various alkaloid, sterol, and flavonoid constituents that act together to safely optimize nervous system functions while stabilizing the highs and lows between nervousness and mental lethargy. For instance, when fed in moderation to animals with chronic nervousness, oatstraw tends to have a calming effect, but when fed to debilitated animals, it tends to stimulate the nervous system. Oatstraw tea or tincture is an excellent choice for animals recovering from exhaustion or suffering from depression disorders. It is known to improve nerve transmission and can be useful for problems such as epilepsy, tremors,

paralysis, and twitching. It is a good tonic for nourishing the body and strengthening nerve function following periods of sedation or anesthesia.

Dried oatstraw brews into a delicious tea that can be poured directly onto dog or cat food as a quickly assimilated tonic supplement. Infuse a heaping teaspoon of oatstraw in 8 ounces of hot water. Feeding 1 ounce of the cooled tea daily is a good amount for cats and animals of similar size. Give 2–4 ounces to most dogs. Glycerin tinctures are also good and can be added to your companion's diet at a daily rate of ¼–½ teaspoon (1–2 milliliters) per 20 pounds of the animal's body weight. Oatstraw is highly water soluble, so there is no point in using an alcohol-based tincture if nonalcohol alternatives are available.

Of course, oats are a well-known feed for horses and other herbivores and should be included as part of their daily diet. In terms of tonic value, fresh oat greens are vastly superior to what is purchased in grain bags, but the greens must be fed in moderation. A few large handfuls can be added to the daily diet, but too much may cause hyperexcitability.

Oatmeal can be included as part of your companion's natural diet. It can also be used externally as a soothing bath for skin problems.

Availability: Oatstraw is available through health food stores

Propagation and Harvest: Oat is easy to grow, but it takes up a great deal of garden space. If you opt to grow it, harvest the top 6–12 inches of the plants after the seeds have formed but before the plants begin to dry.

Alternatives and Adjuncts: For depression disorders, oatstraw can be combined with Saint-John's-wort, passionflower, or chamomile (but consider changing you companion's diet first). For treating epilepsy, oatstraw combines with skullcap, valerian, or kava kava. In animals who are recovering from anesthesia or sedation, alterative and diuretic herbs should be combined with oatstraw in order to help cleanse and nourish the blood and eliminate systemic waste. Possibilities include red clover, dandelion leaf, alfalfa, garlic, and nettle. For older animals who need continuous nervous system support, oatstraw combines especially well with nettle, red clover, alfalfa, and spirulina.

Cautions and Comments: Too much oatstraw may cause excitability or vomiting. If this occurs, simply reduce the amount being fed to the animal.

OREGON GRAPE

Mahonia aquifolium   Barberry Family

Appearance: At first glance, Oregon grape looks similar to American holly (Ilex opaca)—the stuff we deck the halls with during the Christmas season. The almost plasticlike leaves of this perennial evergreen plant are divided into several opposing pairs of oval to lance-shaped, ½- to 3-inch-long leaflets. The leaf edges have conspicuous sharp spines. Flowers are yellow and are borne in clusters at the end of a sturdy central stalk. By midsummer, the flowers develop into clusters of juicy, purple, ¼-to ½-inch fruits that resemble tiny grapes. The fruits are edible but very sour.

Habitat and Range: Three species of Oregon grape are common in the coniferous forests of western North America, ranging through the mountains of central California and New

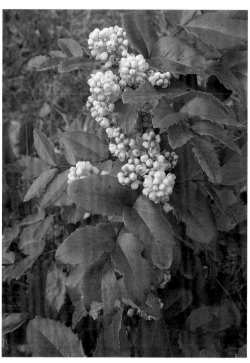

Mahonia aquifolium

Mexico northward into Canada. Tall Oregon grape (*Mahonia aquifolium*) is a variety that grows up to 6 feet tall and is abundant in the coastal forests to the west slopes of the Rocky Mountains. *Mahonia repens* and *M. nervosa* are smaller (up to 12 inches tall), ground-hugging versions that are widespread throughout their range. A fourth less-common species (*M. pinnata*) inhabits the mountains of Baja Mexico and California. All share similar appearances, the primary differentiating factor being their size.

Cycle and Bloom Season: Perennial evergreens that bloom in late spring

Parts Used: Roots

Primary Medicinal Activities: Antimicrobial, stimulates bile production, anti-inflammatory, tonic, antiparasitic

Strongest Affinities: Liver and digestive system, mucous membranes

Preparation: Tincture, tea, decoction, oil infusion, powdered root

Common Uses: For most purposes, Oregon grape serves as an excellent alternative to goldenseal (*Hydrastis canadensis*), an herb that is currently at risk of going extinct from the pressures of overharvest and loss of habitat. Fortunately, Oregon grape remains common and abundant over a much wider range than the overharvested goldenseal and is much easier to cultivate. So unless you have access to a cultivated source of goldenseal, please use Oregon grape instead.

As is the case for goldenseal, a bitter yellow alkaloid called berberine is primarily responsible for the strong antimicrobial activity of Oregon grape. The antibacterial properties of berberine have been shown to be more effective than some forms of prescription antibiotics, including chloramphenicol, when used against various forms of staphylococci. Berberine has also been shown to be active against *E. coli* and other gram-negative-type bacteria. It is even effective against *giardiasis*, a parasitic infestation of the digestive tract that is reputedly difficult to remedy. Like goldenseal, Oregon grape extract is especially useful in the ears, eyes, and the mucous membranes of the vagina and urinary tract, where it combats various fungal infections as well.

For bacterial ear infections or ear mites, an oil infusion of the fresh or dried root works best. To make an oil infusion, cut up the root as finely as possible and place it into a food processor or blender that has a glass or stainless steel blending vessel. (The roots are tough and might cause plastic to crack.)

Cover the chopped root with enough olive oil to leave a ½-inch-thick layer above the herb. Put the lid on and blend until the oil is a vibrant, goldenrod-yellow color (about ten minutes). Strain the chopped root out through a fine sieve, and you'll have a nice, antimicrobial ear oil. If you don't wish to use your blender, you can let the chopped herb and olive oil mixture stand in a covered jar at room temperature for one month before straining. The finished product keeps for several months, sometimes years, if refrigerated. To use the oil, apply 1–10 drops at a time in each ear one to two times a day until the infection is gone. It is also good as a general topical antibiotic for stings, insect bites, cuts, abrasions, puncture injuries of the paws, and other injuries.

Oregon grape is effective in treating conjunctivitis, where it fights infection and reduces inflammation. To treat your companion's eyes with Oregon grape, dilute 4 drops of the alcohol tincture (available at your favorite herb store), or 8 drops of a root decoction, into 1 ounce of sterile saline (available anywhere contact lens supplies are sold). Place a few drops into the infected eye, taking note of any discomfort that may result from the berberine or the alcohol content of the tincture. Some animals are more intolerant than others. If the solution appears to irritate the eyes, dilute it with more saline and flush the eye with plain saline before applying more solution.

Oregon grape root is also noted for its ability to stimulate liver function. It is particularly helpful in cases of chronic constipation associated with poor protein or fat metabolism, situations that often lead to itchy, flaky skin and a dull coat in animals. Used under these circumstances, Oregon grape extract can bring fast and dramatic results, and it does so by addressing an underlying cause of the problem. Generally speaking from a holistic perspective, many forms of dermatitis are symptoms of an underlying liver dysfunction. If the liver cannot eliminate excess toxins or is functionally compromised by blockages that reduce bile flow or production, the digestive tract fails at its job of eliminating waste. One of the first places the body tries to force elimination is through the skin. Oregon grape works in the liver much like a strong version of dandelion—bile production and flow is increased, and digestive efficiency is improved. But Oregon grape stimulates liver function much faster than does dandelion, irritating the organ into working harder. For this reason, Oregon grape should not be used in animals with acute liver disease or existing liver injuries without the supervision of a trained professional. And although Oregon grape is safe when used properly, it is likely to overexcite the liver of most animals if used excessively. If this occurs, your animal will probably vomit because of excessive bile in the stomach; you should stop using Oregon grape and consider a gentler herb such as dandelion. In any case, it is best not to give any herbal medicine every day of an animal's life. Instead, give whatever herbs you are using four to five days per week, then let the animal's system rest for two or three days before proceeding. This break time also gives you an opportunity to monitor changes that may be occurring as a result of your therapeutic efforts.

The bitter tonic action of the alkaloid constituents in Oregon grape make this herb a useful digestive aid. When a drop or two of the root tincture is placed on the tongue, or when a leaf is chewed, an instantaneous salivary response occurs. At the same time, mechanisms are triggered that release bile and various other enzymes and acids into the digestive tract. The digestive system is therefore primed into action before the food arrives. Giving this bitter tonic daily is an excellent holistic approach to safely treating chronic indigestion and malabsorption. If you or your animal has problems with excess gas or with foods that tend to pass through undigested, try using a small dose of Oregon grape before each meal. The results will probably amaze you.

Oregon grape can also be used as an antibacterial in the urinary tract and is regarded by herbalists as an effective remedy for infections of the bladder, kidneys, and urethra. Again, the antibacterial effect of Oregon grape in the urinary tract is attributable to berberine, which stays effective long enough to reach deep into the body. Since most infections of the urinary tract are associated with uncomfortable inflammation, combining this herb with the soothing effects of marshmallow, licorice, or plantain is a good idea. Generally, a formula made with one part Oregon grape to two parts of other soothing herbs is a good infection-fighting, pain-relieving approach.

When combined in small proportions with echinacea, Oregon grape combats the infection directly while the immune system plays catch-up with invading pathogens. At the same time, Oregon grape helps to support the liver at its job of keeping the body clean through elimination of waste, a critical process of maintaining balanced body functions while the body heals. And while conventional antibiotic therapies tend not to discriminate between beneficial microbes and bad ones, the body is allowed to fight infection by natural mechanisms with a properly proportioned berberine-containing herbal support formula without compromising its own microbial warriors. Instead, it receives a measured degree of outside support and is gently stimulated into working harder toward victory. A formula consisting of 10 percent Oregon grape and 90 percent echinacea is generally appropriate for this purpose.

In addition to its liver and disinfectant benefits, berberine is known to possess mild but useful sedative qualities and may be effective as an anticonvulsive remedy. It has also been shown to help lower blood pressure and is believed to slightly elevate blood sugar levels in hypoglycemic animals.

Availability: The plants are available through landscape nurseries. Oregon grape root is available in a variety of forms from herb retailers.

Propagation and Harvest: Oregon grape is widely adaptable to gardens throughout most of North America. Tall Oregon grape (*M. aquifolium*) is the most common variety in commerce and is becoming popular as a landscape shrub. It is quite easy to grow from root cuttings, seeds, or transplants. These plants are drought tolerant and winter hardy. All they essentially need is slightly acidic soil and plenty of redwood compost, but they flourish when afforded at least three hours of shade each day and a good weekly watering. Roots can be dug from mature plants anytime during the year. They can be dried and kept in plastic bags for two or three years.

Alternatives and Adjuncts: In ear oils, combine with garlic and vitamin E oil. To aid in liver congestion and to improve digestion, dandelion root serves as a weaker alternative. For *Giardia* and worms, Oregon grape combines with garlic. In eyewashes, Oregon grape combines especially well with raspberry leaf. For urinary tract infections, marshmallow, plantain, or licorice serve as soothing adjuncts.

Cautions and Comments: Oregon grape should not be used in animals with acute liver disease or existing liver injuries without the supervision of a professional. It has been theorized that too much berberine may inhibit vitamin B assimilation.

OXEYE DAISY

Chrysanthemum leucanthemum   Sunflower Family

Appearance: It brings us satisfaction to tell you about useful plants that can be easily grown in any garden, but it brings us special joy to tell you about useful plants that already grow on the edges of driveways and in vacant lots. Oxeye daisy is such a plant. To the herbalist, a weed is simply a plant with attributes that have yet to be realized. When the usefulness of such plants is brought to light, people reconsider their approaches to weed control. This usually means a reduction in the use of toxic herbicides, which end up in the environment.

Oxeye daisy is a wild relative of pyrethrum daisy (genus *Pyrethrum*), which is cultivated for its insecticidal properties. Oxeye daisy looks similar to the pyrethrum daisy; in fact at first glance it looks like any other white daisy. But close examination of this plant's unique leaf characteristics makes it easy to differentiate from all others during any stage of its perennial growth cycle. The basal leaves of oxeye have proportionately long petioles (leaf stems) and are spoon-shaped with rounded teeth along the edges. The leaves of the upper plant lack petioles, and the flowers are typically daisylike: white with yellow centers and up to 3 inches wide. The entire plant may reach 3 feet in height.

Habitat and Range: Oxeye daisy is a Eurasian import that is now common to roadsides and dry waste areas throughout the northern half of North America, up to about 6,000 feet in elevation.

Cycle and Bloom Season: Plants bloom first in early summer, then often remain in bloom until fall.

Parts Used: Leaves and flowers

Primary Medicinal Activities: Antihistamine, insecticidal (used for fleas), diuretic, stops bleeding

Strongest Affinities: Respiratory tract, skin

Preparation: Tea, tincture, or dried powdered herb

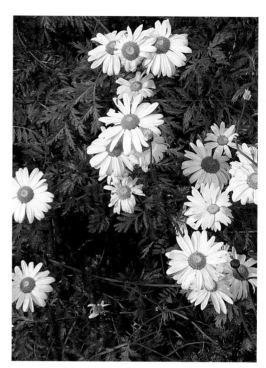

Pyrethrum roseum

Common Uses: The leaves are recognized by some contemporary herbalists for their diuretic and hemostatic qualities, and clinical research suggests that the leaf tea may also be effective as an antihistamine medicine that slows the body's responses to allergens while helping to reduce excess secretions of mucus. The flower tea is especially useful for helping to relieve seasonal hay fever characterized by sneezing and watery discharges from the nose and eyes. At the onset of symptoms, 1 tablespoon of the strong tea can be fed to dogs as part of their daily diet throughout the crisis period. Cats and other small mammals need only 1 teaspoon. Horses and other herbivores can be allowed to eat the fresh plants from their pastures, and rabbits can be given a stem or two of the flowering plant each day.

As is true of its cultivated cousins, the flowers of oxeye daisy contain useful amounts of pyrethrin, a natural insecticide that is useful for controlling fleas. To use oxeye daisy in this capacity, make a skin rinse from the fresh chopped flowers or apply the dried flowers as a mildly effective but safe and natural flea powder.

As a diuretic, oxeye daisy can increase urinary output and dilute urine that is over-concentrated, strong smelling, and too acidic, and it lends weak but measurable astringent and antimicrobial properties to inflamed urinary membranes.

Oxeye daisy is often abundant on the margins of horse and stock trails, making it readily available as a first aid remedy for minor cuts, fly bites, and such. The fresh-leaf poultice can be applied directly to the site of injury to help stop bleeding. Combine it with one of many antimicrobial herbs that grows nearby (such as yarrow or bee balm), and you'll have an excellent, broad-spectrum field dressing.

Availability: A widely distributed weed, oxeye daisy is available through nurseries.

Propagation and Harvest: Oxeye daisy is easy to grow from seeds or transplants. It is drought tolerant, winter hardy, and adaptable to any soil. All oxeye daisy really needs is full sun.

Alternatives and Adjuncts: As a flea-fighting alternative, try feverfew. For seasonal allergies, oxeye daisy can be combined with or replaced by nettle. Dandelion leaf is a much more effective diuretic.

Cautions and Comments: Some animals may be highly allergic to this plant—test a small amount of the tea on your companion's skin before using. If redness or any other response occurs, don't feed it to your animal!

PARSLEY

Petroselinum crispum   Parsley Family

Appearance: There are numerous cultivars of this familiar herb—their primary differences being leaf size and root variations. The most common varieties have tightly curled leaves, whereas Italian parsley (*P. crispum* var. *neapolitanum*) has leaves that are more like those of celery. Hamburg parsley (*P. crispum* var. *tuberosum*) has a thick turniplike taproot and fernlike leaves. All produce terminate umbel flowers, and most will grow to about 3 feet tall.

Habitat and Range: Originally a native of southeast Europe and west Asia, parsley is now cultivated worldwide.

Cycle and Bloom Season: A perennial that blooms in midsummer

Parts Used: Leaves, seeds, and roots
Primary Medicinal Activities: Expels intestinal gas, lowers blood pressure, nutritive, diuretic, helps reduce arthritic inflammation, promotes menstrual discharge, insecticidal, antimicrobial

Strongest Affinities: Digestive and urinary tracts, joints

Preparation: Tea, tincture, or fresh or dried herb

Common Uses: Parsley is much more than a plate garnish. In fact, it is one of the most versatile medicinal plants around—it is an absolute "must have" in the home herb garden.

Parsley root is known by herbalists as an excellent diuretic that is especially beneficial in the treatment of rheumatoid conditions. For humans, it is considered a specific remedy in the treatment of gout; it is believed to help with the elimination of uric acid that would otherwise contribute to the buildup of painful crystals in the joints. For animals, parsley root is useful in cases of arthritis that are compounded or perhaps even caused by poor waste elimination, a problem that is often the result of a poor diet. For these purposes, dogs and cats can be given a strong tea of the dried or freshly grated root (1 teaspoon of the strong tea per day for cats; 1–2 tablespoons for dogs), or a tincture can be used (1–2 milliliters per 30 pounds of the animal's body weight). Horses can be fed a few handfuls of the entire fresh plant (leaves, roots, and all) each day, or a cup of the dried herb daily. Parsley root is especially effective when combined with alternatives, hepatics, and anti-inflammatory herbs.

Parsley leaves and stems are very nutritious, containing up to 22 percent protein and impressive amounts of vitamins A, C, B_1, B_2, and K, as well as fiber, calcium, riboflavin, potassium, iron, magnesium, niacin, and phosphorus. This makes parsley an excellent nutritive in the treatment of anemia. The leaves also contain apiol and several other volatile oils that have antiseptic qualities, making the herb useful for urinary tract infections. And because parsley is a diuretic, it may help boost kidney function in cases of noninflammatory, early-onset renal failure. Apiol also has a stimulant and strengthening effect on intestinal and uterine muscles, making it suitable for improving uterine muscle tone after a difficult pregnancy. In the digestive tract, this tonic activity combines with parsley's carminative properties, making it effective in the treatment of flatulent dyspepsia and colic.

Perhaps the best way to use parsley leaf for gastric or urinary disorders or for its nutritional qualities is to juice it. If you don't have a vegetable juicer, pack an electric blender halfway full with fresh leaves and add just enough water to liquefy the leaves into a dark green soup. The juice, or "blender soup," can be fed directly to an animal with an empty stomach (the best option) or added to your companion's drinking water (second best) or food (the last resort)—1 teaspoon per 20 pounds of the animal's body weight. The juice (or a few drops of the leaf tincture) also serves as an excellent breath freshener.

Availability: Plants are available through nurseries. The herb is also available in various forms through health food and herb retailers everywhere.

Propagation and Harvest: Parsley is easy to grow from seed or transplants. If given rich, well-drained soil, it will return year after year. If allowed to go to seed, it will sprout up all over the garden.

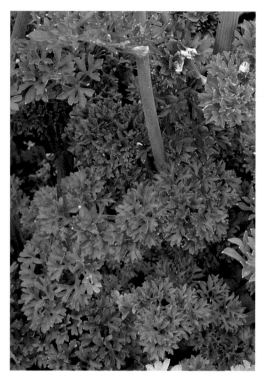

Petroselinum crispum

Alternatives and Adjuncts: For rheumatoid conditions, shepherd's purse serves as an effective substitute. For urinary infections, consider corn silk, couch grass, echinacea, uva ursi, and horsetail as alternatives or adjuncts. For colic and other digestive disorders, fennel, dill, slippery elm, plantain, marshmallow, cleavers, and licorice should all be investigated. Raspberry leaf or nettle serves as alternative uterine tonics or nutritives.

Cautions and Comments: Parsley, in dried, fresh, or tea form is very safe. However, highly concentrated preparations of the seed, such as parsley essential oil, are rich in volatile oils that can be absorbed into the placenta, so don't use the essential oil internally or externally during an animal's pregnancy. While it is thought to aid the healing process after birthing, it may reduce lactation and should be used conservatively in nursing mothers. Parsley should not be used if inflammation of the kidneys exists.

Parsley seeds contain the highest concentration of volatile oils, including a considerable amount of myristicin. Myristicin can have strong hypotensive and hallucinogenic effects, especially in cats, and may cause liver damage or photosensitivity if ingested in large enough quantities. Although such instances are rare, and it's unlikely that an animal could eat enough parsley seed to cause such problems, it's best to be safe by using only parsley leaves, stems, and roots, which contain much lower concentrations of myristicin.

PLANTAIN

Plantago sp.   Plantain Family

Appearance: Common plantain (*Plantago major*) is characterized by its low-growing rosette of broad leaves and its rather drab but distinctive flower cluster. The sturdy succulent leaves are on proportionately long petioles and have distinct parallel veins that contain strong fibers. Flowers are small and inconspicuous, borne in tightly arranged sausage-shaped spikes atop leafless stalks that reach well above the rest of the plant. Ten or more species of the *Plantago* genus inhabit western North America, with common plantain by far the most widespread and abundant.

Habitat and Range: Common plantain is frequently found in high impact areas, growing in the center of dirt roads, walkways, and even the cracks in highways. It is widespread throughout most of North America.

Cycle and Bloom Season: An annual or perennial that blooms March through August

Parts Used: All parts of the plant

Primary Medicinal Activities: Lubricates, soothes, and protects internal mucous membranes; emollient; astringent; anti-inflammatory; stops bleeding

Strongest Affinities: Digestive and urinary tracts, skin

Preparation: Tincture, tea, poultice, or dried seed husks

Common Uses: Plantain is one of many useful plants that have been forgotten by virtue of its abundance and its reputation as a weed. Many of us step on it while en route to the vegetable garden, unaware that it may be more nutritious than the vegetables we tend. Plantain is high in vitamins C, A, and K.

In essence, plantain can be used in the same ways as slippery elm. The mucilaginous and astringent qualities of plantain make it an excellent remedy for reducing inflammations inside and on the body. The aucubin and saponin constituents of plantain have been shown to have antibacterial properties, especially against *Micrococcus flavus, Staphylococcus aureus*, and *Bacillus subtilus*. All of these activities combine to make plantain useful in a wide range of urinary, digestive, and respiratory ailments.

In the urinary tract, plantain can help stop minor bleeding, reduce inflammation, and relieve pain that is secondary to bacterial infection or the passing of small stones (gravel). In the digestive tract, plantain relieves diarrhea and the symptoms of various types of inflammatory bowel disease. Its lubricating properties and anti-inflammatory activities make it useful for treating irritations of the stomach and intestinal tract that occur when an animal eats something that is difficult to pass such as pine needles, a bottle cap, or a brand-new sequined handbag. *Plantago psyllium* is widely known for its seeds and husks, which are used as an effective laxative and a source of dietary fiber. In the upper respiratory tract, plantain helps soothe raspy coughs such as those caused by inhaled dust or canine tracheobronchitis (kennel cough).

Plantain is best used fresh. If you have an electric juicer, liquefy the entire plant, roots and all. Otherwise, chop the washed plants as finely as you can, pack them loosely into a blender, add just enough warm water to cover the herb, and blend the mixture into a dark-green gooey soup. Don't use boiling water because it destroys hydrolytic enzymes that have antibacterial properties. You might end up with a tangle of the strong leaf fibers wrapped around the blades of your machine—this is normal. Strain the liquid through a sieve and refrigerate it in a sealed glass jar until you need it. It will keep for about two weeks in a very cold refrigerator. To use the juice for internal problems, 1 teaspoon can be fed for each 20 pounds of a dog's body weight, once or twice daily. Cats can take up to a teaspoon of the juice twice daily. It's best to administer the juice before a meal and with as little added water as possible. If this isn't possible, the juice can be added to your companion's food. For colic, the removal of sand in the digestive tract, and other digestive problems in horses or other large animals, a handful or two of the fresh plants can be fed as part of a daily diet.

A poultice of plantain is one of the best topical first aid remedies for insect bites, stings, minor burns, and site-specific contact dermatitis (such as minor bouts with stinging nettle). An oil infusion or salve of the fresh or dried plant can be used for the same purposes.

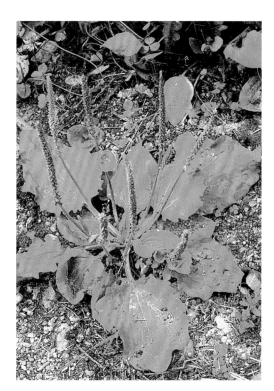

Plantago major

Availability: A widely distributed weed. The husks of *P. psyllium* are available through any respectable health food store, and several psyllium products are now being produced specifically for use in animals. The seeds of several varieties can be purchased through specialty catalogs.

Propagation and Harvest: Plantain is easy to grow—all it needs is ample water during its germination. Sow the tiny seeds as sparsely as you can under ⅛ inch of soil, and keep them wet until they sprout. The plants can be harvested and used anytime, but the mature second-year and older plants make the best medicine.

Alternatives and Adjuncts: Plantain can be used as a substitute for slippery elm, a hardwood tree that is being overharvested for its medicinal inner bark. Marshmallow root contains far more mucilage than plantain does, and it serves as a more effective alternative in cases in which digestive or urinary tract lubrication is needed. In situations in which the astringency and mucilage content of plantain are not enough to bring relief to urinary irritations, try combining marshmallow with a stronger astringent such as uva ursi or rose bark.

Cautions and Comments: Side effects are rare with this plant, but some animals may be allergic to it. If your companion is predisposed to plant allergies, test for sensitivity by applying a small amount to the skin. If no reaction occurs, proceed with a small internal dose (a few drops), and watch for sneezing, watery eyes, or other signs of allergic response.

RASPBERRY

Rubus sp.   Rose Family

Appearance: Raspberries are generally categorized by color—red or black. Leaf and stem characteristics vary between species of this widespread genus of shrubs. Most have divided leaves and five-petal flowers that range from white to crimson in color. The plants are generally found as tangled masses of thorny trailing biennial stems that yield a tasty reward to those brave enough to reach the choicest berries. All species are medicinally useful.

Habitat and Range: As one travels northward through the Rocky Mountains and the coastal states of the West, the diversity of species and the number of roadside bramble patches encountered progressively increases. Many species of *Rubus* are regarded

as invasive weeds. They are common and often abundant inhabitants of pastures, roadside ditches, and riparian habitats. This genus often cross-pollinates, making exact identification of species difficult in many areas. And many species have escaped cultivation, making it anybody's guess where one of these plants will pop up next. Red raspberry (*R. idaeus*—illustrated) is one of the most common indigenous species found throughout North America.

Cycle and Bloom Season: Perennials that bloom and produce fruit from second-year plants, known as canes

Parts Used: Dried leaves and, of course, the delicious fruit

Primary Medicinal Activities: Astringent, strengthens the uterus (uterotonic), nutritive, diuretic, laxative, mild sedative

Strongest Affinities: Female reproductive system, eyes, skin

Preparation: Infusion, poultice, or tincture

Common Uses: Raspberry leaf is a safe and gentle medicinal food. Aside from its nutritional value (it is especially high in vitamin C), raspberry leaf tea has mild astringent qualities that make it useful for a wide variety of remedial and tonic therapies. Taken internally, the tea is useful for treating minor digestive tract inflammations and can be used as a remedy for mild cases of diarrhea. In such instances, a strong infusion can be fed at a dose of 2 ounces per 20 pounds of an animal's body weight (or 1 ounce for cats), twice daily as needed for relief. Alternatively, the dried leaf can be used—1 teaspoon per 20 pounds of the animal's weight, sprinkled onto food daily. For bleeding or inflamed gums, the powdered leaf can be applied directly to the site of the problem, or the tea can be applied to the gums with a cotton swab.

Traditionally, the leaf tea is perhaps the most widely used "female tonic" in existence. It acts to improve the tone and elasticity of smooth muscle tissues in and around the uterus. It is useful as a prepregnancy tonic and in pregnant or postpartum dogs, cats, horses, and other animals during the final weeks of pregnancy. The dried leaf can be sprinkled onto your animal's food (at the previously mentioned doses) as a daily tonic, or it can be fed as a tea. Make the tea by steeping 1 teaspoon of the dried leaf (in a tea ball) in 8 ounces of hot water. The tea can be added to your animal's drinking water until the water is noticeably colored. The animal can then drink at will.

Raspberry leaf is especially beneficial in the form of a saline eyewash for symptomatic relief of conjunctivitis. To make an eyewash, infuse 1 teaspoon of dried raspberry leaf in 8 ounces of hot distilled water. Allow the tea to cool, strain it through a coffee filter, then combine it with enough sterile saline solution to produce a slightly tinted solution. The cooled full-strength tea can also be used as a soothing scalp or skin rinse—its astringency helps to relieve minor itchiness.

Availability: Raspberry leaf is available at health food stores. The canes are available through most nurseries.

Propagation and Harvest: Raspberries are easy to grow. Transplanted canes produce an abundance of leaves, and they produce their first fruit during their second year of growth and every year thereafter. The plants like moist, potassium-rich soil and full sun. Harvest the leaves just before the plants bloom in spring or early summer. Dry them

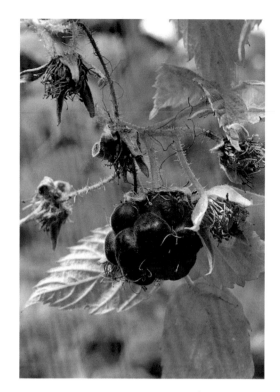

Rubus idaeus

on a clean nonmetallic surface until they are crispy dry. The dried leaves can be stored in plastic bags for a year or more.

Alternatives and Adjuncts: Raspberry serves as a less-threatened substitute for eyebright (*Euphrasia* spp.), a plant that is currently at risk of disappearing because of overharvest. The leaves of strawberry (*Fragaria* spp.) can be used as a substitute for raspberry leaf. As a female tonic, nettle leaf tea serves as a better substitute because it contains a much richer array of vital nutrients. Nettle can also be used in eye and skin washes. For conjunctivitis or inflammation of the mouth that is secondary to bacterial or fungal infection, raspberry leaf combines well with Oregon grape and echinacea. If the problem appears to be of viral origin, mullein leaf or Saint-John's-wort may serve as an effective adjunct. For diarrhea and internal bleeding, stronger alternatives include uva ursi, horsetail, plantain, and cayenne.

Cautions and Comments: Never use raspberry leaves that are not completely dry. As the leaves wilt, they temporarily develop toxins that can be nauseating to your animal.

Despite old claims of raspberry leaf causing uterine contractions, no qualified reports of toxicity have been recorded for this herb.

RED CLOVER

Trifolium pratense   Pea Family

Appearance: Red clover was introduced to the U.S. from Europe as a feed crop for livestock and has since escaped cultivation to make itself at home throughout North America. It is characterized by the predominantly three-lobed leaves of the *Trifolium* genus, of which dozens of species and cultivars are distributed throughout the West. The differences among these many species may be minute, and positive identification of a specific *Trifolium* sp. can be challenging. First, the identification of red clover can begin by recognizing its red, globe-shaped flowers and its soft, hairy stems. Second, we can see that the flower stems (pedicels) are shorter in length than each of the leaf stems (petioles). And finally, red clover has a small carrotlike taproot, whereas many clovers have horizontally creeping roots systems (rhizomes). If all of this fails to answer the question of identity, cheat—find some red clover that has been cultivated and formulate personalized notes for future reference.

Habitat and Range: Red clover is widespread in cultivated fields, road margins, gardens, and other disturbed areas where the plant has been introduced largely through agricultural activities.

Cycle and Bloom Season: A short-lived perennial that blooms in early summer

Parts Used: Flowering tops

Primary Medicinal Activities: Helps with blood cleansing, diuretic, expectorant, tonic, antispasmodic, nutritive, antitumor, effects estrogen production in the body (estrogenic)

Strongest Affinities: Liver, blood, and skin

Preparation: Tea, dried or fresh herb, or tincture

Common Uses: Although traditionally red clover has been used and highly acclaimed as a blood-purifying alterative and anticancer agent for hundreds, perhaps thousands, of years, few scientific studies have been conducted to substantiate these claims. Regardless, thousands of herbalists and an equal number of people who have witnessed red clover's potential as a healing agent and preventative seem to know something. At the root of red clover's attributes is an impressive array of protein, magnesium, calcium, potassium, and vitamin C and B complex. All of these nutrients are joined with a complex assortment of medicinally active chemical compounds. In the mind of a holistically oriented herbalist, all of these components synergistically amount to an excellent remedy for psoriasis, eczema, and other skin disorders, especially those believed to be secondary to excess waste materials in the bloodstream. For such disorders, red clover may be used internally or externally. Internally, a flower tea or tincture gently stimulates the liver and gallbladder to help optimize digestion and replenish the blood. Externally, a cooled tea or poultice can be applied to flaky dry, itchy skin for symptomatic relief. Added to an animal's daily diet as a preventive measure, you can give a pinch of dried red clover to a dog; a tinier pinch to a cat; and a handful to horses, llamas, and sheep. A rabbit can be fed a flower or two a day, and for other animals, as with any herb, moderation is the single-word golden rule.

In horses, red clover is sometimes fed to speed recovery from viral infections of the respiratory tract, particularly when a persistent cough or excessive secretion of thick mucus from inflamed mucous membranes (catarrh) seem to be slowing the healing process by adding stress to a run-down animal. Feed ½–2 cups of the flower heads daily as part of the animal's feed. If tea is a better option, 3 or 4 heaping tablespoons of the dried flowers steeped in a pint of water can be fed daily.

Much of red clover's reputation as an anticancer herb stems from its inclusion in the famed Hoxsey Formula and the still popular Essiac Formula, although skeptics argue that the effectiveness of these formulas are without validation. Both of these formulas have been used extensively during the past seventy-five years, and many cancer sufferers, practitioners, and pet owners have claimed near-miraculous results from them. In addition to these formulas, red clover is often used by itself—again with many favorable claims. As mentioned, scientific evidence to support these claims is scarce but certainly exists. In 1988, a study published in *The Journal of Cancer Research* indicated that the anticancer activity of red clover may in fact be a scientific reality. Specifically, it was found that the flavonoid constituents in red clover blossoms inhibit the harmful activities of a

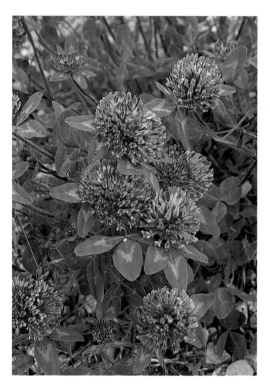

Trifolium pratense

carcinogenic substance called benzopyrene, a compound present in charbroiled foods. In an earlier 1970 study that was published in the same journal, the flavonoid quercetin found in red clover was shown to prevent benzopyrene from becoming active in the liver and small intestines. While these studies fall short of identifying the breadth of red clover's activity against various other carcinogens, they certainly indicate that further research is warranted and add credibility to what holistic practitioners have been telling us all along.

In animals with cancerous lesions of the skin or extremities, a poultice of red clover flowers can be applied in the form of a compress for several hours each day until the animal's condition (hopefully) improves. Internal doses of the flower tea or tincture can be used in dogs, cats, horses, and other animals as well. In the fight against cancer, anything that can be applied safely and without contributing stress to an already stressed body is certainly worth a try. In our minds, red clover is at the top of the list.

Availability: Seed catalogs, feed stores, health food stores, and other herb retailers

Propagation and Harvest: If you have rich, moist soil and a section of garden you wish to delegate to the spreading, strong-rooted nature of this plant, red clover can be easily propagated from seed. Harvest the flowers during dry weather in early summer. Use them fresh or dry them indoors on a piece of clean paper. The dried flowers keep for a year if properly stored.

Alternatives and Adjuncts: For skin problems that are secondary to poor liver metabolism or excessive systemic waste, red clover combines well with yellow dock, alfalfa, burdock, dandelion root, and nettle.

Cautions and Comments: When properly used, red clover is a safe herb, but, as is true for many plants, its use does demand some attention and respect. First, do not use red clover for animals with clotting disorders or in the presence of internal or external bleeding. This plant contains the compound coumarin, which is cited in many toxicology texts as having blood-thinning qualities. However, recent studies suggest that the coumarin alone do not really possess blood-thinning properties. Instead, it is now thought that blood-thinning properties may only occur when certain molds or fungi develop on the herb as result of improper drying. Red clover is also known to contain estrogenic isoflavone constituents that may prove toxic to

livestock and other animals if fed in large quantities. Cases of acute skin and digestive disorders have been reported in horses, sheep, cattle, and other animals who have been allowed to excessively overgraze on fresh red clover. Red clover also possesses some phyto-estrogenic principles that contraindicate this herb's use in pregnant or lactating animals.

ROSE

Rosa spp.   Rose Family

Appearance: Most people are familiar with roses. Hundreds of cultivars adorn flower beds to please the senses and stir the emotions of millions of people worldwide. In addition to the healing power of their beauty, all roses are medicinally useful. The wild species (of which there are dozens in North America) offer the best-tasting, most nutritional hips. Wild roses look and smell very much like their domesticated counterparts except that they have smaller flowers and leaves. Characterized by their white-to-pink (sometimes yellow), five-petaled flowers, thorny stems, and bright red to purplish fruit (hips), these plants represent a safe, easy-to-identify, delightful introduction to nature's pantry and apothecary.

Habitat and Range: Wild roses like consistently moist soil and are often found standing in dense thickets at road margins, in irrigation ditches, and especially as the "defensive edge" of riparian habitats up to about 6,000 feet in elevation. Several species are native throughout North America. Wood's rose (*Rosa woodsii*) represents one of the most widespread pink-flowered species to be found in western North America. Multiflora rose

(*R. multiflora*) grows profusely throughout the midwestern U.S. and eastern Canada, where it forms dense thickets and is often considered a troublesome weed.

Cycle and Bloom Season: A perennial that blooms June through August

Parts Used: Hips, flower petals, leaves, stems, and bark

Primary Medicinal Activities: Nutritive, astringent, bacteriostatic

Strongest Affinities: Digestive system, urinary tract, skin

Preparation: Fresh or dried hips, petals, leaves, and bark; tincture, tea, or decoction

Common Uses: When we think of roses as medicine, we tend to remember reading "Vitamin C with Rose Hips" on product labels. But actually, the nutritive value of rose hips represents only a small fraction of the healing attributes this plant has to offer.

Native Americans used all parts of *Rosa* spp. in a wide variety of applications. The seeds were cooked and ingested for relief from muscular pains. The roots were used as a general purpose astringent for diarrhea, sore throat, conjunctivitis, and to stop bleeding. The flower petals were employed as a bacteriostatic protective bandage on burns and minor wounds and as a treatment for colic and heartburn. A poultice of the leaves was used for insect stings and bites. All of these uses can be safely applied to animals.

Each part of a rose plant represents a different level of astringency. The flower petals are mildly to moderately astringent and can be made into a sweet-smelling

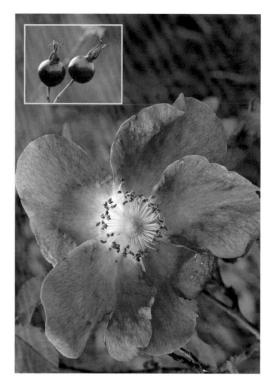

Rosa woodsii

rinse for animals with dry, itchy skin. Petal tea is also useful for mild to moderate cases of colic and diarrhea or for minor irritations of the mouth and stomach. Making a tea is simple—infuse a handful of fresh petals in a cup of near-boiling water. After the tea has cooled, it can be fed to dogs and cats at a dose of 1 tablespoon per 20 pounds of the animal's body weight, as needed. If necessary it can be added to your companion's drinking water. The cooled and strained tea is also useful as an anti-inflammatory eyewash, especially in cases where redness and eye rubbing is attributable to dust or other environmental irritants.

The leaves are stronger than the flower petals and can be decocted for use as a rinse for contact dermatitis or inflamed fleabites or fly bites. Internally, the leaf decoction is useful for cystitis and acute digestive tract inflammations that may be secondary to bacterial or parasitic infection. A typical dose is a ½ teaspoon for each 30 pounds of the animal's weight, once or twice daily, for no longer than four days. The bark and stems offer the strongest astringency and may be useful for acute cases of urinary or digestive tract inflammation that involve labored or painful urination, gushing diarrhea, or minor bleeding. Care must be taken to avoid feeding sharp rose thorns to your companion. The dose is the same as for a leaf decoction, but the maximum duration of use is shorter—the bark and stem decoction should not be used internally for more than two days.

Rose hips are high in vitamin C and serve as a tasty and nutritious treat for animals. Our dogs harvest and eat them as trail snacks! The whole hip can be fed either fresh or dried. Dried hips can be ground in an electric coffee grinder and added to your companion's food as a nutritional supplement. Dogs and cats can be fed ½–1 teaspoon of the ground hips per cup of food. Horses and other large herbivores can be fed a handful or two each day. Because of the ascorbic acid content, too much rose hip causes stomach upset or diarrhea. If this happens, cut back on the amount in the daily feedings.

Availability: Hundreds of rose varieties are available through nurseries. The best are the smaller-flowered wild species that are available through nurseries that specialize in native plants.

Propagation and Harvest: Roses are easy to grow. They prosper in moist, slightly acidic soil. Leaves and flowers can be harvested any time as long as they look healthy. The hips are harvested in the fall after they turn bright red but before they shrivel. The hips can be dried indoors on a clean piece of paper. They keep for several years if stored in a glass jar and kept away from direct sunlight. Don't grind the hips until you need them, otherwise you greatly shorten their shelf life. Harvest the stem bark when you prune your roses each year. Most domesticated varieties have large thorns that can be snapped off. If this isn't possible, you can use the small thornless end stems and peduncles (the stem part just beneath the flowers and hips). The stems can be cut into small segments with pruning clippers or chopped with a sharp knife. They can then be decocted, just like the bark.

Alternatives and Adjuncts: Raspberry leaf, nettle, and chamomile serve as alternatives where a mild urinary or digestive astringent is indicated. For acute cystitis or colic, rose leaf or bark combines with marshmallow, licorice, or slippery elm. Skin rinse alternatives include calendula, chamomile, uva ursi, and juniper. For conjunctivitis, raspberry leaf serves as a replacement, and Oregon grape serves as an excellent antimicrobial adjunct.

Cautions and Comments: The high tannin content in the bark can irritate the urinary tract and kidneys and can trigger uterine contractions, therefore rose bark is best avoided in pregnant animals or those with preexisting kidney problems. Internal use should be limited to acute disorders and short-term therapies (two days or less). Call your veterinarian immediately if internal bleeding is evident, diarrhea is persistent, or urination is labored.

ROSEMARY

Rosmarinus officinalis   Mint Family

Appearance: A creeping or erect shrub that can grow to 6 feet tall, rosemary is characterized by its piney fragrance; narrow, leathery, and densely arranged opposite leaves; and white, pink, or blue 3/8-inch-long flowers.

Habitat and Range: Rosemary is a native of the Mediterranean region, but several cultivars of rosemary are grown worldwide.

Cycle and Bloom Season: A perennial that blooms anytime from early spring to late summer, depending on climate

Parts Used: Leaves, stems, and flowers

Primary Medicinal Activities: Tonic, antidepressant, stimulant, analgesic, expels intestinal gas, antispasmodic, promotes menstrual discharge, astringent, antioxidant, antimicrobial, insect repellent

Strongest Affinities: Nervous system, digestive tract, circulatory system, respiratory tract, and skin

Preparation: Tea, tincture

Common Uses: Rosemary is an extremely useful herb. At the top of its list of medicinal attributes are nervine, antidepressant, antispasmodic, and carminative properties that combine to make rosemary an excellent remedy for flatulent dyspepsia and other digestive problems that are secondary to general nervousness, excitability, or irritability. Adding to rosemary's utility as a calming agent are borneol and an assortment of volatile oils that are known to

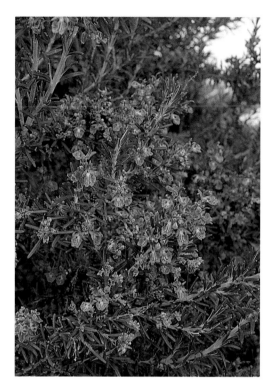

Rosmarinus officinalis

have antispasmodic effects upon the heart and other smooth muscles of the body. These activities not only help moderate cardiac arrhythmia but also serve to strengthen heart function, making rosemary especially beneficial in situations where an animal is recovering from a fearful or traumatic experience, or even shock. The rosmarinic acid contained in the plant is believed to have painkilling properties. In any of the aforementioned instances, about 1/8 teaspoon (0.5 milliliter) of tincture can be given orally as a starting dose for each 20 pounds of an animal's body weight, up to three times daily. Horses and other large herbivores can be fed a handful of the fresh stems and leaves daily.

In addition to its uses as a calming agent, rosemary can be employed as a general cardiovascular tonic, where it not only serves to moderate and improve heart function but also helps to strengthen capillary structures. And when added to your companion's food, rosemary helps mask the flavor of less-palatable herbs and serves as a natural barrier against food-borne bacteria. The ursolic acid and carnisol constituents of rosemary have antioxidant and antimicrobial properties that are effective against *Pseudomonas fluorescens, Rhodoturula glutinius,* and other pathogens that contribute to food spoilage. In fact, rosemary's effectiveness is comparable to that of the more harmful chemical preservatives BHA or BHT. To use rosemary as a preservative, add ¼ teaspoon of powdered herb to each pound of a dog's or cat's homemade diet.

Rosemary also has excellent antimicrobial properties inside or on your companion's body. Scientific studies have shown that it is active against various types of fungi, as well as numerous gram-positive and gram-negative bacteria, including *Staphylococcus albus, Staphylococcus aureus, E. coli, Vibrio cholerae,* and corynebacteria.[6] This makes rosemary useful in antibacterial skin and eye rinses; for minor cuts and burns; and for fighting infections of the mouth, throat, and urinary and digestive tracts.

Ten drops of rosemary essential oil can be diluted with 1 ounce of apricot kernel or almond oil for topical use in the treatment of sprains, arthritic joints, sciatica, and neuralgia. Rubbed into the skin at the site of discomfort, the oil stimulates capillary circulation and helps to relieve muscular and nerve pain. Do not use undiluted rosemary oil internally or externally, though, because it is strong and can cause immediate irritation. The oil is contraindicated for animals who have any type of seizure disorder.

Availability: Rosemary plants are available through nurseries. The dried or fresh herb is available at grocery and health food stores.

Propagation and Harvest: Rosemary is easy to grow from transplants and can be kept as a houseplant in areas where winters are severe. It's not particular about soil and does best in full sun. In the southern and West Coast portions of the U.S., rosemary is often seen as a hedge-forming landscape shrub, which, unfortunately, is unheard of in colder climates.

Rosemary can be started from seed, but germination percentages are poor and the seedlings grow slowly. Rosemary can be harvested anytime, but the leaves' medicinal qualities are strongest in late summer.

Alternatives and Adjuncts: For depressive disorders or nervousness, rosemary can be combined with skullcap or oatstraw. If such a problem is causing digestive disorders, such as vomiting, flatulence, and colic, look toward fennel, dill, flaxseed, parsley, or chamomile as an adjunct. For use as an antimicrobial, rosemary is strengthened by Oregon grape. For topical first aid, rosemary oil combines with arnica, Saint-John's-wort, cayenne, aloe, calendula, or willow bark. For itchy skin and fleas, rosemary and calendula combine as a soothing, healing flea-repellent rinse.

Cautions and Comments: In horses, the volatile oils of rosemary may be detectable in a blood sample;is possible that it may be considered a "prohibited substance" under Jocky Club or other horse show rules. Otherwise, rosemary is a very safeherb.

SAGE

Salvia officinalis   Mint Family

Appearance: Over eight hundred species of *Salvia* exist worldwide, and most are medicinally useful. Most gardeners and Epicureans are familiar with *S. officinalis*, common garden sage. Many of the wild species share the same unique "pebbled" leaf texture and have a similar but much stronger flavor and aroma. Flowers of the *Salvia* genus range from white to deep purple. It's important to know that many wild plants with a sagelike fragrance, or even a common name that contains the word sage are unrelated to the sage we use in the kitchen. One example is sagebrush (*Artemisia tridentata*), a member of the sunflower family that smells like sage but can be harmful if used internally. Given the availability and effectiveness of culinary sage, there's little reason to harvest wild sage for your companion. If, however, you do opt to use a wild sage, learn its Latin name first. If the plant you are considering isn't a *Salvia*, then it's a different medicine as well.

Habitat and Range: Common sage is a native of the Mediterranean region. Dozens of cultivars have been developed and are farmed throughout the world.

In the coastal canyons of southern California, native species such as white sage (*S. apiana*), black sage (*S. mellifera*), Munz's sage (*S. munzii*), and purple sage (*S. leucophylla*) often stand as the predominant flora, growing in dense stands of 2- to 6-foot-high shrubs that may cover the landscape for miles. As one travels north or east, the distribution of *Salvia* species becomes more scattered and less varied, and the plants tend to be small and less predominant. In the deserts of eastern

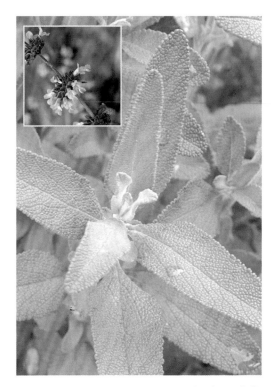

Salvia leucophylla

Washington and Oregon, grayball sage (*S. dorrii*) brings the dry, brushy landscape alive with vibrant hues of purple.

Cycle and Bloom Season: Perennials that bloom in early to late spring

Parts Used: Leaves, small stems, and flowers

Primary Medicinal Activities: Antiseptic, astringent, antispasmodic, expels intestinal gas, inhibits sweating (is an antihydrotic)

Strongest Affinities: Mouth, digestive tract, skin

Preparation: Tea or tincture

Common Uses: Sage is an excellent remedy for infections or ulcerations of the mouth, skin, or digestive tract. Most of its antimicrobial activity is attributable to its content of thujone, a volatile oil that is effective against *E. coli*, *Shigella sonnei*, *Salmonella* spp., *Klebsiella ozanae*, *Bacillus subtillis*, and various fungi—namely *Candida albicans*, *Candida krusei*, *Candida pseudotropicalis*, *Torulopsis glabrata*, and *Cryptococcus neoformans*. A strong sage tea or tincture is useful for treating and preventing gingivitis as well as infection that is secondary to injury or dental surgery. For bacterial or fungal infections of the throat and digestive tract, sage serves as a safe and effective antibiotic and helps to expel gas and ease gastric cramping. Horses and other large herbivores can be fed a handful or two of the fresh leaves or a cup of dried leaves in their daily food ration as a treatment for colic and flatulence that is secondary to bacterial or fungal infection. For smaller animals, the tea can be added to drinking water, or a tincture can be administered directly by mouth. If you choose to make tea, steep 1 tablespoon of the dried leaves in a cup of near-boiling water. Stir the mixture frequently until it has cooled to lukewarm. Strain out the plant material but don't discard it if you're treating a localized infection or ulcer. It can be used as a poultice by directly applying it to an affected area. The tea can be sweetened with honey (which has its own healing properties) and fed at a rate of 1 fluid ounce per 20 pounds of the animal's body weight, two or three times daily. If you choose to use a tincture, a good starting dose is 0.5–1.0 milliliter per 30 pounds of the animal's body weight, twice daily.

In the form of a rinse, poultice, or fomentation, sage tea is useful for treating bacterial or fungal infections of the skin, including ringworm. In such instances, thoroughly soak your companion with the cooled tea once or twice daily. The tea is also a safe and natural disinfectant for turtle or lizard enclosures and may be combined with liquid soap for use as a hand wash after handling animals who may carry salmonella.

Availability: Fresh or dried sage is available at food stores. The plants are available at most nurseries.

Propagation and Harvest: Sage is an easy-to-grow "must have" for the home herb gardener. It likes heavy, slightly acid soil and full sun. It is drought resistant and winter hardy, but in regions where temperatures reach below −10° F, a thick fall mulch is required. Collect the leaves and small stems during midday, when the volatile oils are most concentrated in the leaves, and preferably when the plants are just beginning to bloom. The best way to dry sage is to tie the leaves into small bundles and hang them indoors. When the leaves are crunchy dry, they are ready to store in an airtight glass jar away from sunlight. Properly stored, the herb keeps for two or three years—as long as it smells strong, it's still good medicine.

Alternatives and Adjuncts: For mouth infections, thyme, rosemary, and bee balm are also effective, and consider Oregon grape and myrrh as strong adjuncts or alternatives. For digestive problems, sage combines with Oregon grape, licorice, fennel, parsley, dill, or marshmallow. For infections of the skin, calendula, aloe, chaparral, chamomile, rosemary, and uva ursi all deserve some study.

Cautions and Comments: The undiluted essential oil of sage can cause skin irritation and should not be given internally. Sage is said to inhibit lactation.

SAINT-JOHN'S-WORT

Hypericum perforatum

Saint-John's-Wort
Family

Appearance: Saint-John's-wort is a sturdy perennial weed distinguished by its yellow five-petaled flowers and its small (up to 3/4 inch long) narrowly lance-shaped to elliptical leaves. The flowers and leaves are covered with tiny purplish black dots, each containing hypericin, a medicinally active compound that is often visible as a red stain on the skin after rubbing the foliage between one's fingertips. Saint-John's-wort varies in size among species, but all of them are similar in appearance. The largest and most widespread species, *Hypericum perforatum*, may reach 32 inches in height, whereas *H. anagalloides* (bog Saint-John's-wort), one of the smallest species, grows in mats seldom exceeding 4 inches in height.

Habitat and Range: Habitat varies according to species, but generally the larger species prefer dry to moist open hillsides up to about 6,000 feet in elevation, whereas higher elevations and wetter habitats tend to yield the smaller species. In the Pacific Northwest, *H. perforatum* and *H. formosum* are common and often profuse on open range lands at foothill elevations, where they are considered noxious weeds because of their alleged toxicity to livestock. Saint-John's-wort is a European import that now ranges throughout the Pacific and Rocky Mountain states and in isolated stands through the central and eastern portions of North America.

Cycle and Bloom Season: A perennial that is sometimes referred to as Fourth of July flower, Saint-John's-wort usually blooms from early July through August.

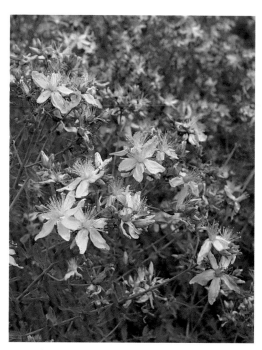

Hypericum perforatum

Parts Used: The top 12 inches of the flowering plant

Primary Medicinal Activities: Wound healing, moderates nerve transmissions (nervine), antiseptic, antiviral, antidepressive, immunostimulant.

Strongest Affinities: Nervous system, skin

Preparation: Tea, tincture, or topical preparation of the fresh herb

Common Uses: It's amazing how our opinions can change by simply looking closer at what we take for granted. Saint-John's-wort has long been regarded as an invasive weed in the western portions of the U.S. Until recently, people wanted to eradicate this plant from the range lands on which it so successfully flourishes, competes with native plants, and threatens grazing livestock with possible toxic side effects. But now, in light of extensive scientific research, Saint-John's-wort has been promoted from the status of a universally hated weed to that of a valued medicine that offers a wealth of curative power. Our awareness of Saint-John's-wort's benefits comes in the midst of an enormous health care crisis and forces us to reevaluate our short-sighted approaches to plants we ignorantly view as our enemies. As well as giving us a valuable opportunity to reconsider the true values in our surroundings, Saint-John's-wort offers new hope in the treatment of AIDS, chronic depression, nervous system disorders, and various forms of herpes virus. A plant is seen as a weed only when we cannot recognize its useful purpose. Because of the lesson we've learned from Saint-John's-wort, we are forced to wonder about the usefulness of all plants and to consider the price we may be paying when we choose to eradicate certain plants in favor of agricultural economics.

Saint-John's-wort has received a great deal of media attention for its demonstrated ability to act as an antidepressant in both humans and animals. Literally hundreds of recent scientific studies have confirmed that it may act as a safe, effective, and natural alternative to antidepressant drugs. In Germany and other European countries, where the most research is being conducted on Saint-John's-wort and its derivatives, the plant has been deemed safe and effective by the government, and millions of people are using the plant daily to treat chronic depression without ill side effects. In fact, one pharmaceutical brand of Saint-John's-wort is being prescribed in Germany at a rate of seven to one over the popular antidepressant drug Prozac. And in the U.S., an increasing number of holistic veterinarians are using the herb to treat separation anxiety and aggression disorders in dogs and cats. Contrary to popular belief, however, Saint-John's-wort does not offer a neatly packaged holistic solution to depressive disorders, especially not for animals.

The antidepressive qualities of Saint-John's-wort represent only a small portion of what this plant has to offer. Saint-John's-wort also has antiviral, vulnerary (wound and burn healing), nerve tonic, and antibacterial activities that are unparalleled by any other herb. And while a great deal of research and marketing has been focused on the hypericin constituents (a red pigment contained within tiny glands that dot the flower petals and leaves of the plant) of Saint-John's-wort, this herb contains dozens of other chemical compounds that have been shown to possess a tremendous range of healing actions. These compounds include various essential oils, flavonoids, tannins, and phytosterol constituents—all of which combine to make Saint-John's-wort active against a wide variety of bacteria, fungi, and even viruses.

For the treatment of burns and wounds, Saint-John's-wort helps speed the healing process while reducing pain at the site of injury. As an antibiotic, preparations of Saint-John's-wort extract have been shown to be as effective as many of their pharmaceutical counterparts, including sulfonamides, a group of general-use antibiotics commonly prescribed for treatment of bacterial infections in dogs, cats, horses, and a wide variety of other animals. Saint-John's-wort is especially useful in instances where soft tissues, joints, or nerve endings have been crushed, crimped, or bruised, a condition that may occur when a cattle dog is stomped or kicked or when a cat expends another of her nine lives in a run-in with an automobile. For first aid purposes, Saint-John's-wort can be applied directly to the site of injury in the form of a salve, a tincture, or an oil infusion, or the tincture can be administered internally. We would probably opt to do both in the described circumstances as the topical application helps to prevent infection and speed healing, while the phytosterol and flavonoid constituents of the internal dose help with nerve pain and repair. Giving 12 drops of the tincture per 20 pounds of the animal's body weight, administered twice daily, is a good starting point in terms of internal dosage.

Saint-John's-wort offers a great deal of promise in the treatment of various forms of viral and retroviral infections, including AIDS, FIV, Epstein-Barr virus, influenza, herpes, and viral hepatitis (particularly in ducks and other fowl). In essence, Saint-John's-wort inhibits reproduction of these viruses, especially if the herb is administered during the earliest stages of disease. In AIDS research, the hope is that Saint-John's-wort will prove to slow the progression of the HIV virus. So far studies have been promising, but it's too early to define the depth of Saint-John's-wort's role in this capacity. Regardless, its use in fighting human or feline AIDS is worth a serious try.

Saint-John's-wort extract may be effective as a preventive measure in dogs who have been exposed to a potentially fatal canine herpes viral infection or in cats, horses, or other animals suffering from a herpes virus. The point to remember is that Saint-John's-wort will not cure the animal of herpes, but it may help keep the virus in check. In our experience with people who suffer from herpes, simultaneous internal and external applications of Saint-John's-wort extract expedites remission of the virus and often helps to lengthen the comfortable period between outbreaks.

Availability: Saint-John's-wort is a widely distributed weed in the western U.S. Seeds are available from specialty seed catalogs. The dried herb and its various preparations are available through herb retailers.

Propagation and Harvest: Saint-John's-wort is easy to transplant or start from seed, but before you plant it, be aware that it is listed as a harmful weed in many areas of the country. If you introduce this plant into your herb garden, be careful that it doesn't escape cultivation. Harvest when the plants are in full bloom, usually in early to mid-July. Clip off the flowering tops, and plan on making tincture or an oil infusion as quickly after harvest as possible—this plant is most effective if made into medicine while it is fresh.

Alternatives and Adjuncts: For anxiety and depressive disorders, lemon balm, skullcap, valerian, and passionflower serve as adjuncts or alternatives. For injuries, Saint-John's-wort combines well with comfrey, calendula, aloe, cayenne, yarrow, or arnica. Licorice, devil's claw, or yucca root all serve as anti-inflammatory adjuncts. Consider oatstraw, skullcap, cayenne, and valerian as possible alternatives or adjuncts for nerve-related problems. As an antiviral or antiseptic, Saint-John's-wort combines with echinacea, Oregon grape, certified organic goldenseal, bee balm, thyme, or sage.

Cautions and Comments: Recent scientific studies have taught us that this herb may strengthen the effects of general anesthesia. Therefore, Saint-John's-wort should not be used within 48 hours preceding surgery. While other adverse side effects are rare, some animals can develop a photosensitive rash from its use. Specifically, people or animals with light skin pigments may be susceptible to sunburnlike effects if they consume too much Saint-John's-wort and subsequently spend too much time in bright sunlight. This side effect has been observed in livestock who have foraged on large quantities of the plants and is one of the main reasons Saint-John's-wort is the subject of herbicidal intervention in some areas of the West. Common sense should preside here—use extra caution if your animal has white hair, white or pink skin pigment, or a short coat. If a rash does develop, get the animal out of direct sunlight and discontinue use of Saint-John's-wort. Consider finding an alternative therapy—it may be that your animal is not a proper candidate for Saint-John's-wort. As always, it is a good idea to consult a holistic veterinarian before diagnosing your pet's condition and self-prescribing any course of therapy.

SHEPHERD'S PURSE

Capsella bursa-pastoris   Mustard Family

Appearance: Shepherd's purse is a common lawn and vacant lot weed that begins its life as a ground-hugging rosette of 1- to 2-inch leaves that are hairy underneath and smooth on top. Later, the upper plant develops one or more slender, erect stems that can grow to about 20 inches tall. The lance-shaped leaves of the upper plant grow alternately, clasping the stem at their bases.

Small, white, inconspicuous flowers are presented at the top of the plant. The flowers develop into seed-bearing capsules that look like tiny (½ inch or smaller), pointed heart-shaped purses—a characteristic that likely earned the plant its common name. These little purses are two-celled, have a single ridge along one side, and are slightly concave along the other. Each cell contains tiny seeds.

Many herbalists take the purse characteristics of shepherd's purse for granted and don't look closely enough when identifying the plant before harvesting. Subsequently, many of them end up gathering and using the wrong plant. Although the impostor is usually another harmless member of the mustard family (Cruciferae), it is often medicinally useless. The seed capsules of the look-alikes have two cells, but each cell contains only two seeds, whereas shepherd's purse always has several seeds.

Habitat and Range: Shepherd's purse is a European import that is widely distributed across North America. It is common in cultivated fields, gardens, lawns, vacant lots, livestock grazing areas, and other disturbed areas. It can be found in almost any environment, from cracks in city streets to remote mountain campsites. It is adaptable to any elevation from below sea level to timberline.

Cycle and Bloom Season: An annual that continuously reseeds itself

Parts Used: Entire plant, including roots

Primary Medicinal Activities: Diuretic, astringent, stops bleeding, tonic

Strongest Affinities: Urinary tract, joints

Preparation: Tea, tincture, fresh or dried herb

Common Uses: Shepherd's purse is especially useful in cases of minor urinary system bleeding. The diuretic activity of this plant is strong enough to increase urinary volume and thus lower the concentration of acidic strong, dark urine, while its mild astringency helps to reduce inflammation in the bladder, urethra, and kidneys. Although it is a relatively weak diuretic, its low volatile oil content makes it a gentle alternative to oil-rich herbs such as parsley root, which are contraindicated in preexisting cases of kidney disease. Shepherd's purse is indicated for arthritic conditions that are believed to be compounded by retention of excess systemic waste materials, where it is believed to help with the removal of fluid and various acid compounds from the joints.

Studies have shown that the hemostatic activity of shepherd's purse in the uterus and urinary tract is attributable to more than just simple tissue-shrinking astringency. The plant contains an assortment of amine and flavonoid constituents that are believed to actually strengthen capillaries and reduce their permeability. This makes shepherd's purse an excellent urinary tonic for animals who exhibit occasional blood in the urine as a result of structural anomalies, scar tissue, or nonspecific atony of the bladder. It has also been found to enhance uterine tone, contract the uterine walls, and lower blood pressure, making it useful in postpartum bleeding and difficult placenta delivery.

Externally, a poultice of the fresh plant can be applied to wounds to stop bleeding. A tincture, poultice, or water or oil infusion can be applied to the skin, as a weak alternative to mustard, to increase subcutaneous capillary circulation at the site of closed-tissue injuries and to help improve the strength and structure of capillaries.

Availability: A widespread weed; available through specialty seed catalogs

Propagation and Harvest: Rather than buy dried shepherd's purse at an herb store, it's

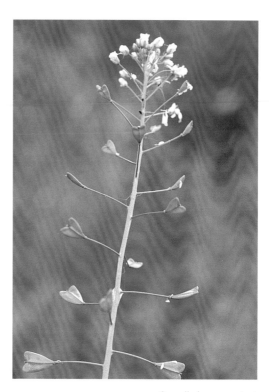

Capsella bursa-pastoris

best to harvest your own fresh herb. The herb loses much of its medicinal potency when it dries and should be used or made into tincture as soon as it is harvested. This plant is easy to grow and spreads all over the garden if allowed. It grows in most soils but grows best in heavily manured soil, which is why it is so common in pastures. Harvest by pulling up the entire plant after the seed capsules have developed but before the plant dries.

Alternatives and Adjuncts: Shepherd's purse can be combined with yarrow in fresh herb tea for bleeding fibroids or as an external first aid remedy (use the two herbs in a poultice). For arthritis, shepherd's purse combines with yucca root, boswellia, devil's claw, licorice, or alfalfa. Dandelion leaf serves as a stronger, yet equally safe, diuretic. For urinary bleeding that is secondary to infection, combine with marshmallow, echinacea, and Oregon grape.

Cautions and Comments: The authors have never witnessed any side effects from the use of this herb, but it has been theorized by others that Shepherd's purse can cause contractions of the uterus and should not be administered to pregnant animals— reserve it for the postpartum period. It is also thought to have hemostatic properties that may interfere with blood-thinning drugs. Therefore, caution and common sense dictates that this herb is best avoided in animals with clotting disorders.

SKULLCAP

Scutellaria lateriflora   Mint Family

Appearance: Skullcap is differentiated from other mints by its blue or white flowers, which are borne (in most species) at the top third of the plant in symmetrically arranged sets of two or more. The flowers are two lobed and tubular; one lobe forms an upper lip, and one forms a larger apronlike lower lip. The lance-shaped, finely to coarsely toothed leaves oppose one another, as in all mints. Like most mints, skullcap has distinctly four-sided stems.

Habitat and Range: Several native species of skullcap grow in North America, most of which live in moist meadows, seeps from springs, and riparian thickets. *Scutellaria lateriflora* and several other cultivars are grown throughout the world.

Cycle and Bloom Season: An annual or perennial (depending on species and climate) that blooms from June to August

Parts Used: Leaves, stems, and flowers

Primary Medicinal Activities: Moderates nerve transmissions, sedative, antispasmodic, anticonvulsant

Strongest Affinities: Nervous system

Preparation: Tea, tincture, dried or fresh herb

Common Uses: For centuries, herbalists have recognized skullcap as one of the most effective herbal nervines available. It is commonly used for acute or chronic cases of nervous tension or anxiety and to help relieve pain from nerve-related injury or disease. Historically, it has been used to treat convulsions, epilepsy, multiple sclerosis, hysteria, and delirium tremens, which is shaking and delirium associated with withdrawals from alcohol (also called d.t.'s). *Scutellaria lateriflora* is still known by many people as "mad dog weed" from its use in the eighteenth century as a cure for rabies. Yet despite its rich history and current popularity among herbalists, very little scientific study has been focused on this plant. From the studies that have been conducted, we have learned that the chemistry of skullcap varies considerably between species, although all species that are marketed and used as herbal medicine contain scutellarin, a flavonoid compound that has been shown to possess sedative and antispasmodic qualities.

We find skullcap especially effective for general nervousness and excitability in dogs and cats and for any condition characterized by oversensitivity of the peripheral nerves. It helps relieve nervous tension related to pain or a traumatic experience, and it is useful as an antispasmodic in nervous irritations of the cerebrospinal system such as sciatica or posttraumatic neuralgia.

Unlike valerian and other herbal sedatives, skullcap by itself does not bring about drowsiness, nor does it dull the reflexes or interfere with motor coordination. Instead, skullcap acts to moderate an animal's responsiveness to physical or nonphysical stimuli and helps to alleviate general restlessness and nervous twitching. This makes it suitable for high-strung felines who are recovering from a frightful experience but who need all of their survival mechanisms intact during their daily outdoor adventures.

Herbalists consider skullcap a specific remedy for grand mal epileptic seizures. We have received several encouraging reports from people who are using skullcap to reduce the severity and frequency of seizures in their epileptic dogs, especially when the herb is combined in equal parts with valerian. Science has not yet revealed exactly how skullcap works in this capacity, but herbalists theorize that it may calm nerve impulses throughout the body, while inhibiting activity in higher brain centers where epileptic seizures might be triggered. Skullcap's effectiveness in moderating epileptic episodes may explain its traditional reputation as a cure for rabies: back in the eighteenth century, little was known about epilepsy, and it's likely that many epilepsy sufferers were misdiagnosed as having rabies.

For epileptic dogs, 0.5 to 1 milliliter of a low-alcohol tincture can be fed two or three times daily, but see your holistic veterinarian for a thorough workup of your companion before proceeding. For generalized nervousness or to help relieve pain in dogs and cats, 0.5 milliliter per 20 pounds of the animal's weight can be fed as needed, up to three times daily for up to a week. It's important to remember, though, that skullcap and other herbal sedatives can only

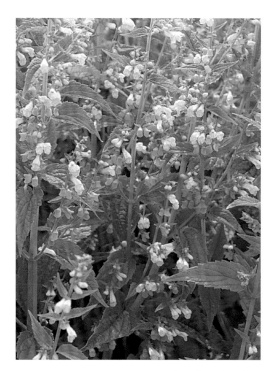

Scutellaria lateriflora

relieve the symptoms of such disorders; they cannot address the underlying causes. For nervousness in a horse, mule, or goat, ½–1 ounce of the dried herb can be added to the animal's feed once per day, as needed.

A study in 1957 showed that skullcap can prevent a rise in serum cholesterol in animals on a high-cholesterol diet, which means that the herb might be useful as a dietary adjunct in animals, such as miniature schnauzers and beagles, who are predisposed to hyperlipidemia.

Availability: Skullcap can be purchased through herb retailers in dried herb form or tinctures. The plants are available through nurseries that specialize in herbs.

Propagation and Harvest: Easy to grow from transplants, skullcap likes consistently moist, rich soil and does best when allowed a few hours of shade each day. Harvest the plants by clipping the upper third of the flowering plant. The plant can be hung in small bunches and dried for later use (the herb keeps for about a year), or the fresh herb can be made into tincture (the optimum choice).

Alternatives and Adjuncts: For epileptic dogs or for use as a nerve-calming sedative, skullcap can be combined with an equal part of valerian. Oatstraw and gotu kola also serve as good adjuncts. For nerve pain and spinal injuries, combine skullcap with an equal amount of Saint-John's-wort.

Cautions and Comments: Some texts and many toxicology databases still claim that skullcap, when used in large quantities, can be damaging to the liver. However, in the years following the first writing of this book, we have learned that such claims are inaccurate. The reports of hepatotoxicity that fueled earlier controversies over the safety of this herb involved skullcap that had been adulterated with germander; an inexpensive look alike that really can be damaging to the liver. Fortunately, the standards by which skullcap is cultivated, processed, and analytically identified are better than ever, and safe, good quality skullcap is in ample supply. Just buy it from a reputable source. This is a very safe herb.

SLIPPERY ELM

Ulmus fulva   Elm Family

Appearance: Slippery elm is a deciduous tree that can grow to 80 feet tall. The outer bark is thick, furrowed, and pinkish brown. The broadly lance-shaped alternate leaves are 4–8 inches long and have toothed margins. The upper surfaces of the leaves feel like sticky sandpaper.

Habitat and Range: Deciduous forests of the eastern half of the U.S. and Canada; slippery elm is at risk of endangerment in many areas.

Cycle and Bloom Season: The tree flowers from March to June and loses its leaves in the fall.

Parts Used: Inner bark

Primary Medicinal Activities: Lubricates, soothes, and protects internal mucous membranes; emollient, astringent, anti-inflammatory, nutritive

Strongest Affinities: Digestive tract, respiratory tract, skin

Preparation: Tea, tincture, dried and powdered inner bark

Common Uses: Slippery elm is best used in the digestive tract, where it serves as a soothing, protecting, and lubricating demulcent and a general astringent at the same time. These effects make slippery elm applicable in a wide variety of circumstances. For diarrhea, enteritis, colitis, and irritations of the stomach, the tannin constituents of slippery elm tighten digestive mucosa to reduce inflammation and inhibit the entrance of excess fluids into the intestines. At the same time, the slippery, oily mucilage constituents of the herb help lubricate the digestive tract to assist in the elimination of waste. In cases of constipation, slippery elm soothes, protects, and lubricates mucous membranes, assisting and relaxing smooth muscles that have been working extra hard to eliminate waste. Higher up in the digestive tract, the mucilaginous astringency of the herb lubricates and helps reduce inflammation in the throat, making swallowing easier and soothing a painful cough. It plays the same roles in the upper respiratory passages, where it relieves the discomforts of kennel cough and other types of bronchitis.

Slippery elm is also nutritious; it was used as a food staple during times of economic hardship in Appalachia. It contains vitamins A, B complex, C, and K and high amounts of calcium, magnesium, and sodium. The fresh inner bark has a slightly sweet pecanlike flavor and was often given to children as a treat to chew on (like chewing gum). It can be fed to convalescing animals as a nutritional digestive tonic—1 teaspoon of the dried inner bark steeped in 8 ounces of hot water to which 1 teaspoon of honey has been added. If constipation is a problem, 1 teaspoon of organic yogurt (a brand that has live cultures) can be added to the mixture. The entire mixture, inner bark and all, is then fed to the animals. Many animals will eat this formula in the absence of anything else, and it is useful for a wide variety of digestive or respiratory problems in dogs and cats. If your companion cannot tolerate honey because of diabetes, allergies, or other problems, eliminate honey from the recipe. If your companion won't eat the bark, strain the fluid through a fine sieve and pour it onto her food. A glycerin-based tincture is also effective and offers the convenience of administering a squirt or two into the mouth. A good starting dose for the tincture is ¼–½ teaspoon (1–2 milliliters) for each 20 pounds of the animal's body weight, once or twice daily.

On the skin, a poultice of slippery elm bark can be applied to wounds, ulcers, boils, or abscesses. In essence, it is used the same way as plantain (*Plantago* sp.), a common weed that is better suited for this purpose

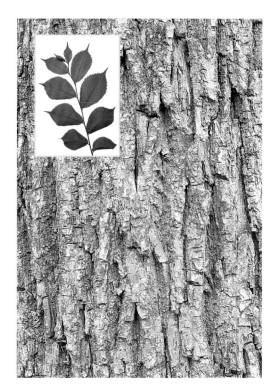

Ulmus fulva

because of its abundance and resilience to human impact.

Availability: Available at herb retailers. When you buy slippery elm bark, make sure that you're getting the inner bark only. The powder or bark should be light, fluffy, and pale pinkish tan in color. If it has darker flecks in it or appears corky, stringy, or woody, it was probably carelessly harvested and the inner bark was not separated from the outer bark. Inclusion of the outer bark dramatically changes the nature of the medicine. The outer bark contains a greater amount of tannin constituents, which may cause digestive or urinary tract irritation.

Propagation and Harvest: Slippery elm is available through nurseries that specialize in native plants. This tree is not difficult to grow, but, like most trees, it grows slowly. If you have room for one of these beautiful shade trees, by all means plant one! You will be doing a dwindling species a great favor.

Alternatives and Adjuncts: Slippery elm has remained quite popular among herb users for centuries. Unfortunately, many of its consumers remain unaware of its declining population in the wild. Slippery elm is being overharvested, and many of the trees are succumbing to Dutch elm disease—a fungal infection that kills trees. Adding to these problems are careless methods by which much of the bark is harvested: the entire tree, which may be one hundred years old, is cut down, stripped of its bark, then used as firewood or hardwood lumber with little regard to sustenance of the species. All in all, consumer demand is currently outstripping natural supply.

We include slippery elm here so that you know to use this herb conservatively, respectfully, and in a proper therapeutic context. Slippery elm should be reserved for circumstances where alternatives are ineffective, and every effort should be made to support the tree's cultivation and conservation in the wild. Fortunately, some effective and accessible alternatives exist for slippery elm. In many instances, slippery elm can be substituted with the common weed plantain (*Plantago* sp.). If a more mucilaginous remedy is needed, marshmallow root (*Althea officinalis*) is an excellent alternative, especially when it is combined with an astringent such as goldenrod or raspberry leaf, or a tincture or decoction of uva ursi or juniper.

Cautions and Comments: With the rare exception of possible allergic reactions, slippery elm is generally safe for animals. The outer bark, however, (which shouldn't be in the slippery elm you buy) can cause irritation to the digestive and urinary tracts and may induce abortion in pregnant animals.

THYME

Thymus vulgaris   Mint Family

Appearance: Most species of thyme are ground-hugging plants with strong sprawling stems, small (1/8 inch) opposite leaves, and tiny cylindrical flowers that range in color from white to pale purple. There are countless variations of leaf color, fragrance, and even flavor available to the gardener. In fact there are so many variations of *Thymus* spp., it is possible to dedicate an entire garden to them.

Habitat and Range: Thyme originated in the Mediterranean region. Over 350 species of *Thymus* exist worldwide most of which are cultivated as a seasoning herb or landscape shrub.

Cycle and Bloom Season: Most of the species of thyme are evergreen perennials. Blooming occurs from early spring to midsummer.

Parts Used: Leaves, stems, and flowers

Primary Medicinal Activities: Antimicrobial, expels intestinal gas, antispasmodic, cough suppressant, expectorant, astringent, expels worms

Strongest Affinities: Digestive and respiratory tracts

Preparation: Tea or tincture

Common Uses: Most of thyme's medicinal activity is attributable to its volatile oil constituents, which are thymol and carvacrol.

Thymol is a good antiseptic for the mouth and throat and is useful for fighting gingivitis in dogs and cats. In fact, it is used as the active ingredient in many commercial toothpaste and mouthwash formulas.

Combined with thyme's infection-fighting qualities are cough suppressant and expectorant properties, which make the herb effective against raspy, unproductive coughs that are secondary to fungal or bacterial infection. As an antispasmodic, thyme helps to ease bronchial spasms related to asthma. A glycerin tincture, or an alcohol tincture that has been sweetened with honey, serves well for most internal applications—¼ teaspoon (1 milliliter) for each 30 pounds of an animal's body weight (12–20 drops for cats), fed to the animal as needed up to twice daily. A cooled tea works too, provided it has been brewed with near-boiling water to draw out the volatile oil constituents—1 teaspoon per 30 pounds of body weight for dogs, ¼ teaspoon for cats, fed directly into the mouth two to three times daily. For infections of the mouth or as a preventative against gingivitis, the tincture or a strong tea can be directly applied to the gum lines or infected sites with a swab. In the digestive tract, it is a useful carminative and antispasmodic in cases of dyspepsia, irritable bowel, and colitis. It also helps expel parasites, especially hookworms. In these cases, the dried or fresh herb can be fed with your companion's food—1 teaspoon per pound of food fed to dogs, a sprinkling for cats. Horses and other large herbivores with digestive problems can be fed a ½ cup of the dried herb or a handful of the fresh plants daily. Rabbits, birds, and other small animals can be fed a couple of fresh sprigs daily. On the surface of the body, thyme tea (skin rinse) or an oil infusion is appropriate for various fungal or bacterial infections of the skin. In the urinary tract, the tea or

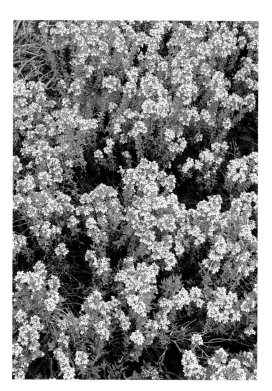

Thymus vulgaris

tincture serves as an antimicrobial as well as a mildly astringent tonic that is said to treat urinary incontinence. Use the tincture doses we have suggested for respiratory problems.

Availability: Thyme can be purchased at any food market. The plants are available at nurseries.

Propagation and Harvest: Thyme is easy to grow from seeds or transplants. It prefers light soil with neutral acidity but can be grown just about anywhere. It is an excellent choice for rock gardens and walkway borders.

Alternatives and Adjuncts: For infections of the mouth, thyme combines with myrrh, Oregon grape, certified organic goldenseal, bee balm, or sage. For respiratory infections, combine with garlic, echinacea, bee balm, or sage. For asthma, thyme works best when used in conjunction with elecampane, mullein leaf, nettle, or lobelia. For digestive problems, fennel, parsley seeds, chamomile, and peppermint are all good herbs to combine with thyme. For worms, try combining thyme with equal amounts of garlic and raw pumpkin seeds.

Cautions and Comments: Thyme is safe, but when it's ingested in large amounts, it has been known to affect menstrual cycles. Therefore, it should be used with moderation in pregnant animals. When isolated from the rest of the plant, thymol is toxic. Do not use an essential oil of thyme in or on your animal.

In horses, the volatile oils of thyme may be detectable in a blood sample, and it may be considered a "prohibited substance" under Jockey Club or other horse show rules.

UVA URSI

Arctostaphylos uva-ursi   Heath Family

Appearance: Also known as kinnikinnick (an American Indian word meaning "smoking mixture"), uva ursi is a mat-forming, densely branched ground cover with woody trailing stems. Several other species of *Arctostaphylos* are small to medium (up to 10 feet tall) erect hardwood shrubs. In mountainous areas of the southwestern U.S., *A. manzanita* is often seen as a predominant shrub. Despite their size differences, all species present leaf, flower, and fruit characteristics that distinguish them as members of the *Arctostaphylos* genus, and all are medicinally useful despite the fact that A. *uva-ursi* is the species of

primary interest among herbalists. The leathery leaves are spoon to lance shaped, with upper surfaces darker green than their undersides. Flowers are pink and urn shaped, and they are arranged in nodding, few-flowered terminal clusters. The fruits are mealy red berries that look like tiny apples.

Habitat and Range: Open forest clearings from the montane zone up to the timberline. *Arctostaphylos uva-ursi* is the predominant species, ranging throughout the northern third of the U.S., Canada, and Europe. In the mountains of Washington, Oregon, Nevada, Arizona, New Mexico, and especially California (where *A. manzanita* is protected by law), several of the larger shrub varieties are predominant.

Cycle and Bloom Season: Blooms April through June. Fruits begin to develop in midsummer.

Parts Used: Leaves and twigs

Primary Medicinal Activities: Astringent, antimicrobial, diuretic

Strongest Affinities: Urinary tract and skin

Preparation: Decoction or tincture

Common Uses: Uva ursi contains a considerable amount of tannins (up to 40 percent), making it one of nature's most powerful astringents. It also contains hydroquinones—an assortment of chemical compounds that are active against a wide variety of pathogens, including *Mycobacterium smegmatis*, *Staphylococcus aureus*, *Bacillus subtilus*, *E. coli*, and various *Shigella* species. Each of these pathogens are often implicated in urinary tract infections.

It's important to know, however, that for uva ursi to be an effective treatment for urinary tract infections, an alkaline reaction is necessary to release the hydroquinone into an active form. This means that uva ursi cannot contribute antibacterial activities to a urinary system in which urine is acidic, a condition that is common in animals, especially cats, with chronic urinary tract problems. In these circumstances, it is necessary either to elevate urine pH into a healthier alkaline state or to combine uva ursi with other antibacterial herbs (the easier option). Regardless of urine pH, uva ursi serves as an effective astringent to stop bleeding and reduce urinary tract inflammation.

Uva ursi is a strong herb, and its high tannin content can irritate the kidneys if used for more than a few consecutive days. Therefore, it is best reserved for situations in which quick intervention is needed.

To use uva ursi internally, make a decoction from the fresh or dried leaves and stems. Use 1 cup of the dried herb for each 3 cups of water. The leathery, almost plasticlike structure of this plant makes it nearly impervious to water, so a simple tea is not an option. For dogs, 1 teaspoon of the cooled decoction can be fed once daily for no more than three days. Cats and ferrets require only ¼–½ teaspoon. Have the animal drink as much water as possible when using this herb, even if you must resort to using a meat broth. The idea is to course the herb through the urinary tract so it can quickly alleviate infection and reduce inflammation. Then, after a day or two, gentler astringent herbs can be used to finish the therapy safely and effectively. Horses and other large herbivores can be fed 1 cup of the dried leaves daily for up to three days. For contact dermatitis, seborrhea, and fleabites, the decoction

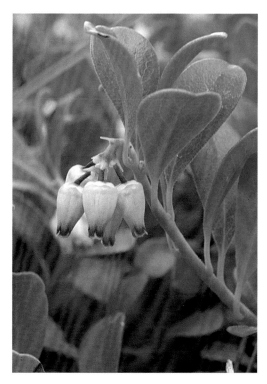

Arctostaphylos uva-ursi

can be diluted (1 cup decoction to 1 quart of water) and used as an antibacterial and astringent skin rinse.

Availability: Uva ursi is available through herb retailers. The plants are available through nurseries that specialize in native plant landscaping.

Propagation and Harvest: Uva ursi is hardy northward to central Canada and serves as an excellent antierosion ground cover. It's not particular about soil but prefers slightly to moderately acid conditions. Uva ursi and other members of the *Arctostaphylos* genus are especially good landscape choices in mountain areas of the western United States and Canada. The leaves and trailing stems can be clipped, dried, and used anytime during their evergreen growth.

Alternatives and Adjuncts: When treating most forms of urinary tract infection, it's a good idea to help flush the animal's system with the use of diuretic herbs. Dandelion leaf, chickweed, cleavers, or shepherd's purse serves this purpose well. For animals with overly concentrated acidic urine, uva ursi can be preceded (by an hour or so) by a dose of mullein leaf tea, which is moderately effective at alkalinizing the urine. Uva ursi also can be combined with antimicrobials such as Oregon grape, sage, thyme, or echinacea. Marshmallow serves as a soothing and lubricating adjunct in urinary tract therapies and is especially useful in the passage of stones and gravel. Corn silk, couch grass, horsetail, raspberry leaf, and cleavers all serve as weaker urinary astringents that are suitable for minor to moderately severe urinary ailments.

Cautions and Comments: Uva ursi is believed to inhibit oxygen delivery to the uterus and therefore should not be used in pregnant animals. Like all strong astringents, long-term internal use of uva ursi may irritate the kidneys, bladder, and urethra. Uva ursi may be contraindicated in cases of preexisting kidney inflammation or renal failure. See your veterinarian in these circumstances.

VALERIAN

Valeriana officinalis   Valerian Family

Appearance: Many people relate the strongly aromatic roots of valerian to the odor of dirty gym socks. Once you have experienced the odor of this plant, identification becomes as simple as probing a finger into the soil to scratch a root. The foliage of this plant is unique as well—the plant first emerges as a cluster of loosely arranged lance-shaped leaves that usually remain larger than the leaves of the mature upper plant. Upper leaves are divided and become progressively smaller toward the top of the plant. Flowers are borne in branched clusters of small white to pink blossoms at the top of the plant. Roots are stringy, brown, and pungent. Several native species of *Valeriana* occur throughout North America, with size being the primary difference among species. Most wild valerians remain under a foot in height, while domestic valerian can grow in excess of 5 feet tall.

Habitat and Range: Valerian is generally found in soils that retain moisture well into summer. Look for it on north-facing banks or hillsides or in partially shaded soils that are high in organic matter. Several native species occur throughout the western third of the U.S. and Canada. It is less common in the midwestern and eastern portions of North America, but in some areas, especially in New England, *V. officinalis* has escaped cultivation and is thriving.

Cycle and Bloom Season: A perennial that blooms from May to July

Parts Used: Primarily the fall root. The upper parts of the plant are useful, too, but make weaker medicine.

Primary Medicinal Activities: Sedative, antispasmodic, anticonvulsive, expels intestinal gas, lowers blood pressure

Strongest Affinities: Nervous system, digestive tract

Preparation: Tincture, tea, fresh or dried root

Common Uses: Valerian is without doubt the most widely recognized herbal sedative. As a sedative, valerian works safely and gently to help calm the nerves and achieve physical relaxation. It does not induce an altered state like one would expect from a prescription sedative or from consumption of alcohol. Contrary to what many people believe, valerian is not a precursor of the tranquilizer Valium. Valium is the brand name for diazepam, a prescription drug that shares no chemical relationship with valerian.

Herbalists use valerian for insomnia and nervous anxiety and to help the body relax in the presence of physical pain. It is useful in calming animals during thunderstorms and on trips to the vet or groomer or to help your companion rest after surgery. For epileptic animals, it sometimes helps to reduce the frequency and severity of seizures.

Animal studies have concluded that valerenic and valerenal acid work similarly to the drug phenobarbital, a central nervous system depressant that is used as an anticonvulsive. And the herb has been shown to inhibit production of an enzyme that breaks down gamma-aminobutyric acid (GABA), an amino acid that is responsible for inhibiting and regulating neurotransmissions in the brain. The theory is this: by preventing the breakdown of GABA with valerian, the increased neural activity that precedes an epileptic seizure is circumvented, and the triggering mechanism is disabled.

When employed as a sedative, valerian is most effective when small doses are fed several times daily over a period of several days. This is especially true when it is used in anticipation of a high-anxiety event, such as a planned interstate trip or a show. In these circumstances, dogs can be fed 5 drops of the tincture three or four times daily, starting three days prior to the event. Cats need only 1 or 3 drops two or three times daily.

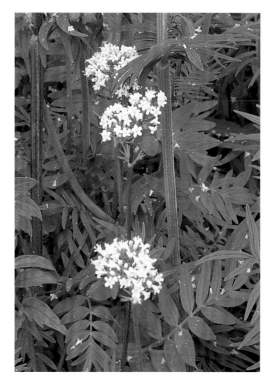

Valeriana officinalis

In the digestive tract, valerian is a useful antispasmodic for situations in which nervousness is compounded by a spastic colon or an upset stomach. But because of valerian's soaplike content, large amounts of this herb may cause nausea and vomiting. For digestive and antiepileptic uses, 0.25–0.5 milliliter of the tincture can be fed for each 30 pounds of an animal's body weight two to three times daily. In horses, valerian helps to reduce anxiety and nervousness without inducing drowsiness or affecting physical performance. Add ½ ounce of the dried and chopped herb or 2 tablespoons of the tincture to the horse's daily feed.

For reasons that remain a mystery, a small percentage of human or animal subjects experience completely opposite effects from valerian—it acts as a stimulant rather than a sedative.

Availability: Various forms of valerian preparations are available through herb retailers. Plants are available through nurseries.

Propagation and Harvest: Valerian can be grown from seeds or transplants. It likes rich, consistently moist soil and full sun or partial shade. It is best to plant valerian early in the spring, when the seedlings and young plants can fully benefit from cool temperatures and precipitation. The roots are dug in late fall of the second year of growth. The fresh roots can be made into tincture or they can be chopped and dried for later use. When properly stored in plastic bags, the dried roots keep for up to three years.

Alternatives and Adjuncts: For epileptic animals, valerian combines well with skullcap. For anxiety and nervousness, valerian can be combined with skullcap, passionflower, hop, oatstraw, or catnip. These herbs also serve as alternatives for animals who have an opposite response to valerian.

Cautions and Comments: Valerian can cause digestive upset if used in large doses, and it should not be used in pregnant animals. Otherwise, it is a safe herb.

WORMWOOD

Artemesia absinthum   Sunflower Family

Appearance: Wormwood is attractive to the eyes and intriguing to the nose. It has silky, finely divided, gray-green leaves and a strong fragrance that is reminiscent of both sage and pine. The tiny yellow ball-like flowers of the plant are presented in loose clusters on the upper branches of the plant. The entire plant may grow to the size of a small bush up to 4 feet tall.

Habitat and Range: A native of Europe, wormwood is cultivated as a garden plant throughout the Northern Hemisphere and has found its way into wild areas throughout most of North America.

It is most commonly found along roadways, in vacant lots, on the edges of cultivated fields, and in other waste areas.

Cycle and Bloom Season: A long-lived perennial that blooms from June to August

Parts Used: Leaves

Primary Medicinal Activities: Antiseptic, antifungal, astringent, expels worms

Strongest Affinities: Skin and digestive tract

Preparation: Tea or dried leaves

Common Uses: As its common name implies, wormwood is among the most well-known herbal worming agents. Hundreds of years of successful use stand in testament to its ability to expel tapeworms, threadworms, and especially roundworms from the intestinal tracts of dogs, cats, horses, goats, sheep, cattle, and humans. We seldom use it, however.

Although wormwood makes life miserable for intestinal parasites, it can also be hard on the host. This is because wormwood contains an assortment of strong volatile oils, bitter principles, and tannins. If used excessively, these constituents can be irritating to the liver and kidneys, and in extreme cases may even damage the nervous system. This is not to say that wormwood can't be used safely, but an extra measure of care and moderation is certainly warranted. The problems with using wormwood are multifaceted: too small a dose is ineffective, but a larger dose might be toxic. Small doses administered over a long period might be effective, but at what cumulative cost to the animal's kidneys, liver, and nervous system? Our conclusion is this: wormwood is useful when the absolute necessity of quick parasite intervention outweighs the risk of toxicity. In holistic animal care, this circumstance is a rarity because therapeutic focus is placed upon the whole animal, not just one or more symptoms of disease.

To use wormwood, up to ¼ teaspoon of the dried powdered herb or about ⅛ teaspoon (0.5 milliliter) of a low-alcohol tincture can be administered daily at mealtime for each 30 pounds of a dog's body weight. Cats can receive up to ⅛ teaspoon daily. Do not administer wormwood internally for more than three consecutive days. Wormwood has an extremely bitter flavor, making it a difficult herb to use. To ease the process of getting it into a hissing cat or tight-lipped dog, the powder or tincture can be placed in a small gel capsule and wrapped with cheese, meat, or other special treat. Externally, wormwood is an effective skin rinse (see chapter 1) for bacterial or fungal infections of the skin, including various forms of dermatophytosis.

Availability: Wormwood is available through herb retailers. Plants and seeds are available from nurseries that specialize in herbs.

Propagation and Harvest: Wormwood is easy to grow, requiring average soil, full sunlight, and only occasional watering. It is hardy northward to central Canada, and plants often live in excess of ten years. The leaves can be harvested anytime, but they are most potent when gathered on a hot summer afternoon.

Alternatives and Adjuncts: For intestinal parasites, garlic, pumpkin seeds, black

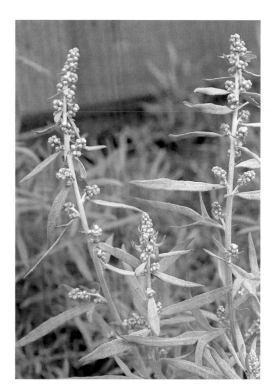

Artemesia absinthum

walnut hulls, sage, thyme, and Oregon grape all serve as effective and safer substitutes. For infections of the skin, wormwood combines with calendula, gotu kola, or aloe. Sage serves similar purposes as a topical antimicrobial.

Cautions and Comments: The volatile oil thujone, which may be present in alcohol extractions of this plant, can be damaging to the liver, kidneys, and nervous system if used excessively. Alcohol preparations of this herb should never be used in animals who suffer from seizures, kidney problems, or liver disease. Wormwood is generally safe when used in dried herb form, or when prepared without alcohol in the form of water infusions (teas) or as a glycerite. However, all forms are best avoided in pregnant or lactating animals.

YARROW

Achillea millefolium   Sunflower Family

Appearance: Yarrow is characterized by its flat-topped terminal clusters of small white to pinkish white flowers and its alternate, finely dissected, featherlike leaves (millefolium translates to "thousand-leafed"). The entire plant is strongly aromatic, with a pungency much like that of mothballs. Stems are often woolly haired. Several cultivars of yarrow have been developed for the floral industry, and many have escaped cultivation. These plants are usually not as cold hardy as their wild cousins and can be identified by their yellow, peach, or red flowers.

Habitat and Range: Yarrow is a native of Asia that has made itself at home throughout the northern hemisphere from sea level to above the timberline. The density of plant populations increases as one travels north through the western U.S.

Cycle and Bloom Season: A perennial that often remains in bloom throughout the spring and summer

Parts Used: Flowers, leaves, and stems

Primary Medicinal Activities: Antiseptic, analgesic, dilates blood vessels, promotes sweating, expectorant, anti-inflammatory, stops bleeding, tonic, lowers blood pressure, fever reducing (febrifuge), insect repellent, expels worms

Strongest Affinities: Circulatory and respiratory systems, urinary and digestive tracts, skin

Preparation: Dry or fresh herb, tea, tincture, or oil infusion

Common Uses: Yarrow is one of the most versatile and well-known herbs in nature's apothecary. In ancient Europe, yarrow was known as "wound wort" by warriors who used the plant (presumably for their horses as well as themselves) to stop bleeding and disinfect wounds on the battlefield. The genus name, Achillea, is derived from the name of the ancient Greek warrior Achilles.

The powder or poultice of the dried or fresh plant is useful for treating less deliberate open wounds such as a barbed wire cut or a foot pad laceration caused by a broken bottle. To effectively stop bleeding and inhibit bacteria, simply crush the herb as finely as possible and apply it directly to the wound. A cooled tea of the plant can be used as a pain- and itch-relieving antiseptic skin rinse, and the aromatic nature of the plant may be of help in repelling fleas, mosquitoes, and biting flies.

Yarrow is a unique peripheral vasodilator and vascular tonic. When taken internally, the flavonoid constituents of yarrow act to dilate and strengthen peripheral blood vessels and help clear away small blood clots, thus increasing circulation to the skin and extremities. Combined with this are anti-inflammatory qualities, making yarrow helpful for problems such as arthritis, navicular syndrome in horses, and severe cases of dermatitis in which peripheral circulation has been impaired by inflammation. It is also useful for subcutaneous blood clots of the ears and the skin, especially when internal doses of the tincture are used simultaneously with external applications of an oil infusion.

In the urinary tract, a yarrow tea or tincture serves as a bacteriostatic agent in the treatment of chronic or acute cystitis. It is useful in the early stage of a kidney infection. In the lungs, yarrow's bacteriostatic and expectorant properties help the body in its effort to eliminate invading microbes and other foreign bodies. At the same time, the herb dilates and tonifies respiratory blood vessels to improve pulmonary efficiency. Because of this remarkable combination of activities, yarrow is among the first herbs we reach for in cases of pneumonia. Yarrow also may be beneficial for racehorses who suffer from hemorrhagic pulmonary edema (bleeding from the respiratory tract) as a result of too much strenuous exercise.

In the digestive tract, yarrow is marginally effective at expelling worms and is useful for inflammations, bleeding, and bacterial infections of the stomach and colon. The bitter principles stimulate digestion and appetite. And yarrow is well known among herbalists as a fever-reducing remedy. It is especially effective when taken as a tea at the onset of a fever.

Scientists once thought that yarrow's therapeutic qualities were chiefly attributable to tannins and a volatile oil called azulene. The chemical makeup of yarrow is extremely complex, however, and recent studies have found that the plant contains sterols and various other compounds that possess a much wider range of medicinal activities than originally thought. One study suggests that yarrow may be a useful antitumor agent and may play an active role in the treatment of certain types of leukemia.

To use yarrow internally in dogs and cats, a tincture is usually preferable over a tea because the herb is bitter and hard to feed in appreciable quantities. For dogs, about ¼ teaspoon (1 milliliter) of the tincture can be fed for each 30 pounds of an animal's body weight, two to three times daily. Cats and similar-sized animals need only ⅛ teaspoon twice daily. Horses and other large herbivores can be allowed to eat the plants from their pastures as they wish, or they can

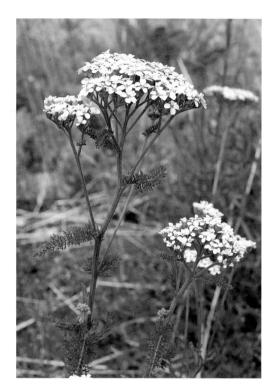

Achillea millefolium

be fed 1 ounce of the dried herb as part of their daily ration.

Availability: Yarrow is a widely distributed weed that is also available through herb retailers and nurseries.

Propagation and Harvest: Yarrow is easy to grow from seed or transplants. True yarrow (*A. millefolium*) is hardy down to at least -30° F and is drought tolerant as well. The yellow and hybrid varieties (of which there are several colors) are less hardy but are still easy to grow in most areas of North America. Moderately rich, slightly acid soil and full sun yields healthy plants, which usually don't bloom until their second year of growth. Harvest the upper third of the flowering plant (stems, leaves, and flowers) in midsummer on a dry, warm day—this is when the highest concentration of active constituents are found in the plant.

Alternatives and Adjuncts: To stop bleeding, nothing compares with a first aid powder made from a fifty-fifty mix of dried yarrow and cayenne. For situations requiring a vascular tonic or peripheral vasodilator, yarrow combines well with garlic, cayenne, ginkgo, hawthorn, or ginger.

For urinary tract infections, marshmallow, couch grass, horsetail, echinacea, and Oregon grape combine well with yarrow. For infections of the digestive tract, combine yarrow with Oregon grape. For topical treatment of inflammations and infections of the skin, consider sage, rosemary, calendula, chamomile, and juniper as adjuncts or alternatives. For topical treatment of closed injuries, yarrow combines especially well with arnica.

Cautions and Comments: Allergic reactions to yarrow are fairly common, and the volatile oils of the plant may cause dermatitis when they are applied to the skin of sensitive animals. This plant contains thujone, a substance that is poorly water soluble but may be present in alcohol extractions of the herb. Any herb preparation that contains appreciable amounts of thujone has a potential of being toxic, especially if large quantities are consumed over an extended period of time (meaning that moderation is the key to safe long-term use). Like most herbs that are rich with volatile oils, yarrow should be used with caution in pregnant or lactating animals, as these constituents have been shown to cross the placenta to the fetus and are known to have stimulant effects upon the uterus if they are ingested in sufficiently large quantities.

YELLOW DOCK

Rumex crispus   Buckwheat Family

Appearance: Yellow dock is a hearty perennial that may grow up to 5 feet. The elongated lance-shaped leaves at the base of the plant grow up to 12 inches long and 4 inches wide. The leaves are often curled at their margins (hence another common name for the plant: curly dock). The alternate stem leaves are smaller but more numerous. The single stout stem is often red and bears long clusters of small, greenish white flowers above the rest of the plant. As the flowers mature and dry, they turn a rust-red color that often stands in bold contrast to the surrounding flora.

Habitat and Range: Widely distributed in disturbed areas throughout North America. The entire Rumex genus is imported from Europe.

Cycle and Bloom Season: A perennial that blooms May through August

Parts Used: Roots

Primary Medicinal Activities: Stim-ulates bile production, helps with blood cleansing, laxative, antimicrobial, nutritive

Strongest Affinities: Digestive tract, skin, and liver

Preparation: Tincture, tea, and dried root

Common Uses: Yellow dock is well described as a quick-cleansing herb. The root contains a combination of anthraquinone, small amounts of oxalic acid and oxalates, and other constituents that stimulate liver function and contractions of intestinal smooth muscles (peristalsis). In effect, the body is prompted to work harder at eliminating waste from the bloodstream and digestive tract. This makes yellow dock especially useful for treating chronic or acute dermatitis that may be attributable to toxic excesses and elimination deficiencies in the body. It is also beneficial in treating rheumatoid arthritis that is secondary to similar circumstances. Because of its ability to quickly flush the body of systemic waste, yellow dock is sometimes used in the herbal treatment of cancer. Because the root is extremely high in iron, it is considered a traditional remedy for anemia.

Yellow dock is effective when used within the parameters we have just described. It is somewhat of a "heroic remedy," an herb that forces quick, dramatic responses in the body, much like an allopathic drug. Therefore, its use in the holistic care of animals should be limited to short-term applications at the onset of detoxification therapies that are focused on long-term holistic results. Alternatively, it can be used as a potentiating adjunct in combination with tonic herbs such as burdock, dandelion, red clover, slippery elm, and alfalfa. Using yellow dock as a symptomatic quick fix (such as for constipation) amounts to little more than substituting an herb for a drug.

Externally, yellow dock can be used as an itch-relieving, alterative skin rinse or poultice in the treatment of skin disorders such as seborrhea, pyoderma, and contact dermatitis. To use yellow dock internally, consult your holistic veterinarian.

Availability: A widely distributed weed. Available through herb retailers and seed catalogs that specialize in medicinal plants.

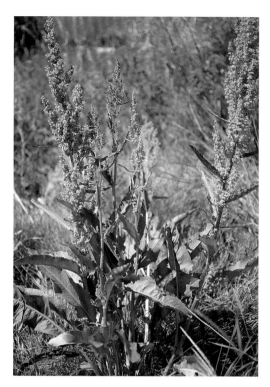

Rumex crispus

Propagation and Harvest: Yellow dock is easy to grow once it's established, but the seeds can remain dormant in the soil for several years before germinating. However, the plants grow in just about any soil and need little care. The roots are dug in fall after the plant has gone to seed and the leaves have begun to die back for winter.

Alternatives and Adjuncts: For situations that require stimulation of the liver, consider dandelion root and Oregon grape as less "heroic" alternatives. For anemia, yellow dock combines well, in proportionately small amounts, with alfalfa, garlic, red clover, spirulina, and nettle.

Cautions and Comments: Even though yellow dock is a much gentler laxative than most herbs that contain considerable

Materia Medica

amounts of anthraquinones, yellow dock should not be used in situations involving either intestinal bleeding or preexisting obstructions such as intestinal tumors. When it is used in moderation, yellow dock is quite safe, but excessive use of the herb is likely to result in intestinal cramping, diarrhea, and vomiting, and it may lead to laxative dependency. Like all stimulant laxatives, yellow dock should not be used during pregnancy.

YUCCA

Yucca schidigera   Lily Family

Appearance: Although argument exists among botanists over yucca's specific family classification, yucca is not a cactus. Essentially, "old scholars" consider yucca a member of Agavaceae, the agave family, while current botanists refer to yucca as a member of Liliaceae, the Lily family. We opt for the latter. Once you see yucca's beautiful cream-colored flower clusters, you will likely agree that it's a lily. The showy 1- to 3-inch flowers are presented in dense clusters atop a proportionately tall central stalk.

The rest of the plant is characterized by its sharply pointed, swordlike leaves. The various species differ primarily by their size, but the most distinguishable of them is *Y. brevifolia*, commonly called Joshua tree, which grows up to 20 feet tall. This large yucca is an inhabitant of the high southwestern deserts of Arizona, Nevada, western New Mexico, and especially California, where it is protected by law. Most yucca species, however, share similar appearances with *Y. schidigera* (Mojave yucca), a long-leafed variety that grows as a 1- to 6-foot-high clump of pain-inflicting puncturing green swords.

Habitat and Range: *Yucca schidigera*'s natural habitats are the dry coastal canyons of California and the inland deserts of the western U.S. This is the primary variety of commerce, and it is widely harvested and marketed by the natural products and landscape industries.

Several other species of yucca range throughout the deserts and plains of North America. Although most of us associate plants such as yucca with hot, dry desert environments, the true definition of desert pertains only to rainfall limitations, and various species of yucca have adapted to dramatically contrasting temperatures. For example, *Y. glauca* (small soapweed) thrives in many areas of the northern plains states and Canada, where summers are excruciatingly hot and dry, but winters are subarctic in average temperature.

Cycle and Bloom Season: A perennial, yucca's bloom frequency and duration depend largely on available precipitation. Cultivated plants may bloom once every one to three years, while wild plants may remain dormant for decades.

Parts Used: Roots

Primary Medicinal Activities: Nutritive, anti-inflammatory, and antitumor

Strongest Affinities: Digestive tract, musculoskeletal system

Preparation: Chopped and dried herb or tincture

Common Uses: Yucca contains notable quantities of vitamin C, beta-carotene, calcium, iron, magnesium, manganese, niacin, phosphorus, protein, and B vitamins, but its greater healing powers are chiefly attributable to its impressive content of saponin compounds. Saponins are a group of soaplike plant glycosides that are characterized by their tendency to dramatically foam up when agitated with water. While dozens of saponins are present in hundreds of useful plants, two root-borne saponins stand out among others as yucca's primary active constituents: sarsasapogenin and smilagenin. These two compounds are irritating, cleansing, and penetrating to the mucous membranes of the small intestine. It is theorized that these actions aid in the assimilation of important minerals and vitamins by allowing increased passage of critical nutrients through the intestinal walls. This in turn optimizes the nutritional value of an animal's food.

Although many of the specifics of yucca's medicinal actions remain unclear to scientists, the results of feeding yucca can be astounding. In studies conducted at Colorado State University, cattle who received a small quantity of yucca in their feed showed greater weight gain than those who didn't. Other trial accounts have concluded that chickens who are fed yucca have a tendency to lay more eggs, and dairy cattle tend to produce more milk.

Another reason you may find yucca in dog, cat, horse, or cattle feed is because it has been found to reduce the emission of unpleasant odors in urine and feces. In studies that examined the chemical breakdown of urea (the body's final by-product of digested proteins), it was found that the anhydrous ammonia that is largely responsible for the less-than-delightful odor of animal excrement is caused by a single microbial enzyme called urease. Further studies concluded that food supplements of *Y. schidigera* inhibit the production of urease, and as a result, fecal and urine odors are reduced by up to 56 percent in dogs and 49 percent in cats.

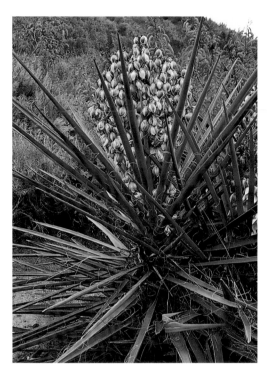

Yucca schidigera

Believe it or not, this attribute has brought about tremendous market appeal for yucca, as millions of people find the notion of less offensive animal waste an attractive alternative to promptly cleaning it up. The holistic question is, What are the deeper purposes of the urease enzymes we wish to suppress? Urease is a natural by-product of a natural metabolic process, and we can only speculate about the long-term results of our interference. People who accept this concept without question simply don't realize (or don't care) that poor-quality proteins produce excess urea and larger, more offensive stools. If an animal is fed a balanced natural diet, excess fecal and urine odor shouldn't occur.

Although much of yucca's nutritive value is likely attributable to its actions upon the intestinal membranes, the mystique surrounding this plant's impressive track record as a medicine becomes much clearer when we take a close look at its active ingredients. Sarsasapogenin and smilagenin are known by the scientific and herbal community as phytosterols, or more specifically steroidal saponins, which are compounds that act as precursors to the corticosteroids naturally produced in the body. Both of these compounds are extracted from yucca and various other herbs as starter substances in the production of pharmaceutical corticosteroid drugs. If this sounds ominous to those of you who are seeking natural alternatives to such drugs, please rest assured.

The differences between a phytosterol and a synthetic steroid drug are extreme. The process by which phytosterols are used to manufacture pharmaceutical steroids starts with a simple plant compound and proceeds from there into a complex scientific process that would have given Einstein a headache. Comparing yucca to a corticosteroid drug is like comparing a single chemical compound in a packet of active dry yeast with a loaf of finished twelve-grain bread. The terms *plant steroids* and *plant hormones* are erroneous—no known plant actually carries steroidal hormones into the body. In essence, phytosterols stimulate and assist the body in using and producing its own corticosteroids and corticosteroid-related hormones. Furthermore, steroidal saponins work with the natural immune functions of the body, whereas synthetically produced counterparts such as the prescription drug prednisolone are designed and introduced into the body with the intent of suppressing immune functions to attain the desired results.

Although this theory has not been proven as fact by the scientific community, it can be reasonably hypothesized that the natural corticosteroid-like actions of yucca may play a role in the body's natural production of growth hormones. This in turn may contribute significantly to the accelerated growth and production we see in animals who receive this plant in their food. We do know, however, that yucca is safe when fed in moderation.

A water extract (tea) of Y. glauca (small soapweed) has been shown to have antitumor activity against certain melanomas in mice. Its mechanism in this context is believed to stem from polysaccharide constituents, not necessarily steroidal saponins.

In a study conducted at the beginning of the twentieth century, the "saponin extract" from the "desert yucca plant" was found to bring about safe and effective relief from pain and inflammation in human arthritis patients who were given the extract four times daily over an extended period. Although this study has been repeatedly discredited by the American Arthritis Foundation because of the controversial manner in which it was conducted, the beneficial effects of yucca in humans and animals remain clearly validated in the minds of holistic practitioners who have used it repeatedly and have witnessed positive results. Several contemporary naturopaths, veterinarians, and animal nutritionists who use yucca in their practices claim that yucca has a 50 to 80 percent success rate in bringing relief to patients suffering from either osteoarthritis or rheumatoid arthritis. Again, yucca's effectiveness here is likely attributable to the plant's nutrition-assisting and anti-inflammatory actions of its steroidal saponin constituents.

To stimulate appetite and increase absorption of nutrients or to relieve the pain and inflammation of arthritis, add a ½ teaspoon of the dried and powdered root to each pound of a dog's daily food ration. Cats need only ¼ teaspoon daily. If you opt to use a tincture, find or make one that contains less than 5 percent alcohol because high-alcohol preparations of this herb may nauseate animals. A good tincture dose is about ⅛ teaspoon (0.5 milliliter) for each 20 pounds of an animal's body weight, once daily before a meal. Half a cup of the dried, chopped root is a sufficient daily dose for horses and other large animals.

Availability: Herb retailers and landscape nurseries

Propagation and Harvest: Because of their moderate size, attractive flowers and foliage, and low water and maintenance requirements, *Y. schidigera* and *Y. glauca* have become popular as landscape plants in areas with moderate temperatures and low to moderate precipitation. These plants do well in depleted soils, and once established they require little care.

Alternatives and Adjuncts: For arthritis, yucca combines well with alfalfa, licorice, dandelion, or shepherd's purse.

Cautions and Comments: If used in large dosages or over an extended period of time, yucca may become irritating to the stomach lining and intestinal mucosa, which may cause vomiting. This problem can be especially dangerous in horses and other large animals who are unable to vomit (instead they bloat). Many Indian tribes of the American Southwest used yucca preparations to induce vomiting in cases of food poisoning. For this reason we would not use any food additive that contains in excess of 15 percent yucca root unless instructed to do so by a veterinarian or trained animal nutritionist. We do not recommend feeding yucca every day in an animal's diet either; rather, give the animal at least a two-day break from the herb each week. Many holistic practitioners believe that if the plant is used constantly over an extended period of time, the saponins in yucca actually begin to have a reverse effect, slowing nutrient absorption (especially fat-soluble vitamins such as vitamin D) in the small intestine. Allowing breaks in your animal's diet helps to alleviate the possibility of a cumulative irritating effect in her digestive tract.

Ashwaganda

Withania somnifera

Primary Medicinal Activities: Strengthens the body's resistance to stress (adaptogenic), anti-inflammatory, antitumor, lowers blood pressure

Common Uses: Coughs, debility, nausea, fever, tumors, wounds, senility

Safety/Cautions/Contraindications: None found

Bilberry

Vaccinium myrtillus

Primary Medicinal Activities: Antispasmodic

Common Uses: Eye problems (given internally)

Safety/Cautions/Contraindications: None found

Blue Cohosh

Caulophyllum thalictroides

Primary Medicinal Activities: Uterine tonic, antispasmodic, promotes menstrual discharge, antirheumatic

Common Uses: Can be used during pregnancy in humans anytime there is threat of miscarriage. It eases false labor pains. It can be used in cases of coughs, colic, and asthma and to ease rheumatic pains.

Safety/Cautions/Contraindications: Blue cohosh should be taken only in small doses during pregnancy and used only under professional guidance.

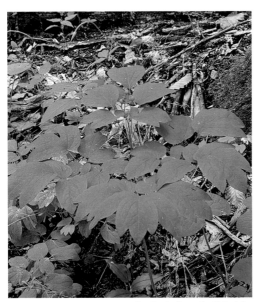

Caulophyllum thalictroides

Boneset

Eupatorium perfoliatum

Primary Medicinal Activities: Relaxing to mucous membranes, antispasmodic, expectorant, mild laxative, tonic, increases perspiration

Common Uses: Pain reliever, upper respiratory tract, bronchitis

Safety/Cautions/Contraindications: Some *Eupatorium* spp. may contain PAs. They should not be taken by pregnant or lactating individuals.

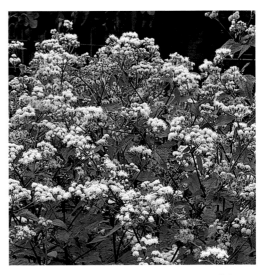

Eupatorium perfoliatum

Boswellia

Boswellia serrata

Primary Medicinal Activities: Anti-inflammatory; diuretic; lubricates, soothes, and protects internal mucous membranes; helps with blood cleansing; appetite stimulant;

helps reduce arthritic inflammation; promotes menstrual discharge; analgesic, antifungal
Common Uses: Liver disorders, bronchial asthma, ringworm, arthritis, lung diseases, and diarrhea. Researchers found that the resin was as effective as sulfasalazine, the standard drug treatment for ulcerative colitis. (I. Gupta et al., "Effects of *Boswellia serrata* gum resin in patients with ulcerative colitis," *Eur. J. Med.* Res. 2, no. 1 [1991]: 37–43.)
Safety/Cautions/Contraindications: None found

Caraway
Carum carvi
Primary Medicinal Activities: Expectorant, expels intestinal gas, antispasmodic, stimulates milk production, aromatic, astringent, promotes menstrual discharge
Common Uses: Stimulates appetite; helps to ease diarrhea, flatulence, and colic; bronchitis; helps increase milk in nursing mothers
Safety/Cautions/Contraindications: None found

Cascara Sagrada
Rhamnus purshiana
Primary Medicinal Activities: Bitter tonic, purgative
Common Uses: A strong laxative that should be reserved for situations where immediate relief from constipation is necessary and where other, less purgative, measures have failed
Safety/Cautions/Contraindications: Should not be used in pregnant or nursing animals as its laxative effects are passed on through the milk. (Varro E. Tyler, *Herbs of Choice: The Therapeutic Use of Phytomedicinals* [Binghamton, N.Y.: Pharmaceutical Products Press, 1994].)

Cat's Claw
Uncaria tomentosa
Primary Medicinal Activities: Antiarrhythmic, anti-inflammatory, antitumor, antispasmodic,

antiarthritic, reduces fever, helps with blood cleansing, immunostimulant, antimicrobial
Common Uses: Abscesses, arthritis, asthma, cancer, chemotherapy side effects, contraception, fevers, gastric ulcers, hemorrhages, inflammations, kidney cleanser, recovery from birthing, rheumatism, urinary tract infections, wounds, boosts the immune system at the onset of viral infection.
Alternatives: Organically cultivated echinacea serves as a more earth-friendly alternative because cat's claw is harvested from the wilds of imperiled South American rain forests.
Veterinary Common Uses: Allergic reactions to insect bites (hair loss and itching); dull coat, hair loss, lethargy, poor skin; inflammation of the muscle, prostate, stomach; mammary tumors; osteoarthritis; parvovirus; dermatitis; inflammation of the vertebrae (spondylitis); arthritis. (Kenneth Jones, University Mayor de San Marcos, Lima, Peru, *Cat's Claw—Healing Vine of Peru* [Seattle, Wash.: Sylvan Press 1995].)
Safety/Cautions/Contraindications: None found

Celery
Apium graveolens
Primary Medicinal Activities: Diuretic, sedative, expels intestinal gas, antirheumatic
Common Uses: Arthritis, rheumatism
Safety/Cautions/Contraindications: Celery seed should be used with caution and moderation in pregnant animals or those with preexisting kidney disease.

Coriander
Coriandrum sativum
Primary Medicinal Activities: Aromatic, expels intestinal gas
Common Uses: Flatulence, spasms from colic pain, stimulates digestive secretions and increases appetite
Safety/Cautions/Contraindications: None found

Cranberry

Vaccinium macrocarpon

Primary Medicinal Activities: Antiseptic

Common Uses: Prevents urinary tract infections caused by *E. coli* by preventing the microorganisms from adhering to the epithelial cells of the urinary tract. (A. E. Sabota, *Journal of Urology* 131 [1984]: 1013–6; M. S. Soloway and R. A. Smith, JAMA 260 [1988]: 1465.)

Safety/Cautions/Contraindications: Use with caution in animals with kidney inflammation

Devil's Claw

Harpagophytum procumbrens

Primary Medicinal Activities: soothes pain (anodyne), anti-inflammatory

Common Uses: Reduces inflammation in cases of arthritis but may not always be effective

Safety/Cautions/Contraindications: Devil's claw is not to be taken by diabetics because it has a hypoglycemic action. Excessive doses may interfere with treatment for cardiac disorders and with hyper- and hypotensive therapies. It should not be taken during pregnancy because it is oxytocic (induces contractions) in animals. (R. Mabey, *The Complete New Herbal* [London: Elm Tree Books, 1988].)

Eyebright

Euphrasia officinalis

Primary Medicinal Activities: Anti-inflammatory, astringent

Common Uses: Conjunctivitis, astringent, nasal catarrh

Availability: Use only organically cultivated eyebright (or grow it yourself).

Safety/Cautions/Contraindications: It is best to avoid eyebright during pregnancy and lactation. This herb may be compromised in the wild. Please use only organically cultivated sources, or use other herbs instead.

Evening Primrose

Oenothera spp.

Primary Medicinal Activities: Sedative, astringent

Common Uses: Asthmatic coughs, gastrointestinal disorders, psoriasis, excess cholesterol in the blood (hypercholesterolemia), arthritis, diabetic neuropathy

Safety/Cautions/Contraindications: May have the potential to manifest temporal lobe epilepsy in those receiving epileptogenic drugs. (Melvyn R. Werbach and Michael T. Murray, *Botanical Influences on Illness*, a *Sourcebook of Clinical Research* [Tarzana, Calif.: Third Line Press, 1994], 112.)

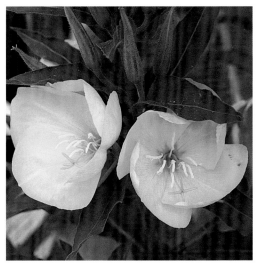

Oenothera sp.

Eucalyptus

Eucalyptus globulus

Primary Medicinal Activities: Antiseptic, reduces inflammation of respiratory mucosa

Common Uses: Flea prevention, bronchitis, asthma (inhaled through a vaporizer)

Safety/Cautions/Contraindications: Eucalyptus may antidote homeopathic treatments or remedies, so it should not be used with homeopathic remedies. The oil should not be used unless suitably diluted. The oil should not be used at all during pregnancy because it may interfere with existing hypoglycemic therapies.

Fenugreek
Trigonella foenum-graecum
Primary Medicinal Activities: Antiseptic; lubricates, soothes, and protects internal mucous membranes; tonic; expectorant; stimulates milk production; reduces fever; laxative; nutritive; lowers blood sugar
Common Uses: Antidiabetic and anticholesterolemic activities; stimulates milk in lactating mothers
Safety/Cautions/Contraindications: May interfere with hypoglycemic therapies. The absorption of drugs taken concomitantly may be affected because of the high mucilaginous fiber content. It is reputed to induce contractions (oxytocic); in vitro uterine stimulant activity has been documented. (Carol A. Newall, Linda A. Anderson, and J. David Phillipson, *Herbal Medicines, a Guide for Health Care Professionals* [London, England: Pharmaceutical Products Press, 1996], 118.)

Fleabane
Conyza canadensis
Primary Medicinal Activities: Stops bleeding, possible flea repellent
Common Uses: This common weed traditionally has been used as a broad-spectrum insecticide. The plant contains considerable amounts of limonene, a compound known for its flea-killing properties. However, little is known about the totality of the plant's chemistry or the safety of this herb. Aside from what we know about the limonene content of fleabane, scientific study is still lacking.
Safety/Cautions/Contraindications: Fleabane may cause spontaneous nasal and upper respiratory irritation in horses. It is highly allergenic.

Gentian
Gentiana lutea
Primary Medicinal Activities: Bitter, promotes salivation (sialagogue), stimulates bile

production, and is a gastric stimulant
Common Uses: Stimulates the digestive secretions in the mouth and stomach to aid digestion and increase appetite. Helps with flatulence and dyspepsia.
Safety/Cautions/Contraindications: Gentian may cause headache in certain predisposed individuals (Varro E. Tyler, Herbs of Choice: *The Therapeutic Use of Phytomedicinals* [Binghamton, N.Y.: Pharmaceutical Products Press, 1994]). Gentian should not be used in individuals who have high blood pressure.

Ginger
Zingiber officinale
Primary Medicinal Activities: Expels internal gas, stimulant, increases perspiration, causes redness of the skin
Common Uses: Indigestion (dyspepsia), flatulence, and colic. Used to increase peripheral circulation. May help in some cases of motion sickness. In small animals, the pungent constituents have been shown to be cardiotonic, fever reducing, analgesic, antitussive, and sedative.
Safety/Cautions/Contraindications: It has been reported to tend to increase the tone of the heart muscle and blood vessels (cardiotonic) and to inhibit blood clotting in vitro. It also has hypoglycemic activity in in vivo studies. Excessive doses may interfere with existing cardiac, antidiabetic, or anticoagulant therapies. Doses that greatly exceed those normally found in foods should not be administered during pregnancy or lactation.

Ginseng
Panax spp.
Primary Medicinal Activities: Increases physical and mental performance, antidepressive
Common Uses: Raises low blood pressure, helps to eliminate exhaustion and weakness
Safety/Cautions/Contraindications: Ginseng should not be used in cases of high blood pressure and may, on occasion, produce

headaches. It is contraindicated during acute illness, any form of hemorrhage, and during the acute period of coronary thrombosis. It should be avoided by those who are highly nervous, energetic, and tense.

Kava Kava
Piper methysticum
Primary Medicinal Activities: Antispasmodic, sedative, hypnotic, anticonvulsive
Common Uses: It may be useful for epileptic animals and as a sedative or antispasmodic for animals who have nervous disorders that involve muscle spasms and general tightness.
Safety/Cautions/Contraindications: Preliminary studies indicate that this herb can be damaging to the liver if used in excess. Kava kava appears to be safe if used prudently and in moderation, but little is known about its effectiveness or safety in animals.

Kelp
Fucus vesiculosus
Primary Medicinal Activities: Antihypothyroid, antirheumatic
Common Uses: Obesity, goiter, arthritis, and rheumatism
Safety/Cautions/Contraindications: Prolonged ingestion may reduce gastrointestinal iron absorption resulting in a slow reduction in hemoglobin, packed cell volume, and serum iron concentrations. Prolonged ingestion may also affect absorption of sodium and potassium ions and cause diarrhea. (Carol A. Newall, Linda A. Anderson, and J. David Phillipson, *Herbal Medicines, a Guide for Health Care Professionals* [London, England: Pharmaceutical Products Press, 1996], 125.)

Lemon Balm
Melissa officinalis
Primary Medicinal Activities: Slows thyroid function, lowers blood pressure, increases perspiration, anti-spasmodic, antidepressive, expels intestinal gas
Common Uses: Lemon balm is believed to block

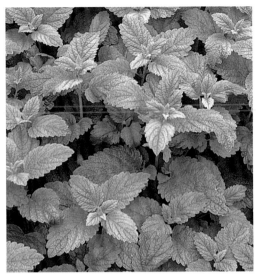
Melissa officinalis

iodide uptake and inhibit antibody attachment at thyroid cells, therefore it may be useful for decreasing thyroid output in felines with overactive thyroid glands (hyperthyroid). Also, it is useful in some cases of depression, anxiety, indigestion, and for lowering blood pressure.
Safety/Cautions/Contraindications: Use with caution and moderation in pregnant animals. Contraindicated in animals with hypothyroid conditions.

Lobelia
Lobelia inflata
Primary Medicinal Activities: Antiasthmatic, respiratory stimulant, antispasmodic, expectorant, induces vomiting, increases perspiration
Common Uses: Used in bronchitis and asthma. Lobelia has a general depressant action on the autonomic and central nervous systems, as well as on neuromuscular action.
Safety/Cautions/Contraindications: Lobeline, a nicotine-like constituent of lobelia, may stimulate respiration in animals; in higher doses it causes vomiting. It should not be used during pregnancy or lactation. Lobelia is similar in action to nicotine.

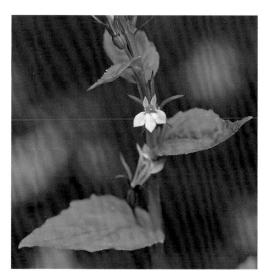

Lobelia inflata

Lovage

Levisticum officinale

Primary Medicinal Activities: Diuretic, expels intestinal gas

Common Uses: Relieves gas pains

Safety/Cautions/Contraindications: Lovage should not be used in cases of kidney disease. Furocoumarins, chemical compounds that may cause photosensitization, are present in the oil. (Varro E. Tyler, *Herbs of Choice: The Therapeutic Use of Phytomedicinals* [Binghamton, N.Y.: Pharmaceutical Products Press, 1994], 78.)

Meadowsweet

Filipendula ulmaria

Primary Medicinal Activities: Anti-inflammatory, stimulates the stomach, alleviates vomiting, astringent, antirheumatic

Common Uses: Protects and soothes the mucous membranes of the digestive tract, reduces acidity, and eases nausea. Meadowsweet can be used for fever and the pain of rheumatism. It has been reported to increase bronchial tone in cats. (O. D. Barnaulove et al., "Preliminary Evaluation of the Spasmolytic Properties of Some Natural Compounds and Galenic Preparations," *Rastit. Resur.* 14 [1978]: 573–9.)

Safety/Cautions/Contraindications:
Meadowsweet contains salicylic acid compounds (spiraein and gaultherin), so it should not be used for cats or other animals who are allergic or sensitive to aspirin. Other than that, no side effects are documented. Meadowsweet should be avoided during pregnancy and lactation.

Myrrh

Commiphora molmol

Primary Medicinal Activities: Astringent, antimicrobial, expels intestinal gas, expectorant, wound healing

Common Uses: Mouth ulcers, gingivitis, sinusitis, respiratory problems, brucellosis, and wounds and abrasions

Safety/Cautions/Contraindications: None found

Oregano

Oreganum vulgare **or** *O. heracleoticum*

Primary Medicinal Activities: Antispasmodic, expectorant, digestive, mild tranquilizer

Common Uses: May assist in expelling parasites from the digestive tract

Safety/Cautions/Contraindications: May stimulate the uterus if used in medicinal quantities

Passionflower

Passiflora incarnata

Primary Medicinal Activities: Mild hypnotic, sedative, antispasmodic, and pain reliever

Common Uses: Seizures, hysteria, neuralgia, insomnia, spasmodic asthma

Safety/Cautions/Contraindications: No reported side effects. Excessive doses may cause sedation and may potentiate MAOI therapy. Uterine stimulant activity in animal studies has been reported. (Carol A. Newall, Linda A. Anderson, and J. David Phillipson, *Herbal Medicines, a Guide for Health Care Professionals* [London, England: Pharmaceutical Products Press, 1996], 206.)

Materia Medica

Pennyroyal

Mentha pulegium

Primary Medicinal Activities: Promotes menstrual discharge, increases perspiration, expels intestinal gas, stimulant

Common Uses: The weak tea as a flea repellent in nonpregnant, nonlactating animals

Safety/Cautions/Contraindications: The oil should be avoided in animals because it is strong and can cause death. The abortion inducing effects are reliable only in near-lethal dosages. (Varro E. Tyler, *Herbs of Choice: The Therapeutic Use of Phytomedicinals* [Binghamton, N.Y.: Pharmaceutical Products Press, 1994].) It is toxic to dogs and cats at high doses. (M. Sudekum et al., "Pennyroyal Oil Toxicosis in a Dog," *Journal of the American Veterinary Medicine Association.* 200, no. 6 [March 15, 1992]: 817–8.) It should not be used in animals with existing kidney disease. Use the herb (not the oil) topically with great caution only in nonpregnant, nonlactating adults. Pennyroyal herb teas have been reported to be used without side effects. (J. B. Sullivan et al., "Pennyroyal Oil Poisoning and Hepatotoxicity," *JAMA* 242 [1979]: 2873.)

Peppermint

Mentha piperita

Primary Medicinal Activities: Alleviates vomiting, expels intestinal gas, moderates nerve transmissions, antiseptic, increases perspiration, analgesic, astringent, stimulates bile production, stimulates the stomach

Common Uses: Flatulence, intestinal colic, irritable bowel syndrome, nausea, vomiting, motion sickness

Availability: Peppermint is easily grown in the garden but may take over, so plant it in a container. It can be purchased readily at most stores, in tea, or dried in bulk form.

Safety/Cautions/Contraindications: It may antidote homeopathic treatments, so it should not be used with homeopathy.

Pineapple Weed

Matricaria matricarioides

Primary Medicinal Activities: Expels intestinal gas, expels worms

Common Uses: Similar but weaker in action to chamomile. It may be effective in treating roundworms.

Safety/Cautions/Contraindications: Use with caution and moderation in pregnant animals.

Pipsissewa

Chimaphila umbellata

Primary Medicinal Activities: Astringent, antibacterial, tonic, diuretic, strengthens kidney function

Common Uses: Urinary tract astringent, infections, and inflammation of the kidneys

Safety/Cautions/Contraindications: This herb may be compromised in the wild. Use only organically cultivated pipsissewa or use other herbs such as pyrola instead.

Saw Palmetto

Serenoa repens

Primary Medicinal Activities: Diuretic, urinary antiseptic, strengthens and nourishes the prostate and smooth muscle tissues of the urinary tract

Common Uses: Cystitis, testicular atrophy, prostatic enlargement, and sex hormone disorders

Safety/Cautions/Contraindications: Human studies report that saw palmetto is well tolerated. It may effect existing hormonal therapies. Avoid during pregnancy and lactation.

Senna

Cassia angustifolia **or** *C. senna*

Primary Medicinal Activities: Cathartic, strong laxative

Common Uses: Powerful cathartic to relieve constipation

Safety/Cautions/Contraindications: Long-term use can cause dependence and can be

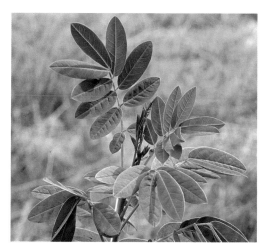

Cassia sp.

detrimental. Prolonged use or over dosage can result in diarrhea with excessive loss of potassium; an atonic nonfunctioning colon may also develop. Senna should not be given in cases of intestinal obstruction or with undiagnosed abdominal symptoms. Care should also be taken by those with inflammatory bowel disease. (J. E. F. Reynolds, ed., Martindale: *The Extra Pharmacopeia*, 28th ed. [London: Pharmaceutical Products Press, 1982]; DeSmet PAGM, ed., et al., *Adverse Effects of Herbal Drugs* vol. 2. [Berlin: Springer-Verlag, 1993].) Excessive use of senna may have an adverse effect on cardiac function due to excessive potassium loss. Anthraquinones, the laxative component of senna, may cause discoloration of the urine, which may interfere with diagnostic tests (J. E. F. Reynolds, ed., Martindale: *The Extra Pharmacopeia*, 29th ed. [London: Pharmaceutical Products Press, 1989.)

Siberian Ginseng

Eleuthrococcus senticosus

Primary Medicinal Activities: Improves the body's resistance to stress, circulatory stimulant, dilates blood vessels

Common Uses: Debility; helps the body to deal and adapt to stressful situations and some types of depression

Safety/Cautions/Contraindications: Siberian ginseng is safe but should be avoided in animals that have been diagnosed with hypertension.

Spirulina

Spirulina spp.

Primary Medicinal Activities: Nutritive, helps with blood cleansing, tonic

Common Uses: A complete and digestible source of vitamin B complex, beta-carotene, protein, and a wide variety of minerals. It serves as an excellent nutritional supplement for dogs, cats, and other animals.

Safety/Cautions/Contraindications: Spirulina is safe for daily use in animals, but its nutrient content is so concentrated that it can cause diarrhea and digestive upset if fed in excessive quantities. A daily dosage of ¼ teaspoon per pound of food is generally acceptable for most animals (1/8 teaspoon for cats).

Turkey Rhubarb

Rheum palmatum

Primary Medicinal Activities: Astringent, purgative, bitter

Common Uses: Constipation

Safety/Cautions/Contraindications: Turkey rhubarb may color the urine yellow or red. It should be combined with carminative herbs to prevent intestinal cramping.

Turmeric

Curcuma longa

Primary Medicinal Activities: Helps with blood cleansing, analgesic, anticoagulant, antifungal, anti-inflammatory, antiarthritic, antioxidant, antimicrobial, antiseptic, aromatic, astringent, stimulates bile production, circulatory, promotes menstrual discharge, strengthens liver function, stimulant, wound healing

Common Uses: Arthritis, asthma, blood clot inhibitor, cancer, candida, inflammation of the mucous membrane, eczema, gastritis, excess cholesterol in the blood, jaundice, nausea, restorative after birth, trauma, uterine tumors

Safety/Cautions/Contraindications:
Infrequently turmeric may cause gastric disturbances. Turmeric is contraindicated in cases of bile duct blockage or gallstones. (Varro E. Tyler, *Herbs of Choice: The Therapeutic Use of Phytomedicinals* [Binghamton, N.Y.: Pharmaceutical Products Press, 1994], 62.)

Usnea
Usnea barbata
Primary Medicinal Activities: Antibiotic, immunostimulant
Common Uses: Infections, mouthwash, wounds
Safety/Cautions/Contraindications: Care needs to be taken that Usnea barbata is used and not some other types of lichen that can be toxic.

Vervain
Verbena officinalis
Primary Medicinal Activities: Sedative, nerve tonic, antispasmodic, supports liver functions
Common Uses: Seizures, for hepatic and gallbladder inflammation
Safety/Cautions/Contraindications: None found

White Oak Bark
Quercus sp.
Primary Medicinal Activities: Antiseptic, astringent, anti-inflammatory, stops bleeding, pain reliever, diuretic, fungicide
Common Uses: Can be used in small frequent doses in cases of acute diarrhea
Safety/Cautions/Contraindications: Excessive doses of white oak bark should be avoided, and it should be avoided by pregnant and lactating adults.

Wild Cherry Bark
also known as Chokecherry
Prunus virginiana
Primary Medicinal Activities: Cough suppressant, astringent, expectorant, sedative
Common Uses: Helpful in reducing symptoms of respiratory distress due to its powerful sedative action on the cough reflex. Used as a respiratory sedative in acute conditions with hectic coughing, heat, rapid breathing, and rapid pulse. It is used in many over-the-counter cough medicines.
Safety/Cautions/Contraindications: Avoid during pregnancy. The seeds, bark, and leaves of this plant contain hydrocyanic acid, which can cause severe diarrhea and vomiting if ingested.

Willow
Salix spp.
Primary Medicinal Activities: Anti-inflammatory, fever reducer, astringent, analgesic, and antiseptic
Common Uses: Pain after surgery, rheumatism, connective tissue inflammation, and arthritis
Safety/Cautions/Contraindications: Willow should not be given to cats without professional guidance because it contains salicylic acid (aspirin), which can be fatal to cats.

Witch Hazel
Hamamelis virginiana
Primary Medicinal Activities: Astringent
Common Uses: Swelling or dilation of veins and capillaries (varicosities), bleeding, diarrhea, dysentery
Safety/Cautions/Contraindications: The drugstore preparation is in alcohol and should not be administered internally.

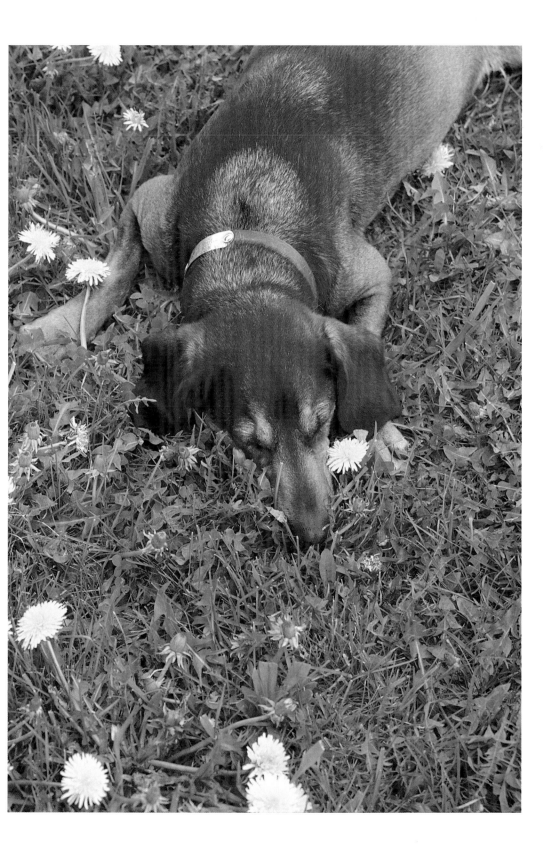

Materia Medica

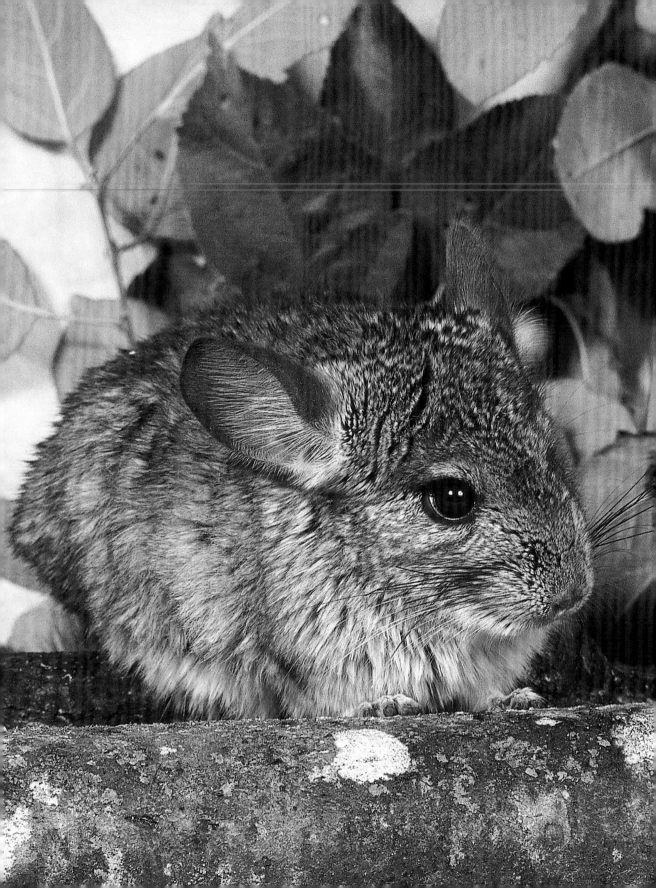

Chapter 3

An Herbal Repertory for Animals: Ailments and Treatments

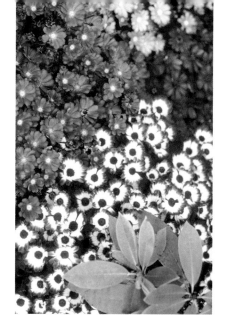

I n this chapter we discuss some of the more common ailments an animal guardian may encounter in the holistic care of animals. Each ailment is categorized by the body system in which it predominates—for example, kennel cough is discussed in the "Respiratory Problems" section, and the issue of fleas is discussed under "Parasite-Related Problems," and so forth. For each ailment discussed, we include a variety of herbal treatments and other holistic measures that you may find helpful in reaching a remedial or curative solution for your companion.

To learn more about the herb choices we present in this chapter, and to determine whether one or more of these choices may be appropriate for your companion, we recommend that you refer to chapter 3. There you will find detailed information such as dosages and parts of the herbs used, preparation and administration options, contraindications, and possible side effects of most of the herbs in the repertory. By no means, though, is this repertory a complete representation of all measures of herbal healing. There are hundreds of potentially useful herbs not discussed here, and we urge you to also access the excellent texts included in the bibliography. This repertory is also not intended to serve as a substitute for the advice and care of a licensed veterinarian. Its purpose only is to express our experiences and opinions. Please keep in mind that we are herbalists, not licensed animal care providers.

Anxiety, Nervousness, and Behavioral Problems

HOLISTIC APPROACHES

It is part of human nature to impose our ideals of acceptable behavior upon our beloved animals. Unfortunately, though, many of us find it difficult to separate these ideals from what makes each animal special, unique, and happy. Thousands of animals are euthanized each year because they were "untrainable" or "uncontrollable," "barked too much," or were simply "too much to bear." Many of these animals were put to death not because there was something untreatably wrong with them but because their identities clashed with their caregivers'.

One of the greatest gifts offered to us by animals comes when we learn to look beyond our own needs to their happiness. Our eight-year-old shepherd/husky dog, Willow, still barks incessantly, whines obnoxiously on trips to the river, and jumps up onto house guests despite our continuing efforts to direct her toward our needs. Sometimes we want to pull out our own hair and tie her snout shut with it, but instead we have developed patience and respect for her personal nature. Willow is simply doing what she must do to be complete and happy, and while we are still working on the guest-mauling issue, we have learned to accept her just the way she is. By reaching this level of acceptance, we

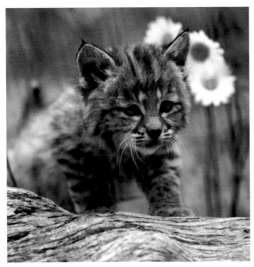

We owe it to our animal companions to look at the world through their eyes.

have been rewarded with the joy she brings to us as we rejoice with her in her rapturous journey through life. Granted, there is a social stigma attached to certain types of animal behavior. However, before we step in and choose what is best for us, we owe it to our animal companions to try to look at the world through their eyes—perhaps even before we bring one of them home.

Anxiety, nervousness, fear, occasional aggression, and depression are normal emotions of each and every animal's life. Some animals may be terrified of thunder, cars, vets, and stairs. Others may dislike children or other animals. Active dog breeds (such as border collies) usually need wide-open spaces to run, and they become anxious if confined. Many cats who would rather sleep than play become nervous wrecks during car rides. But if your animal's behavior changes suddenly or if his nervous tendencies worsen over time, your animal may be ill.

Contrary to conventional standards, holistic treatment of anxiety, nervousness, or behavioral problems does not begin with the use of sedative or antidepressive medicines but with a critical examination of the caregiver's perspective of a situation. Are we really treating anxiety or aggression, or is the problem a symptom of something deeper within the animal or his environment? Perhaps the problem is not really the animal's at all but instead emanates from the caregiver's unfulfilled expectations.

CHRONIC PROBLEMS

Emotional, behavioral, and nervous disorders can result from nutritional deficiencies, endocrine disease, vaccinosis, drug side effects, parasites, neurological disease, or psychological problems. Like humans, animals can suffer from chronic depression that is secondary to chemical imbalances in the brain. But before treating depression with Prozac (fluoxetine HCl) or Saint-John's-wort, you should make a thorough assessment of the animal's diet, health care history, and environment. In most cases, the caregiver is likely to find that the problem is correctable with dietary changes, some loving attention, and perhaps the correct homeopathic remedy.

Our approach toward aggression, depression (which is manifested by a lack of energy, whining, separation anxiety, to name a few symptoms), nervousness, chronic anxiety, or hyperactivity always begins with changing the animal's diet (usually to raw food) and supplementing it with a complement of vitamins, minerals, and EFAs. If this does not effect a positive change, the animal should be checked by a veterinarian for underlying physiological disorders such as thyroid or adrenal gland problems, malabsorption, tumors, parasites, or diabetes mellitus. Once the underlying causes are identified, they can be treated with applicable herbs, homeopathic remedies, aromatherapy, flower essences, or nutritional therapies. Behavioral training, therapeutic touch, or a few sessions with a reputable animal communicator may also yield good results.

In all chronic cases, the sedative herbs (e.g., valerian, skullcap, passionflower) should be limited to temporary control of symptoms during times of added stress such as dreaded car rides to the veterinarian. We do not condone the use of sedative herbs on a daily lifelong basis—not only because of potential side effects but also because they may mask symptoms that are important to recognize in reaching curative solutions. Similarly, Saint-John's-wort and other antidepressants should be reserved for cases in which chronic depression is known to be secondary to brain chemical imbalances.

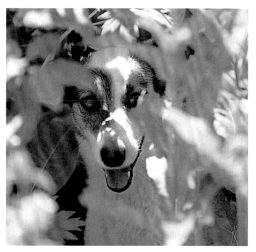

Determine the cause of any emotional or behavioral disorder before treating it.

Adaptogenic herbs such as Siberian ginseng, astragalus, and certified-organic ginseng, may be used continually in moderation to boost the body's functional abilities under stress.

AGGRESSION AND DEPRESSION DISORDERS

As of 1999, the use of Prozac had become almost as fashionable for treating aggressive animals as it had for humans with chronic depression disorders. Likewise, Saint-John's-wort had been touted as "the herbal alternative to Prozac," and it too had become popular for treating aggression and other behavioral and emotional disorders in animals.

Although Saint-John's-wort and psychotropic drugs may have a place in the treatment of certain disorders, they are not the panaceas that some companies would like us to believe they are. Many experts believe that these substances may actually cause a reverse effect in some animals. In Peter Neville's acclaimed book *Do Dogs Need Shrinks?* he cites case histories in which Prozac not only failed to curb aggression but seemingly increased it. One case involved

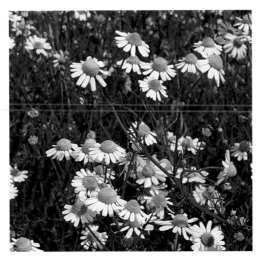
Chamomile can help lift your pet's mood naturally.

The question of what may be missing from the animal's well-being must be answered before anything else. Is the animal receiving all of the nutrients needed for proper brain function? Was the animal abused or neglected in the past? Is there a genetic predisposition to be addressed? Is there anything in the animal's living environment that might be contributing to the problem? Has the animal had adequate opportunities to socialize with other animals and people? Is the animal's behavior related to your own? (This is fairly common—animals often pick up the emotional tone of their living environment.)

After the animal's diet is changed and supplemented, sessions with a good animal behaviorist are highly recommended. Animal behaviorists do not teach "sit-stay" obedience but use their expert knowledge of animal behavior and human-animal relationships to help identify and provide fulfillment of psychological requirements. For instance, most dogs who are "fear biters" do not exhibit aggressive behavior out of hate or neurological disease but because they are insecure in the hierarchy of their "pack." These dogs feel that their human alpha leader is not in charge of their surroundings and therefore feel constantly threatened. The animal behaviorists' job in this situation is to help the guardian and the animal define their positions as leader-protector (the human) and safe-subordinate pack member (the dog). Horses and other herbivores, of course, have completely different psychologies—but they too can find a happier coexistence with their humans with some help from a professional behavior trainer.

Once you have begun a curative, long-term approach toward your animal's aggression or depression, herbs can be used for symptomatic relief during occasions when

a two-year-old Staffordshire bull terrier who was given the drug to stop him from assaulting other dogs. Initially the attacks stopped, but later the dog resumed his hostile behavior—and when he was taken off Prozac, he became more aggressive than ever. Another case involved a three-year-old pointer who was given Prozac to stop her from constantly chasing shadows. After three days she began attacking real dogs instead.

Compounding the potential problems of reverse or other adverse side effects is our limited ability to identify accurately the causes of aggression and depression disorders in animals. The diagnosis needed to prudently prescribe such drugs is severely limited by lack of verbal communication between animal and healer. In other words, psychotropic drugs (and even the safer Saint-John's-wort) are usually prescribed as a speculative "shot in the dark" approach to suppression of symptoms, rather than as part of a curative solution that is based on holism.

From a holistic perspective, treatment of aggression begins in the mind of the human guardian—not the animal.

stress levels are particularly high. Although many herbalists recommend valerian as a first choice herb for anxiety and aggression, it can have a reverse, sometimes stimulating, effect in some animals. It's a depressant and tends to compound irritability and depression. Instead of lifting the subject's spirit, it slows him down and often turns him into a groggy grump. So rather than reaching for valerian, we opt for herbs such as passionflower, lemon balm, chamomile, or catnip that serve more as mood elevators. Rescue Remedy (a flower essence formula) is also one of our first choices.

ACUTE NERVOUSNESS AND ANXIETY

Everyone has his or her own sources of psychological stress. Some people get nervous and tense during airplane landings. Our dogs get anxious and frightened while inside crowded buildings. Stephanie the cat trembles during the first half-hour of long car rides.

Herbs can be helpful for gently calming an animal during stressful occasions. In circumstances in which fear and anxiety prohibit an otherwise passive animal from relaxing, valerian may induce just enough sedation to allow napping. If the animal's anxiety is causing him to hiss, spit, bite, or make other demonstrations of potential violence, a dose or two of passionflower, lemon balm, or catnip may help normalize attitude and defuse the situation. If nervousness is causing trembling or hypersensitivity to touch and sound, skullcap or oatstraw can be very effective—especially if combined with valerian or passionflower. A small dose (0.25 milliliters per 30 pounds of an animal's body weight) of vervain (*Verbena officinalis*) tincture may reduce muscle twitching and restlessness, but too much of this herb may have a reverse effect. In

situations in which nervousness is causing an upset stomach, chamomile, valerian, catnip, or a combination of all three may help induce relaxation and prevent vomiting.

Before you reach for valerian or any other herb, try giving your pet a few drops of Rescue Remedy (flower essence formula), which you can purchase at health food stores. You and your companion may be pleasantly surprised.

Arthritis and Hip Dysplasia

The term *arthritis* is general, referring to the inflammation of a joint. Polyarthritis is the inflammation of several joints. Degenerative arthritis is a term that refers to the condition caused by the wearing of joints as the animal ages. It is also known as degenerative joint disease and is sometimes caused by trauma to the joints, bones, ligaments, or cartilage. Osteoarthritis is usually the result of some type of secondary damage to the joint structures. The damage could result from rupture of ligaments, poor anatomical alignment, or joint dislocation.

Inflammatory arthritis can be caused by an infection or an immune-mediated disease

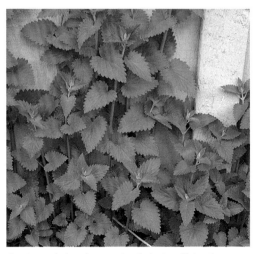

Catnip can help calm an animal who is suffering from anxiety.

that leads to destructive arthritic lesions. In other words, its onset is caused when the immune system actually turns against the body it's supposed to protect.

Arthritis may also take the form of hip dysplasia. Hip dysplasia is the abnormal development of the "ball and socket" joint of the hips of dogs. This condition may vary from a slightly abnormal hip joint to the actual dislocation of the joint. There is controversy among holistic and homeopathic veterinarians regarding the underlying cause of hip dysplasia. Some holistic veterinarians believe that this condition might be caused by vaccinations, specifically the rabies vaccine. Others say it

is caused by heredity—but if this is so, and conscientious breeders are taking care not to breed animals who show signs of it, then why is it not being eliminated? Why is it appearing in an increasing number of breeds more frequently? Despite the evidence, many veterinarians maintain that hip dysplasia is a genetic predisposition in many breeds of dogs. To an extent this may be true, but we believe that there are too many coincidences between hip dysplasia and overvaccination. If your dog is young and may be prone to hip dysplasia, you might want to consider not vaccinating every year.

The belief that hip dysplasia is strictly a hereditary disease discourages many people from growing attached to dogs who are believed to be predisposed. This is truly a shame. Not only can a predisposed breed of dog lead a normal, healthy life but there is a good possibility that hip dysplasia can be prevented by taking some simple, lifelong measures.

In the book *Alternative and Complementary Veterinary Medicine: Principles and Practice*, Wendell O. Belfield, D.V.M., states that hip dysplasia may be caused more by biochemical factors than by genetic inheritance. He believes that hip dysplasia may be an easily controlled biochemical condition in most breeds of dogs caused by insufficient collagen synthesis. He says that if insufficient amounts of Vitamin C exist in affected dogs, they may have difficulty synthesizing enough collagen to assist in maintaining joint stability. Dr. Belfield substantiates his statement with a study he conducted involving eight litters of German shepherd puppies who came from bloodlines that were believed to be afflicted with hereditary hip dysplasia. During their pregnancy, bitches were administered megadoses of vitamin C, and the puppies were maintained on a similar regimen until

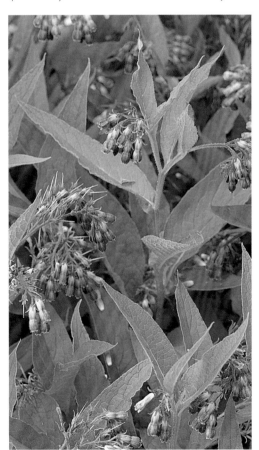

Comfrey can help repair aching bones and joints.

adulthood. As a result, no signs of canine hip dysplasia were noted in any of the offspring.

Unless onset is acute, such as after a joint injury, the first sign of arthritis is usually lameness that may be worsened by cold, inclement weather or exercise. You might first notice that your animal isn't getting around as easily as he once did. You might observe your companion having difficulty getting on or off the couch, climbing the stairs, or perhaps jumping in and out of the car. If you are keenly perceptive of subtle changes in your companion, early onset of arthritis might be signified by abnormal behavior that points to physical discomfort—perhaps your friend just isn't his "old self" or appears irritable for no apparent reason. Watch the daily appearance and behavior of your companion closely. Keep a health care diary for your animal, bearing in mind that nothing you observe is insignificant. If you do keep a diary, you will be much more effective in preventing simple morning stiffness from becoming a crippling disease.

As an animal ages, his joints don't move quite as easily as they once did (Don't we all know that feeling when getting in and out of our favorite easy chair?), but if joint stiffness appears to be progressing ahead of your companion's age, it's time to take remedial measures. But before you start administering herbal remedies, you should know the exact nature of your companion's arthritis. This may require the opinion of a holistic veterinarian who can diagnose the many different kinds of arthritis.

HOLISTIC APPROACHES
If your animal has arthritis, his immune system needs either to be boosted or brought back into balance with the rest of his body. But if the arthritis is related to immune system dysfunction, you may find that immunostimulant herbs such as echinacea

aggravate your companion's condition. Remember that the inflammation associated with rheumatoid arthritis is likely caused by an autoimmune attack upon the joints. If we stimulate the immune system into working harder, we might actually make the arthritis worse.

Instead, holistic efforts should be directed at what is causing the dysfunction. This starts with a critical assessment of the animal's diet, an evaluation of possible food allergies, and a thorough investigation of present and historical influences that may be affecting your companion's immune system. Such influences may include vaccinations, antibiotic or steroid drug therapies, or toxic elements in your animal's environment. Any associated disorders should be identified and corrected as well. For example, does your arthritic companion suffer from chronic constipation, weight problems, hair loss, diarrhea, bladder or kidney problems, chronic infections, or a skin condition? If so, such conditions are likely related to the arthritis. When you have identified as many of these factors as possible, it's time to take remedial action by piecing this holistic puzzle together. It's important to remember that because arthritis is such a complex and variable disease, there is no singular herbal approach to treating it. Instead, holistic treatment is multifaceted, including nutritional supplementation and herbs that are tailored to an animal's individual needs.

If the arthritis is due to wear-and-tear joint deterioration (a frequent problem with working or hard-playing animals), then the supplements glucosamine sulfate and chondroitin sulfate might assist the body in repairing itself. Glucosamine and its related products, glucosamine sulfate and n-acetylglucosamine, have found a use as nutritional anti-osteoarthritic agents by helping protect and regenerate connective tissue and cartilage in affected joints. N-acetylglucosamine has shown promise in the treatment of inflammatory disorders, including inflammatory bowel disease, Crohn's disease, and colitis.

Bovine or shark cartilage, vitamin C, and EFA supplements help repair joint tissue damage. Horsetail herb might be of help too, as it contains a bioavailable form of silicon, an element that serves as the active matrix in connective tissue development. Comfrey is also considered a classic bone and joint repair herb. In addition to their internal uses, these herbs can be effective when applied in the form of an external compress, especially when combined with cayenne and willow bark, which should not be used in cats.

Mineral- and vitamin-rich herbs such as nettle and dandelion provide nutrients that are needed for joint repair along with diuretic activities to help remove excess metabolic wastes from the body, via the urinary tract, that may otherwise contribute to solid buildups in the joints. These herbs also help strengthen kidney function during the ordeal. Another herb to consider is shepherd's purse—this diuretic is believed to have a special affinity toward removal of waste compounds from arthritic joints. Celery seed and parsley root are also excellent choices.

Alterative herbs such as alfalfa, red clover, and burdock are strongly indicated to build up blood structure and to assist with the transport of systemic waste from body tissues. Liver supporting herbs (hepatics) such as dandelion root, yellow dock, and Oregon grape help by strengthening liver and gallbladder function, thus helping with digestion, nutrient absorption, and solid waste elimination. Lymphatic herbs such as cleavers and calendula may be of assistance by aiding the circulation of tissue-cleansing lymph in and around inflamed areas.

Cayenne and ginger also may be useful. Both are vasodilators and may benefit the arthritic animal by increasing blood circulation to affected areas. In some animals, though, these same actions may aggravate an inflammatory condition. For this reason, internal use of these herbs should proceed with caution, and it is best to administer them in small doses that are proportioned as lesser ingredients to a formula composed of other anti-inflammatory and alterative herbs.

Herbs that are useful internally for inflammation and pain of arthritis and hip dysplasia include licorice, yucca, and willow bark (the latter is not for cats). Alfalfa also has a long-standing reputation for relieving the discomforts of arthritis. It should be among one of the first herbs to be considered for internal use because it can be safely fed as a daily food supplement (1 teaspoon per pound of food fed each day).

Tonics as well as herbs can be helpful in treating arthritis. Circulatory tonics such as yarrow, hawthorn, rosemary, and ginkgo are worth considering for internal use. They provide a gentle increase of blood flow in tissues surrounding arthritic joints, so muscles remain oxygenated and more flexible.

On the facing page is a basic tonic formula for arthritic animals. Ingredients can be changed, added to, and proportioned to serve the specific needs of your animal. The arthritis relief compress that follows might also help to relieve the pain of arthritis.

Animals have a reputation for not letting their chronic problems slow them down much. As a result, arthritic joints sometimes become aggravated and inflamed because of physical exertion or injury. Provided that there is no open wound, a simple external application of arnica oil or tincture on the affected joints often brings fast

A Systemic Support Formula for Chronic Arthritis

Combine the following either as dried herbs or tinctures:

2 parts alfalfa
1 part dandelion root
1 part parsley root
1 part cleavers or calendula

This formula can be used as a dry herb food supplement. If you do choose to use dry herbs instead of tinctures, use calendula instead of cleavers because cleavers is almost useless after it is dried. An appropriate dose for each 30 pounds of the animal's body weight is 1 tablespoon mixed into food daily. If you opt to use tinctures, find those that contain little or no alcohol. (They are much easier to feed and much safer on the digestive tract.) You can administer 2–4 milliliters of the tincture for each 30 pounds of body weight directly into the animal's mouth or drop it onto his food daily. This combination is safe for dogs, cats, horses, and most other mammals and can be given over an extended period with no ill side effects. If your companion tolerates its bitter flavor, a one-part portion of yarrow can be added to this formula to serve as a vascular tonic.

Arthritis Relief Compress*

3 parts dried willow bark
3 parts dried comfrey leaf
3 parts dried yarrow
1 part powdered cayenne
  *not for use on cats

To make this compress, first make a decoction from the willow bark by gently simmering in enough water to cover it for about 20 minutes. Remove from heat but do not drain. While the water is still hot, add the other three ingredients. Mix thoroughly, adding just enough boiling water to make a thick paste. Let the mixture stand until it is cool enough to handle but still hot. The poultice is now ready to use as a compress. (See the "Basics of Herbal Preparations" in chapter 1 for further instructions.)

After applying the compress, check it after about 5 minutes to assure that the cayenne is not causing excessive irritation to the animal's skin. If it is, remove the compress and either lower the proportion of cayenne or remove it from the formula (make a new batch). For best results, the compress should be left on the animal for an hour.

symptomatic relief. Some good "strain and sprain" herbal ointments, salves, and liniments are also available on the market, many of which contain time-proven topical analgesics such as eucalyptus, cayenne, or camphor. Olbas oil or tiger balm are among our favorites, but do not use these products if your animal is under homeopathic care as they may antidote the homeopathic remedy. Also, be careful not to apply any undiluted oil or herbal ointment to an animal, especially cats, who can be sensitive to these types of products. Animals also may lick these products off of their fur and skin, and some of these products may prove toxic if ingested.

The discomforts of arthritis can be approached with internal herbal therapies as well, and often the fastest results are reached when topical and internal applications are used simultaneously. See the box on this page for a simple formula for symptomatic relief.

Of course, nutrition is the crux of any of the holistic healing modalities and is the most important factor in the prevention of arthritis. Many times changing to a raw food diet helps the animal and obviates more drastic measures.

Some animals benefit from occasional chiropractic adjustments from a qualified holistic vet who is trained in the proper manipulation of an animal's spine. Acupuncture may also help many arthritic animals who are in pain.

Cancer

When we hear the word cancer, many of us immediately think, "Oh no—this is the end!"

But cancer is not always a death sentence. There are many ways to deal with cancer, and many types of cancer can be treated holistically with the help and advice of a qualified holistic veterinarian.

A Symptomatic Relief Formula

Combine the following tinctures:

1 part alfalfa
1 part yucca
1 part licorice

for dogs, cats, horses, and most other mammals

Feed 1–2 milliliters of this formula for each 20 pounds of an animal's body weight, one to three times daily for up to ten days or until pain and inflammation are reduced.

In traditional Western medicine, we have been taught to believe that the best way to treat cancer is to poison it or cut it out. In holistic medicine, the treatment of cancer goes far beyond the physical nature of the disease to address the emotional and spiritual aspects of the sufferer as well. Many holistic practitioners believe that by cutting out or poisoning the cancer, we are only driving it elsewhere—perhaps deeper into the body where it can progress more insidiously.

For example, when the "check engine" light goes on in your car, you may stop, check under the hood, and add some oil if needed, or you may park the car and not drive it until the problem is identified. You're not going to rip out the wire that controls the light so it won't be a nuisance anymore. Unfortunately, in the case of your car, this quick-fix approach doesn't address the worn-out crankshaft bearing that degenerates and grinds away the engine block as you continue driving down the road—and when the car breaks down next, the damage is far more likely to be irreparable. Ripping out the wire is exactly what traditional Western medicine does in many cases of cancer. Voilà, cut and yank, and the problem has been "remedied."

In holistic medicine, the whole individual is treated, not just the cancer. Cancer is only a symptom of what is going on deeper within the being. In the treatment or prevention of cancer, all components of body, mind, and spirit need to be evaluated and supported. A critical assessment of diet is the first place to look—feeding poor-quality commercial food that is laden with artificial colors, preservatives, and by-products only makes the problem worse. The second step is to eliminate unnecessary vaccinations from the animal's life. A body that is working extra hard to build a cancer-fighting immune system doesn't need the stressful interference of vaccinations.

HOLISTIC APPROACHES
Nothing would please us more than to inform you of a new herbal "silver bullet" against cancer, but unfortunately such a thing does not exist. Although countless studies support the usefulness of herbs and various other holistic medicines in treating cancer, the disease is far too complex, variable, and adaptable for singular therapeutic approaches. In fact, cancer has so many faces that its early symptoms can include anything from a minor cough or excess shedding to occasional diarrhea. Just as varied is the list of possible causes—it seems that everything science looks at closely enough (foods, environmental toxins, natural and synthetic chemicals) carries the potential of causing cancer.

When cancer has progressed to a point where the diagnosis is certain, curative treatment is often less effective. But, if the disease is caught in its earliest stages, the prognosis can be quite positive. Effective prevention and treatment of cancer must begin with the guardian's intimate familiarity with his or her animal. Nobody offers more diagnostic insight into cancer than the person who keeps a detailed observational diary of his or her companion animal.

The diary should include lifelong records of illnesses or odd behavior or appearances. More important, though, it should reflect what the animal is like during times of optimal health. The guardian's capacity to notice minor deviations from perfect health is the most powerful tool in the early treatment of cancer and most other types of chronic disease.

Following are a few common warning signs the Veterinary Cancer Society recommends that pet owners look for in dogs. These symptoms apply to other animals as well. Remember, nothing here represents a conclusive diagnosis of cancer, but any symptoms listed should illuminate a red "check engine" light:

- abnormal swellings that continue to grow, especially in the lymph
- sores that do not heal
- bleeding or discharge from the mouth, nose, urinary tract, vagina, or rectum
- offensive odor
- difficulty eating or swallowing
- difficulty breathing
- difficulty urinating or defecating
- hesitation to exercise or loss of energy
- loss of appetite, weight loss
- persistent lameness or stiffness of movement
- lumps in the mammary glands
- abnormalities or difference in size of testicles

All of these symptoms may represent a cancer that has developed beyond its early stages, and therefore the animal should be taken to a holistic veterinarian immediately.

What might be indicative of the earliest onset of cancer? Well, just about anything out of the ordinary: a chronic cough or skin problem, decreased energy, aggression, pain, or stiffness—the list of early symptoms is endless. This doesn't mean you should live in constant fear of your companion developing cancer, but you should remain aware that a change that appears to be minor can develop into a serious condition. Don't ignore any changes in your animal. If a minor problem persists, consult a veterinarian.

All forms of cancer share a common characteristic: the disease starts when atypical cells begin reproducing and invading other cells. As healthy cells are destroyed and replaced by cancerous ones, lesions and tumors form and the body structures they occupy become dysfunctional.

Many holistic healers theorize that cancer is not really an acquired disease but rather the result of a metabolic imbalance that has progressed out of control. Cancerous tumors begin as small pinpoint lesions that occur off and on throughout an animal's lifetime. In most cases, the immune system is able to stop the tumors before they develop their own blood supply and begin consuming cell structures elsewhere in the body. But if the body is not in homeostasis (a state of balanced, harmonious health), it may not be able to eliminate the tumor before it takes control of its surroundings and a malignancy results. From this holistic perspective, carcinogenic compounds, excess ultraviolet light and radiation, and other substances that are said to cause cancer are not seen as "carriers" of the disease but as triggering or encouraging mechanisms.

The potential for cancer exists within every animal (human and otherwise). The key to preventing it lies inside a healthy body, not only in the outside influences that we consider threats. Perhaps you have noticed (as we have) that a disproportionate number of seemingly healthy people develop cancer despite all external efforts to avoid it. Why is this? It is because despite all the measures they may have taken toward eliminating potential carcinogens from their lives, deeper issues of physical, emotional, and spiritual health have not been addressed, and the people have fallen from homeostasis.

None of this is to say that we should disregard the existence of carcinogenic substances in food, water, and the environment. To the contrary, every effort should be made to become aware of and eliminate cancer-causing factors in our lives and the lives of our animals. But we must also provide our bodies with the proper elements of nutrition and systemic support that are needed to maintain homeostasis and prevent cancer. Furthermore, the immune system must be properly equipped and always ready to respond to a nearly infinite number of cancer-causing influences. It must be allowed to do its job without interference from antibiotics, immune-suppressing corticosteroid drugs, and vaccine therapies. Every time we interfere with natural immune system functions we may be compromising the body's ability to respond to and correct cellular or immune system imbalances that could develop into cancer.

WHEN CANCER OCCURS

The immune system represents the most complete form of disease intervention on earth. If allowed or enabled to function, it is infinitely more efficient than anything human beings can comprehend, much less devise. When cancer takes hold, the body's defenses need all of their resources to fight it. The holistic approach to cancer begins, then, by providing the body with every opportunity to perform optimally. This means supplying it with supplemental measures of nutritional and systemic support.

Several diet programs have been designed to strengthen and support animals with cancer. Many involve foods that are rich in fiber and antioxidant compounds. Intensive vitamin, mineral, and other supplemental therapies are often employed as well. These typically include vitamins A, B complex, C, and E, as well as selenium, iron, coenzyme Q_{10} (CoQ_{10}), EFAs, digestive enzymes, and dimethylglycine. The best anticancer diet for your animal is one tailored specifically to his individual needs by a holistic veterinarian who is familiar with treating the disease.

HERBAL THERAPIES

Herbs play important roles in supporting the body in its effort to rid itself of cancer. Herbal therapies focus on tonic support of organs and systems that have special significance in the fight. Because cancer is so variable, it's difficult to generalize an herbal approach. Every case of cancer is different, as are the metabolic requirements of each animal who has cancer. But a good starting point for herbal treatment of all animals with cancer is to support the liver, kidneys, and lymphatic system—the body's waste filtering and elimination systems. By helping the body cleanse itself, the immune system is less encumbered with cleanup chores and better able to fight cancer. The infamous Essiac and Hoxsey formulas were designed for this purpose. Although the formulas for both have likely been changed several times over the past years, each contains an array of alterative and cholagogue herbs that are targeted toward cleaning the blood, improving digestion, and

eliminating waste (primarily via the digestive tract). The Essiac formula is commonly marketed in health food stores.

The Hoxsey formula is available in various interpretations most of which contain at least six different herbs. Some herbalists, however, believe that the original formula contained only two: red clover and burdock.

Red clover is at the top of our list of anticancer herbs because it inhibits the activities of carcinogenic compounds, helps improve blood structure, and strengthens lymphatic functions that are crucial in cleansing cell tissues throughout the body. It also contains sterol constituents that may inhibit the production of blood vessels that supply and support newly formed tumors. Alfalfa provides similar alterative activities, but we don't know yet if it possesses the same tumor-inhibiting properties as red clover.

Burdock and dandelion root provide gentle stimulation to the liver, thus improving digestion and the removal of waste. These herbs do not cause added strain upon the filtering organs, and therefore they can be used continuously over a long period. In situations in which toxic buildup of systemic waste

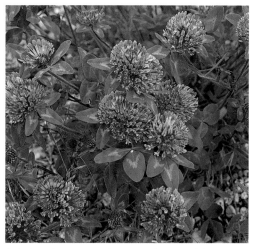

Red clover has many anticancer and tumor-inhibiting properties.

must be eliminated quickly in order to liberate the immune system, yellow dock serves as a much stronger liver stimulant and in fact is known as a traditional remedy for heavy metal toxicity (it is also a laxative). Milk thistle may be helpful for protecting the liver against harmful by-products of the cancer or from damage that may result after protracted drug therapies.

Diuretic herbs may also aid in removal of systemic waste via the kidneys and urinary tract. At the top of the diuretic list are dandelion leaf and nettle. These herbs stimulate urine production and provide potassium and other minerals that need to be continually replaced throughout the cleansing process.

To help remove toxic waste, slippery elm, marshmallow, flaxseed, and plantain serve as useful devices for lubricating, protecting, and reducing inflammation of mucous membranes throughout the urinary and digestive tracts. If poor liver function has caused chronic constipation, frequent small doses of turkey rhubarb tincture (0.25 milliliters per 30 pounds of the animal's body weight, three times daily) serve as an effective laxative. It should be limited to as-needed, short-term use because it can cause diarrhea, intestinal cramping, and other discomforts.

Immunostimulant herbs may help boost your companion's immune response to the cancer. Astragalus is especially well suited for this purpose because it adds energy-boosting adaptogenic qualities to its immunostimulant properties in cancer-debilitated animals. Garlic is another excellent immune system tonic to consider. While boosting production of killer T cells and other immune system components, it has also been shown to trigger enzyme responses that help break down waste materials before they enter the bloodstream.

Once the specific characteristics of the cancer have been identified and correlated with the animal's holistic needs and cancer-fighting abilities, herbal medicines may be administered directly against the cancer. As we mentioned earlier, this approach requires the experience of a trained professional who is used to recognizing and treating cancer. Many herbal devices have shown great promise in combating specific forms of cancer. Acemannan, a compound derived

A Tonic Support Formula for Animals with Cancer

Combine the following low-alcohol (glycerin) herb tinctures:

2 parts red clover
1 part astragalus
1 part dandelion root
1 part garlic

This formula can be fed to the animal continuously over a long period: 0.5 milliliters per 20 pounds of the animal's body weight, three times daily. If constipation is part of your animal's problem, try adding 2 parts marshmallow to the formula. If this fails to bring results, add 1 part yellow dock. If that doesn't work, try substituting the yellow dock with turkey rhubarb. If liver damage is evident or a threat, twice-daily doses of milk thistle may be fed in addition to this formula to help repair and protect the liver. A standardized milk thistle preparation that contains at least 70 percent silymarin constituents is best for repairing an already damaged liver.

from aloe vera, has been shown to be effective against fibrosarcoma and FeLV. It is theorized that acemannan triggers an increase in the immune attack upon the viruses believed to cause these usually fatal diseases. An intravenous drug called Carnivora is derived from the Venus's flytrap plant for treatment of malignant tumors. Although it has not been approved for use in North America as of 1999, Carnivora has shown some incredible tumor-reducing results in Europe. Herbalists have also seen good results from the use of violet leaf extract in the treatment of certain cancers. It, too, is believed to have tumor-reducing qualities.

Cardiovascular Problems

In contrast with the vast array of cardiovascular disorders that loom over their human guardians, animals have little risk of contracting heart or arterial disease during the first three-quarters of their lives. Strokes and heart attacks are almost unheard of in dogs and cats simply because their bodies are naturally designed to metabolize the meat and animal fats that send many of their caretakers to an early grave. This doesn't mean that animals aren't susceptible to the ills of chemical preservatives, excess sodium, and refined sugar. Nor does it mean their cardiovascular systems are more resilient to abuse or neglect. It means only that unhealthy foods, chemicals, and environmental influences may have a different effect on our companion animals than they do on us. Simply put, a dog or cat on a low-quality, poorly digestible commercial diet is far more likely to die from kidney failure than arteriosclerosis. On the same note, an animal's cardiovascular system will fail, just as ours will, unless all requirements of good nutrition, exercise, and environmental quality are met.

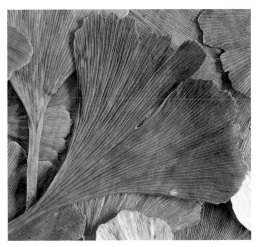

Ginkgo helps to increase circulation.

The heart and vascular system operates continuously and under constant pressure throughout an animal's life. Factors such as excessive body fat, chronic illness, secondhand smoke, and aging add to the stress and inevitable wear and tear of this vital system. Unlike us, however, our companions have little choice in how their cardiovascular health is maintained—that determination is left up to us.

DIET AND EXERCISE: THE HEART OF HEART HEALTH

Cardiovascular health all begins with a complete diet. The heart consists of specially adapted smooth muscles and connective tissues that must perform optimally throughout every moment during an animal's life; therefore, the heart needs to be continually fed and repaired. The vascular system must remain strong, free of obstructions, and responsive to the body's needs. It, too, must be continually supplied with the tools and fuel needed for self-maintenance and flawless function. A big problem arises, however, when an animal is afforded only an average "maintenance diet" for subsistence. The cardiovascular system's nutritional daily requirements are never static but instead are continually fluctuating and changing as challenges arise. This means that no single commercial diet, no matter how complete, organic, or digestible it might be, can contain all of the nutritional elements your companion's heart needs on a day-to-day basis.

The only way to be sure that your animal is receiving the nutrition needed for good cardiovascular health is to provide a diversity of fresh whole foods throughout his life. Supplemental vitamins, minerals, and EFAs also help assure that your companion's cardiovascular system is getting the special considerations it needs. Amino acids are especially important, as they serve as the protein building blocks of smooth-muscle development and repair. Cats must have taurine in their diets, and dogs must have a sufficient supply of l-carnitine, or degenerative heart disease (idiopathic dilated cardiomyopathy) may result. Coenzyme Q_{10} also plays important roles in prevention and treatment of heart problems. It has been shown to help protect the heart muscle from damage secondary to hypoxia, infection, and inflammation.

CARDIOVASCULAR PROBLEMS IN DOGS AND CATS

In cats, the most common form of noninherited (acquired) heart disease is hypertrophic cardiomyopathy, an enlargement of the left ventricular wall and septum that reduces the heart's functional ability to pump blood. In dogs, the most common form of acquired heart disease is valvular degeneration in which the heart valves fail to completely close when they should, causing an audible (with a stethoscope) heart murmur and decreased cardiac output. This condition can lead to poor circulation to the extremities, the formation of blood clots in the veins and arteries, and congestive heart failure. In both dogs and cats, acquired cardiomyopathy is most likely to occur in middle-aged or older animals.

Animals may suffer from inherited forms of heart disease as well. In dogs, one of the most common is patent ductus arteriosus, a congenital defect (most commonly seen in miniature poodles and German shepherds) that essentially amounts to a leak between chambers of the heart. In cats, congenital defects in the mitral and tricuspid valves of the heart are fairly common.

Other forms of cardiovascular disease may be secondary to bacterial, protozoan, or viral infection. Congestive heart failure, a condition in which high pressure in the left atrium of the heart causes a backup of fluid into the pulmonary capillaries and lungs, is common in obese or geriatric animals or those with heart defects or dysfunction.

Animals with heart problems may exhibit shortness of breath, coughing, and diminished physical stamina. Further examination may reveal cardiac arrhythmia, pulmonary edema, or blood pressure problems. If you suspect that your animal companion has a heart problem, you should get him to a holistic veterinarian right away.

HERBAL THERAPIES

The herbal approach to heart disorders is to strengthen and support cardiovascular and pulmonary function and efficiency. Tonic herbal therapies are especially helpful in older animals who need a gentle measure of daily cardiovascular support. In all cases, a daily supplement of hawthorn helps improve coronary blood flow, moderate blood pressure, and strengthen heartbeat. Garlic may also be of benefit. Ginkgo, yarrow, or cayenne should also be considered to help increase circulation in the extremities, brain, and throughout the peripheral capillaries of the body. If rapid, erratic heartbeat is part of your companion's disorder, bugleweed may be useful to safely slow and strengthen the heart. If myocardial inflammation or pulmonary edema is present (such as with congestive heart failure), a daily regimen of strong dandelion leaf tea helps remove excess fluid from the body. At the same time, it supplies the body with potassium, a mineral that is essential to healthy heart function.

Adaptogenic herbs such as astragalus or Siberian ginseng may increase overall energy levels in the animal. Astragalus is also known to have antiviral qualities that are specific to heart infections. Echinacea or other immunostimulant herbs are indicated in circumstances where bacterial or viral infection is involved.

A Cardiovascular Tonic

Combine the following glycerin tinctures:

2 parts hawthorn
2 parts dandelion leaf
1 part yarrow
1 part ginkgo

An appropriate dose for dogs, cats, and other small animals is 0.05–1.0 milliliter for each 20 pounds of the animal's body weight daily. Horses and other large herbivores can receive 20–30 milliliters daily. If more practical, horses and other large herbivores can be fed 1–2 liters of the fresh herbs daily (in lieu of the tincture formula).

In addition to this formula, dietary supplementation of garlic may be of benefit to the animal.

Digestive System Problems

We are all familiar with the sounds and sights of an animal suffering from digestive upset— and with cleaning up the aftermath. This is not a pleasant part of taking care of animals, but it's a fact of life, nonetheless.

It's normal for a healthy animal to vomit or get diarrhea on occasion. Dogs and cats may intuitively induce vomiting by eating grass or other plants. This action serves to cleanse the stomach. Diarrhea may occur if your animal eats something that he is not accustomed to or eats too much of something that his body doesn't need, such as salty food that was sneaked beneath the dinner table. Vomiting and diarrhea are usually harmless and self-correcting, but they could also be symptoms of a much more serious condition.

Digestive upset could be indicative of a parasite imbalance, pancreatitis, colitis, giardiasis, ulcers, liver dysfunction, bacterial or protozoan infection, or even cancer. This leads us back to what holistic animal healing is all about: caring about your animal enough to recognize the difference between an isolated incident and a serious illness.

THE REALITY OF DIGESTIVE UPSET

Human nature dictates that anything unpleasant to any of the human senses must be immediately suppressed or ignored. To think about vomit or diarrhea, much less look at what it contains, is virtually taboo. Humanity's aversion toward secondhand food material is a limiting factor in the holistic care of animals. If we are to care for beloved companions who cannot articulate how they feel, we must learn to set aside this aversion long enough to consider fully what vomiting and having diarrhea might actually mean in terms of their health. Is that mess on the sofa just a wad of grass or a hair ball, or does it contain blood (which sometimes looks like coffee grounds), worms, or thick yellow discharge? Forcing yourself to thoroughly examine the mess rather than covering it up immediately with half a roll of paper towels might make the difference between health and sickness for your companion.

The conventional way of dealing with digestive upset is to suppress the uncomfortable or unpleasant symptoms. For diarrhea, there are stool hardeners. For constipation, there are laxatives. For vomiting, there are antiemetic drugs. But from a holistic perspective, the paramount question of what caused the problem in the first place remains unanswered with these approaches. In fact, stopping the body's efforts to purge itself may do more harm than good.

If your animal is experiencing chronic diarrhea or is vomiting but is exhibiting no other signs of disease, try changing his diet. Oftentimes when an animal is placed on a natural diet, these occurrences are greatly diminished or eliminated altogether. Food supplementation with digestive probiotics and enzymes often helps too. If your animal's stool or vomit looks odd or if the situation is severe or persistent, see your veterinarian immediately.

APPETITE LOSS (ANOREXIA) AND MALABSORPTION

Loss of appetite in animals is seen in many different illnesses. It can be very dangerous for cats, who may suffer from hepatic lipidosis, a degenerative condition where the liver becomes congested and dysfunctional from a rapid buildup of fat. A cat with hepatic lipidosis loses his ability to use stored fat, and as a result, the body utilizes its own muscle mass as a source of protein. About 35 percent of cats with this disease eventually die from it.

If your companion chooses not to eat, don't jump to conclusions and panic. For various reasons, some animals may naturally decide to fast. Fasting should be allowed if it doesn't continue for more than a few days and as long as the animal seems healthy in all other ways. Keep a close eye for signs of weakness, weight loss, fever, runny eyes, or any other signs of ill health. If after a few days of fasting your companion is still turning up his nose to his favorite treats, assume that something is wrong—even if he seems otherwise healthy—and get to a vet!

A gum or tooth infection, ulcers of the mouth, periods of strenuous exercise, or warm weather may cause decreased appetite. Intestinal parasites, digestive ulcers, tumors or other masses, digestive flora imbalances, bacterial or fungal infections, and liver dysfunction are just a few causes of appetite loss. Your companion also may be depressed or simply bored with his diet. In other words, the possibilities are endless and some are life threatening. If your companion isn't eating and you can't pinpoint the cause on your own within a few days, the best course of action is to consult your holistic veterinarian for medical help.

It's difficult to generalize about how to approach appetite loss because the possible causes are too diverse and extensive. It is safe to say, however, that vitamins, probiotics, and enzyme supplements play important roles in animals who aren't cleaning their plates. In addition, a few herbs stand out in their abilities to stimulate appetite and improve nutrient absorption in the digestive systems of some animals. One such herb is yucca, which contains saponin constituents that are believed to increase nutrient permeability in the small intestine while at the same time stimulating appetite. By improving the absorption of nutrients, animals who are eating less are able to make the best use of the food they do eat. Alfalfa is another herb to consider—it is nutritious and is also regarded as an appetite stimulant in animals. Both yucca and alfalfa should be used in moderation (especially with horses), as they may actually cause digestive upset or bloat if fed in too much abundance. Bitter herbs such as gentian, dandelion, and Oregon grape may help get the digestive juices flowing to trigger an increase in appetite, as might peppermint, fennel, or garlic.

COLIC AND FLATULENCE

The term *colic* is generic, referring to any condition that causes pain, inflammation, or other discomfort in the colon. Most commonly, colic is caused by flatulence (trapped gas), which is usually associated with abdominal distention and irritability. Colic is most often caused by something the animal ingested, but bacterial, fungal, or parasitic infection may also be the cause, as could a deficiency in liver or gallbladder functions or an ulcer, a tumor, or an injury somewhere in the digestive tract. Regardless of the onset, colic can be especially serious in horses—so serious that herbs may not act fast enough to prevent a life-threatening situation. If your horse is suffering from colic, call your vet immediately!

To find a long-term solution to colic (especially chronic, recurring cases), you must first identify the underlying causes. Then and only then can a holistic, long-term solution be found. Until you find the answer, it is possible to relieve the uncomfortable symptoms of colic with herbs. The first course of remedial action is to aid in the elimination of excess gas and help reduce pain and spasms in the colon. Chamomile, fennel, dill, catnip, or peppermint are all good choices for this. If inflammation appears to be

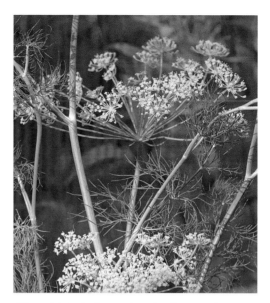

Dill expels intestinal gas and soothes the stomach.

part of the problem, slippery elm, plantain, marshmallow, raspberry leaf, certified organic goldenseal, or nettle may help. If an ulcer is suspected, licorice lends antimicrobial and anti-inflammatory properties that are especially well suited for the problem. If giardiasis, *E. coli*, or some other form of parasitic, bacterial, or fungal infection is part of the problem, consider combining Oregon grape or goldenseal tincture with an equal amount of licorice tincture (0.5–1 milliliter for each 20 pounds of an animal's body weight, twice daily). This helps inhibit the invading microbes while speeding the healing of digestive mucosa. Fresh echinacea can be especially helpful for horses suffering from colic of bacterial origin—allow the animals to eat as much of the fresh plants (roots, flowers, and all) as they intuitively desire.

DIARRHEA

Diarrhea is caused by an overabundance of fluid entering the intestinal tract. This in turn can interfere with the digestion process and may result in malabsorption and severe

A Basic Formula for Colic

Combine the following ingredients either as teas, tinctures, or dried herbs:

1 part fennel seed
1 part marshmallow root
1 part chamomile

An appropriate starting dose for most dogs is either 1 tablespoon of the dried herbs, 1 milliliter of a low-alcohol tincture combination, or 2 tablespoons of a strong tea sprinkled on a small amount of food, twice daily. Cats should receive half of the dog dose. Horses and other herbivores can be fed 2–4 cups of the dried herbs or 4–8 cups of the fresh herbs daily.

dehydration if left unaddressed. From a holistic perspective, diarrhea is a by-product of systemic dysfunction or the body's effort to deal with some form of excess. Normally, nutrients pass through intestinal mucous membranes to enter the bloodstream. To aid in this metabolic process, the membranes allow a measured amount of water, bile, and other digestive fluids to enter the intestinal tract from the opposite direction (from the body). When too much fluid is allowed to enter the intestinal tract for whatever reason, loose stool is the result. Conversely, when too little fluid is allowed into the intestinal tract, constipation occurs.

The standard, symptomatic approach to diarrhea is to inhibit the entrance of fluid into the intestinal tract. This is usually accomplished with the use of astringent herbs or drugs—those that cause contraction (shrinking) of mucous membranes. By quickly shrinking intestinal membranes, excess fluid is prohibited from entering the digestive tract, and the stool firms up. If herbs are the medicine of choice, those containing large amounts of tannin constituents, such as uva ursi, rose bark, or white oak bark, are generally the quickest acting. The problem is that these and most other "tannin heavyweights" can be irritating to the stomach and kidneys and therefore must be used only for a short duration—about a day or two at a time. The better approach is to be patient. Try gentler astringents first, such as chamomile or raspberry leaf. If these fail, try slippery elm or plantain (our favorite)—these herbs combine their tannin constituents with the soothing and protecting effects of mucilage. If these herbs fail, try combining one of the aforementioned astringents with an equal amount of marshmallow root. The soothing, mucilaginous quality of the marshmallow helps moderate the irritating effect of the tannins.

With all of that said, it's now time to reconsider the use of astringents altogether. Remember, the goal of holistic herbal medicine is to assist the body in its abilities to correct and heal itself. When we use astringent herbs to treat diarrhea, we are only suppressing the body's response to deeper problems. Plus, we have to consider that the diarrhea actually might be part of the body's natural healing process. The bottom line is this: if your animal is suffering from a sudden onset of diarrhea, try to make lifestyle arrangements that allow you to live with the situation for a day or two—until it passes. Encourage your animal to drink plenty of water, restrict salt intake, and let nature take its course. If bacterial infection or giardiasis is the suspected cause, Oregon grape or certified organic goldenseal might help solve the problem.

Regardless of what you might suspect, if the problem persists or worsens, take your companion to a holistic vet for a thorough examination. At the very least, have the stool analyzed for the presence of blood, worms, or other evidence of deeper health problems, and be sure that the animal is drinking plenty of water to avoid dehydration. Once the underlying causes are identified, a holistic course of action can be directed at the root cause (not the symptoms) of the problem.

A Tonic Formula for Chronic Constipation

Combine the following as either dried herbs, low-alcohol tinctures, or strong teas:

2 parts dandelion root
2 parts marshmallow root
1 part Oregon grape
1 part yellow dock
1 part fennel (to relieve any associated gas or griping)

*This diet should be supplemented with flaxseed or psyllium husks.

For dogs, try 1 teaspoon of the strong, combined, cooled teas or 1 milliliter of the tincture per 30 pounds of body weight, two or three times daily.

Cats can receive ¼ to ½ teaspoon of the strong, combined, cooled teas or 0.25–0.50 milliliters of the tincture per 15 pounds of body weight, two or three times daily.

CONSTIPATION

Constipation is usually caused when the body is unable to fully digest food or when other materials cause a blockage. If an animal is receiving a healthy, well-balanced diet, constipation should not be a problem, and contrary to what many conventional dog and cat care texts may say, a healthy diet should include fresh raw bones from an organic source, if possible. The idea that raw bones cause digestive blockages in dogs and cats is untrue, at least if the animal is healthy to start with. Carnivores are naturally designed to digest and metabolize bones. If they can't digest them and constipation occurs, it's because their digestive system is not working efficiently (or perhaps they're eating too many bones).

In treating constipation, the first step is to rule out the possibility that your companion ate something he shouldn't have—such as a piece of wood; pine needles; some tough dry grass; or perhaps that heirloom tapestry that was handed down through your family for fifteen generations. If ingestion of "something different" is ruled out, then look deeper for some sort of interrelated problem. Start with a thorough reevaluation of diet and make sure that your animal is receiving the enzymes and probiotics needed for healthy digestive flora. Try feeding your companion some organic, live-cultured yogurt. Eating yogurt activates reproduction of digestive flora and often has quick and natural laxative effects. If the animal is straining to pass stool, then some ground flaxseed, psyllium husk, or marshmallow root might help lubricate the intestines. Feed ¼ teaspoon of any of these herbs for each 20 pounds of an animal's weight along with plenty of water. Fresh chickweed can be fed to horses, goats, llamas, dogs, cats, birds, and other animals for a gentle laxative and soothing effect.

Chronic constipation is often a cumulative effect of liver or gallbladder congestion or dysfunction. If bile production is reduced in the liver, or if the gallbladder or a bile duct is blocked by solid waste or inflammation, then the digestive tract cannot receive the chemicals it needs to effectively break down food materials. The result is constipation. Again, this condition is usually caused by one or more elements of the diet (such as low-grade protein or too much fat) that cannot be effectively digested and metabolized. Aside from a change in diet, the herbal approach is to improve bile production and transport with cholagogue herbs such as dandelion root and Oregon grape. If the problem is believed to be associated with liver damage or inflammation, milk thistle, turmeric, or licorice should be added to the program to help protect and regenerate liver cells. Essential fatty acids, such as those found in the oils of flaxseed, evening primrose, and borage, serve critical roles in liver repair as well.

By now you may have noticed that we have not mentioned the use of laxative herbs. This is because constipation is almost always a by-product of a deeper problem for which a laxative can serve only as a symptomatic quick fix. The strongest laxative herbs are those containing anthraquinone constituents. Anthraquinones stimulate peristalsis—spasmodic smooth-muscle contractions of the bowels. In effect, these spasms force stool out of the body, causing uncomfortable cramping, griping pain, gas, and loss of smooth-muscle tone. With long-term use, laxatives can even cause digestive dependency (i.e., your animal will not be able to pass stool without the laxative). Since the holistic approach to animal health is focused on assisting (as opposed to forcing) the body with its natural functions, strong laxatives such as senna, aloe, cascara sagrada, and turkey rhubarb should be reserved for times when all else fails and bowel movement is an immediate necessity. Before resorting to any of these herbs, give yellow dock a try. Although it too contains considerable amounts of anthraquinones, it tends to be much more gentle, and it imparts liver and digestive stimulating qualities that add to its value in treating constipation. We find it especially effective when used in small proportions with liver tonic herbs, such as dandelion root.

Finally, when encountering constipation in pregnant animals, the safest approach is to avoid anything that contains anthraquinones. Instead, look to marshmallow, chickweed, flaxseed, or psyllium husks to provide colonic lubrication without stressing the reproductive organs or the fetus.

Horses and other herbivores seldom get constipated, but they commonly suffer from various other forms of colic. When these animals do get constipated, it's usually attributable to poor-quality feed or forage or to the ingestion of sand, gravel, and other nonorganic materials. In these circumstances, dietary supplementation with a few tablespoons of ground or finely chopped marshmallow, flaxseed, or psyllium husks usually assist with elimination.

HAIR BALLS

Anyone who has been licked by a cat knows that felines have rough, "barbed" tongues. This makes it difficult for them to spit hair out after each of their hundred or so daily baths, so they must swallow the hair. This in turn may lead to vomiting and the possibility of intestinal obstructions.

One conventional approach to hair balls is to feed the affected cat some petroleum jelly, a practice we feel is especially dangerous because the jelly, being totally insoluble in water, can be aspirated into the lungs of a choking or vomiting cat and cause life-threatening pneumonia. Other approaches employ laxatives, the theory being that the hair balls can be expeditiously eliminated out the opposite end of the kitty. Again we frown—the poor cat is having a tough enough time without suffering a caretaker-induced case of intestinal cramping and diarrhea.

Fortunately, there are some safe and effective actions you can take to help your feline eliminate hair balls more easily. Foremost is a well-balanced, raw food diet. Raw meats, bones, and vegetables contain the fiber and roughage necessary to bind with ingested hair and carry it out of the body. Giving ¼ teaspoon of bran, psyllium husks, or ground flaxseed also provides fiber and lubricating mucilage to help remove hair balls. Giving ½ teaspoon of marshmallow root tea or 12–20 drops of the glycerin tincture will likely help lubricate the process as well. If your cat will eat marshmallow root au natural, ¼–½ teaspoon of fresh or dried root can be finely chopped and added to Kitty's food for a similar effect. Adding a teaspoon of olive oil to the food can be helpful too.

For rabbits who get intestinal obstructions of fur, a common practice by some rabbit caretakers is to feed pineapple juice to "melt" the fur away. The fur passing more easily is probably due to the enzymatic action of the juice, and supplementing with digestive enzymes would most likely work in a similar fashion when used as a preventative.

INFLAMMATORY BOWEL DISEASE
Inflammatory bowel disease and colitis involve mucosal inflammation of the colon. Animals with inflammatory bowel disease often suffer from severe diarrhea, labored or painful bowel movements, gastric distention, and rectal bleeding or mucus discharge. In cats, the problem is sometimes labeled Crohn's disease. Causes are often difficult to pinpoint, even with the best diagnostic methods. Immune system disorders, circulatory impairment in the intestinal tract, parasitic infections, defects in permeability of the intestinal wall, dietary sensitivities, or adverse drug reactions are all part of a long list of causative possibilities.

Conventional approaches to inflammatory bowel disease include feeding a controlled diet that may include supplemental dietary fiber and the use of corticosteroids and other immunosuppressive drugs. In cats, inflammation is often treated with sulfasalazine (Azulfidine), a compound that is also used in humans for similar disorders.

Natural therapies usually start with adjustments in diet and supplementation with vitamins and probiotics that support digestion and moderate immune system activities. A daily regimen of n-acetylglucosamine (250–1,500 milligrams), glutamine (250–3,000 milligrams), *Lactobacillus acidophilus* (20–500 million microorganisms), proanthocyanidin complex (10–200 milligrams), dimethylglycine (50–250 milligrams), and vitamin C (250–3000 milligrams) represents one suggested nutritional therapy for dogs and cats. Papaya supplements may also prove beneficial in improving digestion, but care must be taken to assure that any or all of these supplements do not cause or worsen diarrhea.

The symptoms of inflammatory bowel disease can often be relieved with the same herbs we recommend for treating gastritis. Because reduction of mucosal inflammation is of critical importance, anti-inflammatory and demulcent herbs such as licorice, slippery elm, plantain, marshmallow, flaxseed, and psyllium husks may be

A Formula for Inflammatory Bowel Disease

Combine the following as either teas, tinctures, or dried herbs:

2 parts slippery elm or plantain
1 part marshmallow root
1 part licorice
1 part fennel seed

For dogs, 1 tablespoon of the dried herbs, 1 milliliter of a low-alcohol tincture combination, or 2 tablespoons of a strong tea can be fed twice daily. Cats should receive half the dog dose. Horses and other herbivores can be fed 2–4 cups of the dried herbs or 4–8 cups of the fresh herbs daily.

especially useful. Aloe vera juice or calendula may also relieve the discomforts of inflammatory bowel disease. Certified organic goldenseal may help to reduce mucosal inflammation. Astragalus is well suited for immune support in cases in which infection may be involved because it tends not to overstimulate the immune system when an increased autoimmune response may already be a contributing factor in the inflammation.

LEAKY GUT SYNDROME (INTESTINAL DYSBIOSIS AND HYPERPERMEABILITY)

Leaky gut is a term used for a condition in which food compounds abnormally permeate intestinal barriers to enter the bloodstream. Oftentimes, this leads to an immediate defensive attack by the immune system and severe food allergies. In some cases, systemic infection, arthritis, seborrhea, or other forms of autoimmune disease may result.

Leaky gut syndrome has many causes, any number of which may be secondary to another. Poor diet; excessive use of antibiotic drugs; or bacterial, parasitic, or fungal infections may alter digestive flora to the point that intestinal mucosal barriers will be vulnerable and weakened by certain food-carried chemicals. The problem may also be caused by chronic inflammatory bowel disease—when the intestinal mucosa is inflamed, its structural integrity may be altered in a way that allows unusually large food particles, bacteria, parasites, fungi (such as *Candida albicans*), or protozoa to cross intestine-blood barriers.

The most effective approach to avoid leaky gut is with a natural diet that contains all of the probiotic elements necessary for healthy digestive flora, structure, and function. Research has shown that glutamine, a fatty acid component, plays important roles in maintaining gut tonicity, thus reducing the possibility of leaky gut. One study concluded that animals deprived of glutamine were more likely to suffer sepsis, bacterial infection of the blood.

Leaky gut can be progressive and debilitating shortly after onset. The holistic approach toward correcting the problem is to provide supplemental measures of digestive probiotics to build intestinal flora and strengthen mucosal barriers. Plantain, marshmallow, raspberry leaf, certified organic goldenseal, and chamomile can be used to reduce inflammation, tonify intestinal mucosa, and provide an additional barrier against invading microbes. Flaxseed is also strongly indicated, as it provides soothing, cleansing, and protective mucilage and fiber constituents as well as an added measure of mucosa-strengthening omega-3 fatty acids.

Ear Problems

Ear problems most commonly come in the form of bacterial or fungal infections, mites, fleas, or foreign objects (foxtails, dirt, etc.) lodged in the ear canal. Some other common problems include hematoma of the earflap and tumors of the inner ear.

Mullein flower, Oregon grape, garlic, marshmallow, ginkgo, and yarrow are especially well suited for treating infections and parasite infestations of the ear. Mullein flower, garlic, and Oregon grape are all strong antimicrobials with strong affinities toward

Antimicrobial and Antiparasitic Ear Oil

Combine equal amounts of the following oil infusions:

Mullein flower
Oregon grape
Garlic
Marshmallow

You can add 10–20 drops of vitamin E oil to this mixture to act as a preservative and aid in skin healing. For ear mites or infections of fungal or bacterial origin, 6–12 drops of the oil can be applied to affected areas of the earflap or ear canal. A soft plastic dropper is best for application into the ear canal, while a piece of soft cotton, gauze, or even clean fingertips will suffice as an external applicator.

inhibition of mites and various pathogens that may cause ear problems. The slippery oily mucilage of marshmallow root provides soothing relief and a protective, antimicrobial barrier on inflamed tissues of the outer ear. Yarrow is especially useful for treating small hematomas of the earflap. Used externally, the oil helps strengthen exterior capillary walls, while internal doses of yarrow and ginkgo tea or tincture improve capillary circulation and internal tonicity. Witch hazel may also be effective for external treatment of earflap hematomas, as its strong astringency quickly constricts weak or inflamed blood vessels.

Elderly Animal Care

What is considered old for a pet? We know that to a certain degree longevity varies with the type, size, and breed of an animal. For example, a small dog may live into his teens, while a larger breed of dog may be entering his golden years at only seven or eight years of age. But for those of us who strive to understand what life must be like from the animal's perspective, a different question comes to mind: What would our pets themselves regard as old age?

We all grow old. Various body parts become fatigued from oxidation and wear and tear, systemic efficiency begins to decline, and certain bodily functions simply don't work as well as they used to. But how much of the aging process is actually relative to time and physiological degeneration, and how much is the result of surrendering to the thought of being old and feeble? We raise this question on behalf of the animals who have taught us just how carefree and fun the latter part of life can really be. Unlike humans, animals age without even considering the concepts of mortality and personal vanity, and those of us who pay close enough attention to them can gain some precious insight about what being old really means.

For humans, old age is as much a product of mind-set as it is of physical circumstances. To animals, the entire idea of "yielding to the wheels of time" does not apply—an elderly animal does not live in anticipation of death but in celebration of life. As his human guardians roll their tired old bodies out of bed in the morning and moan, groan, and complain about their hemorrhoids, the elderly dog waits by the door virtually shouting, "Who cares about not having teeth anymore? There's a squirrel out there and it's near my doghouse! Let's go get him!" There are some powerful lessons about life and happiness here.

Chronic diseases are often disregarded as just a part of growing old. In fact, many pet owners see their animals' old age as a

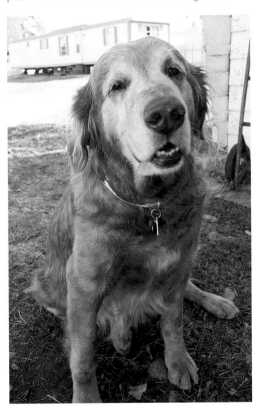

Providing your pet with a healthful diet, holistic lifestyle, and a lifetime of love can help him enjoy his later years.

downhill slide to inevitable suffering and death. As a result of this mind-set, countless numbers of animals are euthanized not because their time has naturally passed but because their guardians are fearful of watching the animals grow old and die a natural death. Granted, it's difficult to live in anticipation of a companion's death, but all things considered, this is really our problem, not theirs.

The fact that an animal is growing old and becoming more susceptible to illness does not automatically predispose him to chronic disease, it just means that he needs some added care and attention. With your loving support, your old best friend can enjoy life right up to his last day.

We are firm believers that animals who receive plenty of love and attention, a wholesome homemade diet, a minimum of vaccinations, and holistic measures of health care throughout their lives can beat the odds of longevity set by genetics, breeding, and physical size. By affording them the elements of sustained health and well-being, animals reward us before and after they pass from our lives. They leave us with the peace of mind that comes from knowing that their lives were totally fulfilled by kindhearted and respectful human beings who cared enough to allow them to live and age gracefully and innocently—as animals do.

HERBAL THERAPIES

Most chronic problems seen in elderly animals are the results of poor or incomplete nutrition. Liver problems, chronic renal failure, diabetes, arthritis and hip dysplasia, and neurological problems (such as canine cognitive dysfunction) are just a few of the conditions that may be prevented by lifelong good nutrition. Tailor a dietary program to your companion's specific needs as early as possible. Each month of nutritional deficiency can trim healthy years from the latter end of your animal's life. A holistic veterinarian can assist you in determining the proper diet and nutrients for the age, physical condition, and lifestyle of your companion.

In older animals, herbs are especially useful for providing added support to body functions and systems that are becoming less efficient. Nothing can compare with spirulina or other forms of blue-green algae for tonic nutritional support of an aging body. Astragalus is an especially well-suited general tonic for older animals because it provides a measured degree of immune system support while also strengthening the animal's resistance to stress. Garlic serves this purpose as well, but added care must be exercised in assuring that it does not cause digestive upset in elderly animals.

The liver and digestive organs endure a lifetime of abusive environmental toxins and systemic waste materials, so it stands to reason that they will eventually begin to fail in the later years of life. To support liver and digestive functions, an animal's diet should be frequently reevaluated and adjusted as needed to accommodate any reduction in these organs' metabolic capacities. Additionally, digestion and waste elimination can be improved with digestive enzymes and mild liver stimulants, such as dandelion or burdock root. These help with the removal of solid wastes from the body while increasing the production of bile and digestive enzymes. Marshmallow root, fed fresh, dried, or in any form of low-alcohol liquid, aids in the passage of stool by providing a protective, anti-inflammatory, and lubricating barrier to the intestinal mucosa. Flaxseed or psyllium husks work in a similar manner as well.

The kidneys have a difficult life too because they must filter and eliminate waste from the blood over the course of a lifetime. Over time they may become scarred and dysfunctional from repetitive infections, stones, and other damaging influences that may or may not have been detected earlier. To increase urinary efficiency and help strengthen mucous membranes in the urinary tract, a tea of dandelion leaf, nettle, cleavers, or parsley leaf can be added to the animal's drinking water—just enough to noticeably tint the water. Giving one of these herbs provides alterative qualities that the animal's body can selectively utilize to eliminate waste and maintain clean, well-nourished blood. This can be done every day for the remainder of the animal's life.

If the animal displays early symptoms of renal failure, twice-daily doses of ginkgo and hawthorn help to improve blood circulation and reduce blood pressure in the kidneys, while corn silk, marshmallow, and plantain help to reduce any inflammation.

Oatstraw serves as an excellent nervous system tonic that can be fed daily to help improve and regulate nerve transmission. In animals who display diminished mental clarity or odd behavior that is attributable to brain dysfunction (e.g., cognitive dysfunction in canines) blood circulation and neurological functions of the brain can be assisted and sometimes improved with the use of ginkgo, gotu kola, or peppermint. In certain cases, Saint-John's-wort may be beneficial as well, but this determination should be made by a holistic veterinarian who is familiar with your animal.

Aches, pains, and loss of mobility that result from joint and connective tissue degeneration may be relieved with supplements of glucosamine or chondroitin sulfate, horsetail, or yucca root. In cases of arthritis flare-ups, licorice, devil's claw, or boswellia may bring symptomatic relief.

Cardiovascular efficiency can be supported with daily supplementation of hawthorn berries. If circulatory impairment is evident in the legs, ears, or tail of the animal, ginkgo, yarrow, or cayenne may be of assistance. The Animal Essentials dry herb and vitamin formula is also a good broad-spectrum daily supplement.

WHEN THE END IS NEAR

If your companion receives a good diet, plenty of exercise, and a lot of loving attention, chances are excellent that he will live happily to a ripe old age. However, any animal guardian must be prepared for the inevitable end. This can involve the need for you to make the weighty and difficult decision of whether your pet's death should be kindly assisted. This choice is ultimately up to you, and there's no easy way around it. Recently, there has been some interest in hospices for animals, similar to the hospices we are familiar with for people. Vets become involved in the hospice-care team and help teach a caregiver how to maintain and care for an animal who is dying in the home. It can make the dying experience much less confusing for both the animal and his guardian.

Endocrine System and Related Problems

The endocrine system consists of glandular organs and structures that are situated throughout the body, each of which produces and secretes specific hormones and other substances for distribution via the blood or lymph. The specific substances produced by the various components of the endocrine system play key roles in activating or regulating organ functions and countless other metabolic activities and balances

throughout the body. If one or more components of this complex and interrelated system fails, a chain reaction of dysfunction can be triggered throughout the body.

Because endocrine system diseases and disorders can affect a wide variety of organs and functions throughout the body, such conditions are easily misdiagnosed and often written off as behavioral disorders or dietary problems. The insidious nature of endocrine disease is compounded by its typically slow progression, and oftentimes a problem is not accurately identified until the animal's condition is irreversible. This is when loving attentiveness and a well-kept diary by a holistic caregiver can really pay off. By noticing and addressing subtle symptoms when they first occur, a guardian can take corrective measures against most endocrine system problems before they become life threatening.

ADRENAL GLAND DISORDERS

The adrenal glands produce various hormones that are important in nervous system functions, regulation of the immune system, and bodily responses to stressful situations. The adrenal cortex (the outer tissues of the adrenal glands) is chiefly responsible for the body's production of corticosteroids, the hormones responsible for natural control of inflammation.

Addison's Disease (Hypoadrenocorticism)

Addison's disease is caused by deficient secretion of cortisone and other hormones from the adrenal cortex. The cause of the disease is unknown, but it may be secondary to an immune system disorder that is responsible for destroying the adrenal glands. Usually the disease progresses slowly, allowing an attentive caregiver to take remedial action early.

Secondary hypoadrenocorticism is

caused when synthetic corticosteroids are introduced into the body, natural adrenal functions are replaced, and the adrenal cortex subsequently begins to shut down. Many animals who are finishing prednisolone or other steroid therapies or animals who have been subjected to excessive vaccinations suffer from this form of hypoadrenocorticism.

Addison's disease occurs most frequently in middle-aged female dogs. It rarely occurs in cats. Early symptoms may be subtle and include occasional lack of appetite, digestive upset, and decreased energy and stamina. In many cases, symptoms may be apparent only during or after an activity that causes physical or psychological stress, such as a car ride, a frightening encounter with a big, mean dog, or a dreaded trip to the vet. Symptoms progressively worsen over time until the slightest measure of stress may result in debilitation.

Degeneration of the adrenal glands is generally irreversible, but if the nutrients needed for maintaining a healthy body and balanced immune system are provided, progression of the disease can be slowed dramatically. An organic raw food diet, free from pesticide residues, antibiotics, and livestock growth or milk production hormones, is likely to yield the best results. Additionally, a high-quality dietary supplement that contains a full complement of vitamins, minerals, and EFAs is strongly indicated. Supplemental feeding of dried nettle, dandelion leaf, or parsley leaf provides the body with an array of vitamins and minerals that are essential in maintaining strong adrenal functions. Any or all of these herbs can be mixed with the animal's food— 1 level teaspoon per pound of food fed daily. Spirulina is also an excellent supplement for adrenal care—¼ teaspoon for each pound of food fed daily. An excellent herb and vitamin supplement called Animal Essentials is well suited for animals that have Addison's disease or diabetes mellitus.

Borage leaf may help gently boost adrenal output, particularly in cases associated with extended steroid therapies. Licorice offers a much stronger boost to adrenal function. It's important to note, however, that these herbs only stimulate adrenal function, they do not repair or adequately nourish the glands. Siberian ginseng or other adaptogenic herbs may be useful for reducing the impact of stress upon the adrenal glands.

Cushing's Disease (Hyperadrenocorticism)

The opposite of Addison's disease is Cushing's disease in which overactive adrenal glands produce too much cortisone and other hormones. This is most commonly caused (in about 85 percent of all cases) by a malignant or benign tumor of the pituitary gland. The tumor causes the pituitary to overproduce a hormone that stimulates the adrenal gland, causing Cushing's disease. The disease may also be caused by excessive use of corticosteroid drugs or by a tumor of one or both adrenal glands.

Cushing's disease occurs in dogs, cats, horses, and other animals. The condition progresses with tumor growth. Symptoms include increased thirst and appetite; increased urination; abdominal distention; increased panting; obesity; muscle weakness; hair loss; and dry, scaly, or wrinkled skin.

Conventional treatment is based on the diagnosis of the cause. In cases that stem from a pituitary or adrenal gland tumor, surgical removal or drug therapies are both options. The prognosis is variable according to the amount of disease progression.

Herbal therapy is limited to tonic support of organs and systems that are subjected to additional stress because of the disease.

Dandelion root, burdock, garlic, and nettle are good choices for supporting an overtaxed liver and digestive system and to help replace potassium that is lost as a result of increased urination. Adaptogenic herbs such as Siberian ginseng or astragalus help buffer adrenal responses to stress. Kelp is especially useful for maintaining iodine and other trace mineral levels that are essential for adrenal function. If your companion has Cushing's disease, avoid licorice, borage leaf, and other herbs that stimulate adrenal activity.

DIABETES MELLITUS

Diabetes comes in many forms, each requiring specific courses of treatment. To simplify, the most common form of diabetes (diabetes mellitus) occurs when the pancreas becomes dysfunctional and produces too little insulin. Because of this deficit, the body is unable to effectively utilize or store the glucose, proteins, fats, and carbohydrates needed to maintain homeostasis. Consequently, serious imbalances are triggered throughout the body. If left untreated, animals with diabetes mellitus suffer and are likely to succumb to kidney failure, loss of vision, or any number of autoimmune, heart, or nervous system problems.

Unfortunately, there is no cure for diabetes. Conventional treatment of advanced cases usually involves insulin replacement therapy. This approach can be effective, but all too often other relative factors are never addressed. These factors include special trace mineral or EFA needs that arise from special demands placed upon overworked organs, as well as kidney damage that has already occurred from the disease.

Diabetic animals should receive regular exercise and good, wholesome food fed in small amounts, several times throughout the day. By ingesting many small meals, the body has an easier time producing, using, and stabilizing insulin and glucose levels. Dietary yeast may be added to the animal's diet to aid in the metabolism of glucose, and 25 to 200 IU of vitamin E each day may help reduce an animal's insulin requirement. For dogs and cats, a daily regimen of 50–300 micrograms of chromium; 500–6,000 milligrams of vitamin C; 4–160 milligrams of digestive enzymes; 200–1,500 milligrams of n-acetylglucosamine; and 10–200 milligrams of proanthocyanidin complex may be of benefit as well. Regular exercise is important for maintaining healthy body weight and cardiopulmonary function and may also help decrease the animal's insulin need.

The primary role of herbs in treating diabetes is to help strengthen and support systems of the body that have been ravaged by the metabolic chaos of the disease. Because a diabetic body has a diminished capacity to utilize critical nutrients, herbs that strengthen digestion and nutrient absorption are strongly indicated. These include bitter herbs such as dandelion leaf, chamomile (both the leaf and the flower), calendula, and hop. In addition, yucca and alfalfa are useful for increasing absorption of nutrients in the small intestine. Dandelion root and burdock root both contain considerable amounts of inulin, a compound that helps moderate and maintain blood sugar levels. Bilberry (*Vaccinium myrtillus*) or huckleberry leaf (*Vaccinium* sp.) may also be effective in moderating glucose levels in the blood, and a few juniper berries added to each feeding may help optimize the body's utilization of insulin. Cardiovascular and kidney efficiency can be improved with the use of hawthorn and ginkgo. Scientific studies have shown that aloe vera and chemical compounds found in fenugreek seeds may also reduce blood glucose levels and stimulate insulin production in diabetic animals. Animal Essentials is an excellent herb and vitamin supplement for diabetic dogs and cats.

PANCREATITIS

The pancreas produces insulin, a substance that enables the body to utilize and store glucose (the body's fuel). It also produces pancreatic enzymes that are essential for digesting food and assimilating nutrients in the digestive tract. It is a delicate organ that is easily damaged and slow to heal.

Pancreatitis, inflammation of the pancreas, can result from a high-fat diet, obesity, traumatic injury, or excessive use of corticosteroid, antibiotic, or diuretic drugs. It can also be related to underlying systemic problems such as liver, gallbladder, or kidney disease; cardiovascular disease; or bacterial infection. Symptoms may include abdominal pain, restlessness, severe vomiting and diarrhea (sometimes with blood present), diminished appetite, and weakness. Onset can occur quickly (acute pancreatitis), or symptoms can progressively worsen over time (chronic pancreatitis). Pancreatitis is most common in middle-aged dogs, especially those who are overweight from being "pampered" with generous junk-food handouts. The disease is less common in cats.

Natural treatment of pancreatitis is centered on diet and nutrition. To ease the inflamed organ's burden, meals should be doled out in small portions and fed three or more times per day. Food should be served with probiotic (e.g., acidophilus, bifidus) and enzyme supplements at room temperature, which make the food easier for the animal to digest. And excess fat and foods that contribute to digestive upset should be eliminated from the diet. In addition to healthy food and food combining, daily supplements of EFAs such as stabilized flaxseed, fish oils and vitamins A and E are said to help repair and strengthen the pancreas.

Meats, grains, vegetables, and fats are digested and absorbed at different metabolic rates, the pancreas must produce different enzymes for each. A diseased pancreas may have difficulty producing all the enzymes needed to digest a meal that includes too many food groups; so therefore, pancreatic efficiency can be optimized if each meal is composed of food types that are of similar digestibility. For example, grains and vegetables can be served together, as can grains and fruits or protein (meat) and vegetables. Meat and grains should not be combined during the same meal, however, because their digestion requirements are different. (For more information on food combining, pick up a copy of *Keep Your Pet Healthy the Natural Way* by Pat Lazarus.)

Herbal therapies are best directed toward supporting organs and systems related to pancreatic function and the onset of pancreatitis. A thorough veterinary examination is needed to determine which therapy to use. In almost all cases, treatment of pancreatic disease requires tonic support of the liver and digestive system. Milk thistle helps to regenerate and restore normal function to a liver that is damaged as a result of drug therapies or infection. Dandelion, burdock root, or Oregon grape can help improve digestion and reduce pancreatic stress by gently increasing bile and enzyme production in the liver. If bacterial infection is present, echinacea helps to boost the immune system's response to the invading microbes. Yarrow is said to help reduce pancreatic inflammation and improve blood circulation to the organ.

THYROID PROBLEMS

The thyroid gland consists of two lobes, one located on each side of the trachea.

The gland secretes important hormones, including thyroxine (T4), triiodothyronine (T3), and calcitonin. Release of these hormones is controlled by yet another hormone, called thyroid stimulating hormone (TSH), which is produced by the pituitary gland.

Thyroid hormones control the intensity of critical functions throughout the body, including heart rate, body temperature, fat and glucose metabolism, digestion, and neurological activities. If the thyroid becomes dysfunctional, some serious health problems occur.

Hyperthyroidism

Hyperthyroidism occurs when a thyroid tumor, a viral or bacterial infection, or environmental or nutritional factors cause the thyroid gland to secrete excess hormones into the blood. Symptoms may include ravenous appetite, weight loss, increased water consumption and urination, aggressive or hyperactive behavior, and rapid or erratic heartbeat and respiration. The problem occurs more frequently in cats than in dogs or other animals.

Conventional treatment of hyperthyroidism ranges from chemotherapy to surgery to radiation therapy. One approach involves destroying the thyroid completely with radiation and then putting the animal on hormone replacement therapy for the rest of his life.

Once the thyroid becomes damaged or dysfunctional, its condition is difficult (some say impossible) to reverse. Therefore, the best holistic approach toward hyperthyroidism is to help prevent it by providing a good natural diet and avoiding unnecessary chemical or environmental hazards, including X-rays, antibiotic therapies, food preservatives, and unneeded vaccinations. Daily supplements of vitamin B complex, vitamin C, CoQ$_{10}$, and EFAs are also important

contributors for maintaining healthy thyroid function.

Herbal therapies include symptomatic treatment and tonic support of systems that are under added stress from an increased metabolic rate. Bugleweed is considered a specific symptomatic remedy for hyperthyroidism because it is known to slow thyroid function by reducing production of TSH. Its use, however, should be monitored by a holistic veterinarian. Hawthorn is helpful for moderating an erratic heartbeat, while skullcap and valerian may help calm and reduce the "jittery jumpiness" of a hyperthyroid animal. Kelp and other rich sources of iodine should be avoided because iodine stimulates thyroid function.

Hypothyroidism

The opposite of hyperthyroidism is hypothyroidism—deficient production of hormones by the thyroid. Hypothyroidism is usually caused by physical degeneration of the thyroid gland, which can be the result of protracted drugs or therapies, radiation such as X-ray exposure, vaccinosis, genetic predisposition, or nutritional deficiencies. Hypothyroidism occurs rarely in cats and horses or other large animals, but it is fairly common in dogs. Destruction of the thyroid is generally irreversible, and animals who are suffering advanced stages of thyroid degeneration may need hormone replacement therapy.

Symptoms of hypothyroidism include weight gain, reduced appetite, mental dullness, lack of energy, hair loss on the trunk and tail, and a dry coat that pulls easily from the skin. If left untreated, the problem can lead to chronic seizures, head tilt, lack of coordination, and other serious neurological disorders.

Iodine is critical in the functions of a healthy thyroid, and many holistic practitioners believe that dietary supplementation of iodine-rich kelp helps stimulate an underactive thyroid. Many researchers and practitioners believe, however, that supplemental iodine may contribute to immune-related factors of the disease and trigger a worsening effect.

Licorice may have a slight stimulant effect on an unproductive but physically intact thyroid, and adaptogens such as organically grown ginseng, astragalus, or Siberian ginseng might help energy levels and the body's response to stress. Otherwise, herb use is limited to treating the discomforts subsequent to hypothyroidism. For instance, related digestive disorders can be treated with dandelion root, Oregon grape, or yellow dock, whereas seborrhea might be relieved by gotu kola, burdock, or red clover.

In our opinion, homeopathy and the use of glandular preparations offer more effective courses of early- to late-term treatment than herbs do.

Epilepsy, Convulsions, and Seizures

A seizure can be frightening if you've never seen one before. Some animals may experience a seizure once in their lives and then never again. On the other hand, some have several seizures every day of their lives.

The causes of seizures are widely varied, ranging from epilepsy to nervous system disease or injury. In dogs, hyperthermia, poisoning, low blood sugar, nutritional deficiencies, distemper, intestinal parasites that have entered the bloodstream, tumors, low blood calcium after birthing, liver or kidney disease, and thyroid problems may be underlying factors. In cats, convulsions may be linked to feline infectious peritonitis (FIP), toxoplasmosis, lymphosarcoma (leukemia), thiamine deficiency, or a heart disorder.

All cases of seizures involve electrical disturbances of the brain that result in muscle contractions of variable intensity and loss of motor control. Many animals lose consciousness and bladder or bowel control during a seizure, and some may exhibit overly affectionate, frightened, or "clingy" behavior immediately before an epileptic episode. Digestive disorders, hair loss, neuralgia, and several other problems may also be associated with chronic convulsive disorders.

Conventional therapies typically involve the use of phenobarbital, potassium bromide, or other anticonvulsant drugs. These measures can prove to be effective, but they cannot address the underlying causes of chronic convulsive disorders.

HOLISTIC APPROACHES

Holistic treatment usually entails a lifelong effort, beginning with a dietary and environmental assessment and adjustment, and continuing with nutritional supplementation and herbal therapies that focus on normalizing and maintaining

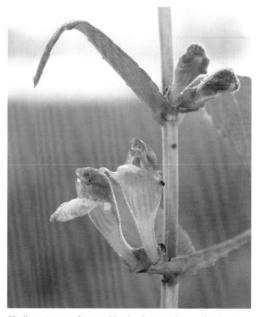

Skullcap is one of several herbs that can be used to treat epilepsy.

nervous system function. All possible environmental causes of or contributors to seizures should be removed from your home. Eliminate all possible contact with antifreeze fluids, household chemicals, pesticides and herbicides, lead-based paints, and other neurotoxins from your companion's environment. (These substances are harmful to humans, as well.)

Animals with epilepsy or other convulsive disorders should be on a natural, whole foods diet. Cats with epilepsy, however, should not be fed raw fish because it contains thiaminase, an enzyme that breaks down vitamin B1 (thiamine). Vitamin B1 is essential for healthy nervous system functions. In all animals, dietary supplementation with omega-3 and omega-6 EFAs is important in the development and maintenance of healthy nervous system structure and function. Animal Essentials makes an excellent EFA supplement for dogs and cats. In addition to EFAs, supplementing your companion's diet with essential and nonessential vitamins, minerals, and digestive enzymes and with probiotics is indicated to assure that the nervous system is getting everything it needs to heal and function optimally. A daily supplementation of 100-300 milligrams of betaine HCl; 50-500 milligrams of dimethylglycine; 200-1000 milligrams of taurine; and 10-200 milligrams of proanthocyanidin complex is said to be helpful for epileptic dogs. Recent studies have shown that a ketogenic diet can be effective for treating severe epilepsy in humans, but at this point we can only speculate about the usefulness of this approach in animals.

We have seen promising results with the use of skullcap in the treatment of epileptic animals. This nervine is believed to moderate overactive synaptic activity in the higher brain centers in which epileptic episodes may be triggered. We have received many good reports about valerian and oatstraw, too, especially when they are combined in equal proportions with skullcap. Although these herbs do not represent a cure for epilepsy, their reported effects include less frequent and less severe episodes. Lemon balm, ginkgo, rosemary, hop, passionflower, and perhaps kava kava (research is promising in the area of controlling seizures in rodents) may also be effective in the treatment of chronic seizures. Additionally, flower essences of vervain or chestnut bud may be helpful in moderating seizures.

FIRST AID FOR SEIZURES

If your animal experiences a seizure, gently protect his head from sharp or hard objects until the episode passes. Don't attempt to restrain the animal's body—the muscle contractions of a violent convulsion can be self-injurious if the animal cannot move and jerk about freely. Never place your hand in or near your animal's mouth during a seizure— your companion may be unaware of your presence and may unknowingly bite you with incredible force! If you are indoors during the episode, dimming the lights and speaking softly to your companion helps reduce the fear and confusion that sometimes precedes and usually follows the episode. Rescue Remedy rubbed on the ears before, during, and after a seizure sometimes helps moderate the episode and calm the animal. Be sure to take a hearty dose yourself!

Eye Problems

Many eye problems are just subtle signs of chronic underlying diseases. You might think your animal is the "picture of perfect health," but if he has runny eyes or the beginning of cataracts, these conditions indicate that there is an underlying imbalance. Many times herbs alone are not enough to correct that imbalance. A vet who is trained well in classic homeopathy can address the underlying disease and help the body heal itself.

In some cases of simple infection or irritation, an herbal wash of saline solution and raspberry leaf tea clears up the problem immediately. In other cases, eye problems mark the beginning of a lifelong course of holistic therapy.

CATARACTS

Cataracts are white opacities that block the passage of light into the eyes. They are caused by loss of water or rearrangement of fibrous tissue in the eye lens. Formation of cataracts (known as senile cataracts) is a normal part of the aging process. They seldom result in blindness and usually cause little or no vision impairment in older animals, even if the pupils take on the blue-white hue that is characteristic of the condition. Cataracts sometimes involve leakage of lens protein into the inner eye. When this happens, an immune response is triggered and the animal suffers serious inflammation of the eye.

Providing a well-balanced natural diet throughout an animal's life is the surest way to prevent the development of problematic cataracts. In cats, cataracts have been linked with vitamin B_2 (riboflavin) deficiency, a problem that stems more from poor nutrient assimilation than it does from lack of vitamin B_2 in the average feline diet. Lactation is also believed to deplete the feline body of B_2. Therefore, dietary supplementation of the digestive enzymes and probiotics necessary to metabolize B_2 is an important part of cataract prevention—especially in nursing cats. Other recommended vitamin supplements include glutathione, vitamin C, CoQ_{10}, proanthocyanidin complex, vitamin E, and dimethylglycine.

A Simple Astringent Eyewash

Using a clean dropper bottle, combine the following:

½ tsp of cooled clear raspberry leaf or nettle tea *
½ tsp of Oregon grape or goldenseal tea *

Add 1 oz of sterile saline (available in the eye care section of supermarkets and pharmacies)

Shake the mixture thoroughly—the finished solution should be tinted yellow.

* Make sure that the tea is absolutely free of particles—you don't want them in your animal's eyes!

If possible, hold the animal's head to one side and use a dropper pipette to thoroughly rinse the eye laterally, from the nose outward, toward the animal's cheek. The idea is to wash any irritating particles away from the animal's eye. This process can be repeated two or three times daily until the condition improves. If the rinse causes further irritation, stop using it—your companion may be sensitive to the herb you are using. Other herbs to consider for use in eyewashes include calendula, chamomile, thyme, bee balm, chickweed, dandelion leaf, or rose petals. Regardless of which herbs you use, be extra careful in assuring that they are free of dust, pollen, or toxic residues (such as herbicides or car exhaust), as the eyes are extremely sensitive to such foreign substances.

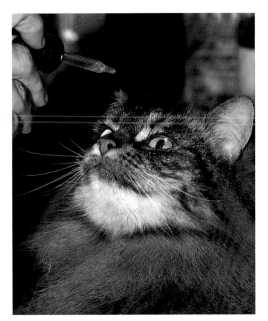

An herbal wash may clear up a simple eye infection or irritation.

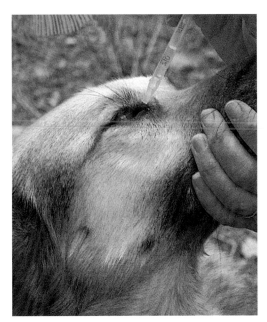

Homeopathic eyedrops may eliminate cataracts.

Both conventional and herbal approaches to treating cataracts are limited. Conventional treatment includes cataract surgery, a procedure that can be very effective. While some herbalists claim that a small dab of eucalyptus honey applied to the inside of the lower eyelid each day for several weeks can reduce the opacity of the eye lens, another approach involves the internal use of an ancient Chinese herbal formula called *Hachimijiogan.* Animal studies have shown that *Hachimijiogan* is capable of slowing the progression of cataracts, especially if therapy commences during early stages of the disease. Bilberry, when used in conjunction with vitamin E supplements, has been shown to help stop progression of senile cataracts in humans. In this approach, a standardized (to 25 percent anthocyanosides) bilberry extract is administered at a dose of 20-40 milligrams per 40 pounds of body weight, three times daily.

According to veterinarian Susan G. Wynn, homeopathic preparation eyedrops made from the juice of *Cineraria maritima* can be effective for eliminating cataracts in animals. Wynn says to dilute the drops by half with artificial tears (sterile saline solution) because the juice stings when used full strength. When using this method, she sometimes sees cataracts disappear in two to three months.

CONJUNCTIVITIS

Conjunctivitis is a generic term that refers to inflammation of the mucous membranes and soft tissues surrounding the eye. The problem occurs when bacteria, fungi, or other foreign substances come in contact with these tissues and tearing fails to eliminate the irritating elements. Most cases are acute and are caused by dust, plant material, or other environmental irritants. In these cases, a simple saline eye rinse usually brings relief. An astringent eyewash using raspberry leaf or nettle tea combined with a tea of certified organic goldenseal or

Oregon grape root offers further assistance by fighting infection and quickly reducing inflammation and soreness.

GLAUCOMA

Glaucoma involves abnormally high inner eye pressure. It can occur in most animals, but it is especially common in cats and in certain breeds of dogs. The disease is often secondary to other intraocular diseases such as inflammatory adhesions and tumors. Signs of glaucoma may include swollen or reddened eyes, dilated fixed pupils, loss of vision, and corneal edema. Conventional approaches to glaucoma usually involve antiglaucoma drugs that help reduce intraocular pressure. In some cases, corticosteroid therapies are used.

Although glaucoma is difficult to treat with herbs, perhaps the greatest success comes from the reduction of intraocular pressure with herbs such as ginkgo and bilberry. *Cannabis sativa* (marijuana) can be effective, too, but, of course, its accessibility is severely limited by legal restrictions.

Coleus forskohlii, an herb that's used in ayurvedic medicine, contains forskolin, a substance that has been shown to significantly reduce intraocular pressure in humans, monkeys, and rabbits. However, its safety and effectiveness in various other animals have yet to be determined.

First Aid

BE PREPARED!

The old scout motto "Be Prepared" really rings true if you're out walking your dog and he is attacked by another dog, cuts himself on barbed wire, or sprains his paw while playing Frisbee. Having a first aid kit specially designed for your animal and knowing how to use it provides insurance for the well-being of your companion.

Taking a course from the Red Cross or a local vet, kennel, or shelter enables you to deal with everything from life-threatening emergencies to minor cuts and sprains.

In addition to the basic first aid necessities (plenty of gauze dressings and bandages,

Ideas for a First Aid Kit

Place some of the following items in a water-resistant carrying case:

- Blankets, extra collars, leashes, muzzles, water bowls

- Gauze, bandages, small flashlight, scissors, tweezers, swabs, Vetwrap™, hemostats, rectal thermometer (with case), ear scope, hydrogen peroxide (for use as an emetic in certain poisonings, as well as an antibacterial wound wash), activated charcoal powder (for poisonings); preserved, sterile saline solution (for washing out wounds and eyes and to wash minor burns)

- Herbal salve, Rescue Remedy, cayenne pepper and yarrow mix (to stop bleeding), herbal tinctures such as Oregon grape and echinacea

- A list of items in the kit and brief descriptions of how they are used

First aid kits for animals are available through many catalogs, and you can add your own items to personalize the one you choose. A catalog company called PetSage carries several nice ones, including one for birds.

tweezers, cotton swabs, a bulb syringe, and a variety of herbal medicines), we also carry a homeopathic travel kit with us wherever we go. Homeopathic remedies are compact, convenient, effective, and especially useful for emergency situations. It's also important to learn canine and feline cardiopulmonary

Echinacea and Oregon Grape Clay Poultice

Combine the following:

4 oz green or bentonite clay
(powder)*
½ oz echinacea tincture
(alcohol based)
½ oz Oregon grape tincture
(alcohol based)

*Be sure to use only supplement-grade clay (available at health food stores)

Bentonite clay that is sold at hardware and feed stores often contains harmful bacteria and other impurities. Alcohol-based tinctures (as opposed to glycerin-based) are preferable because they add astringency to the formula and serve as preservatives in a poultice that is saved for future use. Thoroughly combine the three ingredients, adding just enough distilled water to make a thick paste. The poultice can then be applied to the affected areas and left on to dry, if possible. Leftover poultice can be put into an airtight container and stored in the refrigerator almost indefinitely. If it dries out, just add more water or tincture to soften it.

resuscitation (CPR) and the ABCs of basic first aid. Regardless of how extensive your first aid kit or classroom training might be, everything you compile is functionally useless if you are unable to react properly in a crisis situation. The most crucial aspects of emergency preparedness are proactive study and mental conditioning. An emergency situation is a poor time to read up on what to do or give. During a crisis, time is of the essence, especially if your companion is bleeding severely or having a difficult time breathing. When placed under the stress of an emotional, adrenaline-pumped situation (such as after you watch your cat get hit by a careless motorist), the human mind loses much of its ability to formulate an effective plan of action—the mind begins to race, the knees start to shake, dizziness sets in, and it's difficult to think. Instead of thinking the situation through, the brain must react by instinct. If there is no plan imbedded deep in the mind's subconscious, panic sets in and all control of the situation is lost to a rampant avalanche of emotion and confusion.

Panic is our worst enemy in an emergency situation because the confusion it causes paralyzes our abilities to take effective actions. It's best to prepare for stressful emergency situations before they occur. This is done by visualizing crisis situations so that the mind is better prepared to respond intuitively and effectively when a real emergency occurs. For instance, if you are an avid backcountry equestrian, spend some time each week with your eyes closed, imagining various emergency situations that could occur to you and your companion on your upcoming trail trips. Be creative but realistic in your visualization of each unfortunate event—imagine the fall, your companion's pain and terror, your racing heart, and the initial surge of panic and doubt that starts to envelop you. Then imagine overcoming that surge and taking control of your emotions to assess the situation. Imagine opening your first aid kit and systematically selecting the items your companion needs as you calm him down by softly petting him and assuring him that you are in charge of the situation. Imagine yourself remedying the situation and knowing that everything will be fine.

When we worked in emergency services, we called this exercise "crisis rehearsal"—others call it "creative visualization." To some of you, this may sound like a program

First Aid Oil for Contusions and Blunt Trauma Injuries

Combine equal parts of the following oil infusions*:

Yarrow
Comfrey
Saint-John's-wort

*See "Basics of Herbal Preparations" in chapter 1 for instructions on how to make an oil infusion.

Apply this first aid oil immediately to blunt injuries where subdermal bleeding is evident. After a day or two when the bleeding has stopped and the healing process has begun, arnica oil can be applied sparingly to the injury site for up to three days (any longer might irritate the skin). This will help move congested fluids out of the injured area by opening

for paranoia, but it is quite the opposite. Paranoia is born from fear and a conscious sense of being helpless and out of control. Crisis rehearsal builds confidence and subconsciously prepares the mind for unforeseeable events. Each time you practice this technique, your subconscious mind stores experiential memories from which to act in emergencies. In other words, you don't need to think, worry, or be paranoid of unforeseeable possibilities each time you take your companion on an adventure—instead, you have the elements of effective crisis management stored beneath the enjoyment of your adventure, where instinct can retrieve and use them if the need arises. This is an extremely effective technique for preparing for the worst. It has saved our lives and the lives of others more than a few times. Crisis rehearsal can make the difference between life and death for you and your companion.

BITES AND STINGS

If your companion receives a bite or a sting, the first course of action is to try to identify what launched the attack. Of course, this is not always possible, but if you can learn about the nature of the bite or sting, you will be more effective at treating it. In most cases, the primary course of action is to minimize pain, swelling, and the possibility of infection with the use of astringent and antimicrobial herbs. A poultice or infusion of plantain, sage, bee balm, mullein, calendula, or chamomile can be directly applied to the site of an insect bite or sting for these purposes. To make a poultice, simply mash a few fresh leaves of the herb with a small amount of water to make a crude pestolike paste. In the field, the herb can be crushed and chewed in your mouth, then applied as a paste to the wound. Oregon grape, goldenseal, myrrh, thyme, or echinacea tincture, oil infusion, or salve can be applied to the area if stronger antimicrobial agents are warranted. One or all of these herbal preparations are excellent choices for building a first aid kit. An infusion of rosemary can be used for a bite or sting to gently bathe and soothe the surrounding area. Adding 6–8 drops of tea tree oil diluted in 1 ounce of water is also good for direct application to bites and stings, but be careful with animals who have sensitive skin—the oil is strong.

For severe welts and inflammation, strong astringents such as decoctions of uva ursi, rose bark, white oak bark, or juniper leaves can be liberally applied to affected areas. A clay poultice made with bentonite clay is also effective, especially when herbs such as echinacea and Oregon grape are added to support lymphatic functions and inhibit infection. When applied to the site of a sting or bite, the clay pulls antigens away from the body to reduce swelling and help prevent capillary transport of venom into other areas.

Bites from toxic spiders, such as the brown recluse or black widow, or venomous snakes should be immediately followed with large doses of vitamin C and echinacea to build the body's immune defenses and increase lymphatic cleansing of involved tissues. Immediate administration of the appropriate homeopathic remedy is also highly advisable. In the case of a bee or wasp sting, the homeopathic remedies Apis and Ledum help relieve stinging and swelling. If there is an anaphylactic reaction, or if the airway is compromised in any way, get to a veterinarian immediately. If you already know that your companion is predisposed to acute allergic reactions, you should be carrying a prescription injectable epinephrine and antihistamine kit (Anakit or Epipen) that helps to antidote your animal's reaction to insect or reptile venoms. See your veterinarian about obtaining a kit.

BRUISES, BUMPS, AND OTHER BLUNT TRAUMAS

Contusions (bruises) are caused when blunt impact or crushing pressure causes tissue damage and bleeding beneath the skin. In humans, contusions are usually characterized by their purplish red color. Because animals have different skin pigments and hair, feathers, fur, or scales to hide such evidence of injury, contusions and other forms of traumatic, subdermal hematoma must be identified by other symptoms. Usually there is swelling and tenderness at the site of a contusion. The animal may favor or lick the injured body area. Close examination (beneath the animal's coat) usually reveals discoloration at the site.

Since contusions are contained beneath the skin, the risk of infection is low (provided the animal is healthy to begin with). First aid usually begins with applying an ice pack to slow bleeding and assist the coagulation process. Contrary to what some herbalists may think, arnica oil or salve is sometimes contraindicated in the early treatment of contusions or subdermal hematoma. Arnica, a peripheral vasodilator that works rapidly, may actually increase bleeding at the site of injury. Instead of reaching for your handy first aid vial of arnica oil, reach for an oil infusion of yarrow. Yarrow is remarkable because it acts as a vasodilator when ingested but as a fast-acting vasoconstrictor and hemostatic agent when applied topically. This makes it very useful for reducing the severity of fresh contusions, especially when combined with an oil infusion of Saint-John's-wort. Having a special affinity toward the repair of crushed nerve endings, Saint-John's-wort helps to relieve pain and minimize the possibility of lasting nerve impairment. Comfrey oil, salve, and poultice are also excellent first aid devices for blunt trauma injuries because they gently assist with lymph circulation without contributing to internal bleeding, and they accelerate the regeneration of damaged cell structures.

BURNS AND SCALDS

There are two important considerations to keep in mind when your companion suffers a burn. One is that until the site of the injury cools down, cellular damage can continue for several minutes after a burn first occurs. This is especially true if the burn was caused by steam or scalding fluid, which can penetrate tissues and carry injurious heat deep beneath the skin. Another consideration to keep in mind is that when the skin is damaged, its ability to resist infection is greatly impaired. To defend itself against invading bacteria, the skin relies upon delicate cell membranes and thousands of tiny capillaries to carry lymph, blood, and various antibodies throughout its structure. When a burn occurs, circulation is obstructed within the site of injury, and the deprived tissues are left vulnerable to infection.

The first course in treating a burn is to cool it down. Ideally, the site of the burn should be liberally irrigated with cool sterile saline, which greatly reduces the continued destruction of cells. If sterile saline is not available, clean water (preferably distilled), snow, or ice can be generously applied—just keep in mind that the area you are irrigating is especially susceptible to any infectious microbes that may be in the water (i.e., the cleaner it is, the better). Never apply a salve, oil, or ointment to a burn—these types of preparations can seal in heat and bacteria, making the situation worse. Don't cover the burned area with a bandage either unless you will be able to keep the dressing continually soaked with cool, clean water.

If the burn appears to be deep (second or third degree) or if it involves the mouth, nose, feet, or a large percentage of the animal's body, get the animal to a veterinarian immediately—the situation might be serious.

The second course of action (for minor burns) is to take continuing measures to assure that the burn is kept clean. Irrigate the burn several times each day with sterile saline. Aloe juice can be directly applied to the burn after each irrigation to help fight infection, reduce pain, and speed the healing process. A cooled tea of chaparral, calendula, or gotu kola can be effective for these purposes as well, as might a poultice of fresh chickweed. Comfrey is useful too, but it should not be applied until you are absolutely sure that the risk of infection has passed. Comfrey heals wounds so fast that it can seal bacteria or fungi into the wound! A skin rinse of chamomile, peppermint, catnip, bee balm, or thyme may bring relief from pain. Lavender oil (8 drops diluted into each ounce of clean water) is also good for relieving the pain of burns and scalds.

The homeopathic remedies Apis and *Urtica* spp. (nettle) are effective treatments for burns. We keep a bottle of diluted *Urtica* tincture in our kitchen for use on burns. It takes the sting away immediately and prevents blistering. It can also be given internally.

To help the healing process from inside out, dietary supplements of vitamins C and E are important, as are fatty acids. Gotu kola can be added to an animal's diet to help with skin regeneration, as can horsetail.

FRACTURES

Obviously, herbs cannot be expected to realign and set a broken bone, but a variety of herbs are useful throughout the postclinical healing process. Horsetail, nettle, comfrey, and alfalfa all contain nutritional components that play important roles in the healing of bone tissue. Yarrow and ginkgo help by increasing blood circulation in impaired extremities. Licorice, yucca, devil's claw, Saint-John's-wort, and cayenne are all useful for reducing inflammation and pain. Valerian, skullcap, passionflower, or hop can be used to help a recovering animal rest and relax.

HEATSTROKE, HYPERTHERMIA, AND HEAT EXHAUSTION

Heatstroke or heat exhaustion can occur as a result of too much strenuous exercise or excessive exposure to heat. If heatstroke is not treated immediately the animal's body temperature may rise to irreversible levels and brain damage, kidney failure, or death may quickly follow. Symptoms of heat illness include excessive panting or difficulty breathing, high body temperature (above 104° F for a dog or cat), lethargy or collapse, loss of appetite, bloody diarrhea or vomit, increased heart rate, increased respiratory rate, reddened tongue or eye tissues, hot and flushed skin, and seizures or coma.

Perhaps the most common cause of heat-related illness and death in dogs and cats occurs when they are left in cars on a warm or hot day. Don't ever leave your companion in the car unless the weather is mild, there is ample shade to park under, the windows can be left rolled down, and the animal is left with plenty of drinking water. Even on days that don't seem hot, the temperature in a well-ventilated vehicle can exceed 100° F in a matter of minutes. With the windows rolled up, the temperature can climb to 180° F (a steak cooks at 140° F)! Dogs and cats need to pant and get fresh air to cool themselves. If you find an animal in a car that is closed up, try to contact the owner and offer to give a bowl of water to his or her companion who "looks thirsty." If done in a nonthreatening way, without offending the person, you could save an animal's life. If the person insists on letting the animal suffer, call the local law enforcement agency.

If your companion displays signs of heat-related illness, get to a cool area immediately, wet the animal with water, and if possible, take the animal's rectal temperature. If the animal's temperature seems abnormally high, get to a vet immediately. If you are carrying a homeopathic kit with you, you might try administering a dose of Glonoinum (30C) while en route. Rescue Remedy (a flower essence formula) might be helpful as well. Allow your animal to drink as much cool water as he needs.

After the danger has passed and your companion appears to be recovering, you can begin replacing lost minerals and

All-Purpose First Aid Oil or Salve

Saint-John's-wort oil infusion
Oregon Grape oil infusion
Comfrey oil infusion
1 oz grated beeswax

Combine equal amounts of the oil infusions. Add the grated beeswax to the combined oils. Gently heat the mixture over a low flame, stirring constantly until the beeswax has completely melted and combined with the oils. Remove from heat and pour into salve jars immediately—it thickens as it cools.

nutrients by feeding him herbs such as nettle or chickweed tea.

MOTION SICKNESS

Motion sickness is fairly common among dogs and cats, especially puppies and those who seldom take rides in cars. The causes of motion sickness are varied. The inner ears of puppies and other young animals continue to develop until the animals approach adolescence, which means that their equilibrium may be especially sensitive to motion. Another factor comes into play in animals who are frightened or become hyperactive during car rides. In these animals, extreme nervousness may cause stomach upset, dizziness, or hyperventilation, all of which can result in vomiting.

In most cases, motion sickness becomes less of a problem as an animal matures or becomes accustomed to the feeling of hurtling through space in a "crate on wheels." Have you ever thought about how an animal might perceive such an unnatural occurrence as a car ride? With this in mind, it's important to help your companion to consider car rides to be fun as early in life as possible. Make a point to play with your companion at the destinations of her first couple dozen car trips to replace confusion and fear with anticipation of a good time. For many animals, this approach is effective. We dearly remember riding to our mountain cabin with our dog Mollie on weekends. The winding highway and steep ravines often made her nervous and carsick, so each time we reached the most challenging part of the highway, we would begin saying to her, "Get your Frisbee! Get your stick! Do you want to go swimming? Find the cat (her beloved friend and playmate)!" After a few verses of this, her mind would be so focused on the playtime that would soon follow that she would forget about the frightening ride and car sickness wasn't a problem. Eventually, her nervousness during car rides was completely replaced by the thrill of another adventure.

Of course, some animals may never get over motion sickness, and anything that might help is certainly appreciated, especially if you're sharing a subcompact sedan with a Newfoundland. Ginger, peppermint, catnip, fennel, or dill might help relieve an upset stomach that might lead to vomiting. Ginkgo is known to improve blood circulation in the inner ear and may help with equilibrium problems. Valerian helps calm a hyperactive animal and also eases a nervous stomach. Skullcap, passionflower, and oatstraw are all excellent nervine-sedatives that can help reduce nervous anxiety. Of course, before you try any of these (in combination or singularly), give Rescue Remedy (flower essences) a try. A few drops on your animal's tongue just before you get into the car might make the difference between an unpleasant episode and a fun car ride.

PENETRATING INJURIES (CUTS, SCRAPES, PUNCTURES)

Penetrating injuries are part of life, especially if you have an active outdoor animal. Animals tolerate wounds much better than we humans do, and provided animals have healthy lymph and immune systems and no blood-clotting disorders, minor open injuries usually heal quickly and completely. The primary concern here is that the injury is kept clean and as well ventilated as cleanliness allows. From a holistic perspective, an animal licking his open wound is a natural part of the healing process. This is how animals cleanse wounds, and, in fact, the saliva of dogs and cats contain antimicrobial properties that help fight infection and speed healing.

At the onset of a penetrating injury, the first course of action is to make sure that the bleeding is in no way life threatening. If bleeding is profuse, nothing serves as a better hemostatic agent than a half-and-half mix of powdered cayenne and yarrow. When applied liberally and directly into a wound, these two herbs work amazingly well to stop hemorrhage and inhibit infection. After the powder is applied, gauze compresses can then be placed on top to assist the process and keep the injury clean. Treat for shock, and get your companion to a veterinarian immediately.

If the wound does not appear to be life threatening, allow it to flush and seal itself, and thoroughly clean the site with fresh water (use sterile saline if possible) or some hydrogen peroxide as soon as possible. Oregon grape, goldenseal, Saint-John's-wort, thyme, sage, echinacea, or yarrow tea or liniment can be used to irrigate the wound each day to help prevent infection. Tea tree oil is effective too, but it must be diluted. Add 8 drops into 1 ounce of olive, almond, or apricot kernel oil. Calendula, comfrey, gotu kola, or aloe can be added to the daily regimen after risk of infection has passed to help speed the healing process and reduce scarring. Any or all of the herbs we just mentioned can be used in the form of a first aid salve that is applied between each daily cleansing. The salve is also useful for field treatment of minor wounds.

POISONING

A shocking number of companion animals die each year of poisoning. Some cases involve cruel human intent, others an unfortunate discovery or accident. But most companion animal poisonings are the direct result of carelessness. Improperly stored or disposed of automotive antifreeze fluid represents one of the most frequent causes of accidental animal poisoning. Ethylene glycol, the compound found in antifreeze, has a sweet flavor that is appealing to dogs, cats, and other animals. It destroys the kidneys, and as little as 1 tablespoon can be fatal to a medium or large dog.

Lead poisoning from old house paint, discarded batteries, spilled petroleum products, or industrial waste is also a common cause of companion animal poisoning. Pesticides, herbicides, and household cleaning chemicals are familiar toxins as well.

The mechanisms by which poisons act against the body are as varied as their chemistries. Lead-based poisons cause brain damage, while pesticides, herbicides, and household chemicals may cause nervous system damage, liver and kidney damage, internal bleeding, hypoxic blood disorders, or even cancer. Certain plants may cause poisoning too, although animals are less likely to ingest them, and their effects are mostly limited to digestive upset, photosensitive reactions, rashes, and in a few cases, internal bleeding. Food poisoning is usually limited to the digestive tract and is generally corrected by vomiting.

The chemical structure of a poison and the way it behaves in the body dictates the manner in which an animal is treated. In some cases, vomiting is induced to expel the poison from the body as quickly as possible. But in other instances, such as ingestion of petroleum products or acids, vomiting may further compound the problem by allowing poison to enter the lungs or burn the esophagus on the way out. This makes a general approach to poisoning impossible and illustrates why it's critically important to identify the source of poisoning as quickly as possible.

To prepare for the unforeseeable, keep some activated charcoal on hand. This is fed to a poisoned animal under the direction of a veterinarian to help absorb many forms of poison as the animal is rushed to the veterinary hospital.

If a poisoning does happen, don't waste time with home treatment—get your companion to a veterinarian immediately! If two or more humans are present, one should transport the animal, while the other(s) should confirm the identity of the suspected poison and relay that information to the waiting veterinarian.

Although many types of herbs such as violet root, elderberry, and aloe can be used to induce vomiting in certain cases of poisoning, this action is not recommended unless you know the exact nature of the poison and the proper course of action. Guessing can be fatal. Therefore, herbs are best reserved to support and help rejuvenate an animal's body after the crisis has passed.

To help repair the liver after a poisoning, milk thistle is strongly indicated. If the liver is inflamed, licorice may be of benefit. Mild cholagogue, alterative, and diuretic herbs, such as dandelion (root and leaf), burdock, alfalfa, and red clover, assist the body in efforts to eliminate residual toxins and their metabolic by-products. Yellow dock is believed to help remove heavy metals from the body. Immunostimulant and antioxidant herbs such as echinacea and garlic give the immune system a needed boost, while adaptogens such as astragalus or Siberian ginseng can help improve the body's overall responses to the added stress. If kidney damage is evident, marshmallow, corn silk, ginkgo, hawthorn, horsetail, and couch grass are all candidates for use.

If you wish to learn more about poisonings or need help during an emergency, call the Animal Poison Control Center at 1-888-426-4435. A consultation fee of $60 applies.

SHOCK

Shock occurs when the vascular system is unable to provide adequate blood supply to vital organs. Hemorrhagic shock is caused when blood pressure and volume are reduced as a result of internal or external bleeding. Cardiogenic shock occurs when heart disease or dysfunction causes a reduction of blood delivery to other organs. Septic shock is caused when bacteria invade the heart muscle, other organs, or the blood itself and cause enough injury to cells to interfere with their ability to utilize oxygen. All types of shock create a situation in which various body tissues are deprived of oxygen that would normally be provided by the blood. Shock is therefore a life-threatening situation that demands immediate and decisive first aid attention. Get to a vet! You must stop bleeding and take measures to increase blood volume immediately. If the animal's breathing is labored, try to position his body in a way that appears to make breathing easier. If possible, try to keep the lower half of the animal's body slightly higher than the heart and head—this helps to keep blood volume at the brain, heart, and lungs.

While en route to the veterinarian, Rescue Remedy can be applied to the ears, paws, or lips of a conscious or unconscious animal. TTouch, acupressure, and homeopathic remedies (Aconite and Arnica) may also prove helpful. If you've been trained, be prepared to perform CPR in the event of cardiac arrest.

After a shock crisis is over, cardiopulmonary function can be assisted with the use of cardiovascular tonics. Hawthorn and ginkgo can be fed to strengthen the heart and increase blood circulation throughout the body. Yarrow or cayenne can be used to increase blood circulation and oxygenation in the lungs. Nettle, spirulina, and alfalfa are good nutritives for building healthy blood. Garlic feeds the blood and also has antioxidant, vascular tonic, and immunotonic qualities.

TENDONITIS, SPRAINS, AND LIGAMENT INJURIES

Injuries of fibrous tissues that connect muscle with bone can be extremely painful and slow to heal. Generally speaking, the sooner herbal therapy starts, the faster the animal's recovery will be.

Arnica oil, salve, or poultice should be applied immediately after the injury occurs— this begins the healing process by increasing capillary circulation and lymphatic infusion. However, Arnica should not be used on open wounds. If Arnica is not available, yarrow, cayenne, or Saint-John's-wort may prove beneficial, as will a poultice compress of comfrey. Homeopathic Arnica, Ledum, Rhus toxicodendron, or Ruta (depending on symptoms) may be effective first aid treatments as well.

To continue the healing process, the animal's diet can be supplemented with vitamin C and glucosamine sulfate or chondroitin sulfate. These supplements play positive roles in the reconstruction of connective tissues. Feeding your companion animal horsetail and comfrey can also aid in the reconstructive process. To help minimize pain and inflammation, yucca, licorice, willow bark (but not for cats), devil's claw, and boswellia are all choices to consider. Yarrow and ginkgo can be fed to maintain good blood circulation in the affected extremity.

Immune System Care

To recognize and treat immune system disorders effectively, it's important to have a general understanding of what the immune system is and how it works. The immune system is composed of a complex assortment of various cells and molecules, all of which are joined in an interdependent effort to maintain a balanced state of health. Each and every organ, tissue, and cell of the body has an integral role in this effort—the liver and kidneys, for instance, are responsible for filtering toxins and waste from the blood, and the skin serves as a first line of defense against pathogenic microbes and other environmental threats. Working beneath or within the structures and functions of the various organs and tissues of the body is a sophisticated army of frontline defenders— the millions of special cells, molecules, and microbes we know specifically as the immune system. Each member of this elite army has a special function—some members serve as sentries and detectives with the sole purpose of seeking out and identifying harmful invaders or waste products, while others serve as responding attackers to kill and remove invading microbes and other foreign substances.

Like any army, the immune system must quickly reach each battlefield, or site of infection, to be effective. To allow a rapid response, the blood and lymphatic system serve as the army's transport and incursion system. The blood carries antibodies (specialized proteins that serve to detect and report any foreign presence to the army's soldiers), lymphocytes and monocytes (the first-response assault teams), and interleukins and various other cytokines (messenger molecules that provide communication between other elements of the army), as well as oxygen and nutrients that are necessary to feed tissues and wage a battle wherever the immune army is needed. To clean up the aftermath of battle, the spleen filters the blood and serves as a fatal trap for foreign bodies that were not killed by the body's warriors.

The lymphatic system's purpose is to cleanse and nourish cells and tissues and to carry the immune effort across barriers that cannot be effectively reached by the blood. Lymphocytes are produced in the bone marrow, thymus (hence the "T" in killer T cells), and throughout the body in various mucosal-associated lymphoid tissues. The lymph (a clear, viscous fluid) then carries these warriors via an intricate network of tiny vessels on an endless journey in and out of the bloodstream and the body's various tissues. As the lymphocytes seek and destroy foreign invaders, the lymph picks up their dead bodies and other debris. The waste is then filtered out and surviving invaders are destroyed at lymph nodes that are strategically positioned throughout the body.

Autoimmune disease or dysfunction occurs when one or more elements of the immune system becomes deficient, overwhelmed, or overactive. Holistic treatment of autoimmune diseases (such as lupus, arthritis, FIV, allergies, to name a few) centers on assisting the body in its innate ability to establish and maintain balance and preparedness within the immune system. The use of vaccines, antibiotics, and steroid drugs is contradictory to the holistic healing effort because these substances are antagonistic to the body's natural defense mechanisms. Such measures work by suppressing, confusing, or bypassing natural immune functions, which amounts to an artificially induced state of autoimmune deficiency.

Barring genetic predisposition, animals who are consistently well nourished and properly cared for have strong immune systems throughout their long, healthy lives. On the other hand, animals who are subjected to immunosuppressive drug therapies eventually develop some form of immune dysfunction—perhaps arthritis, chronic seborrhea, allergies, or diminished resistance to certain strains of bacteria, fungi, or parasites.

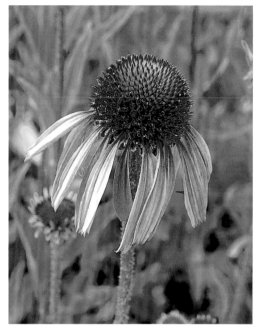

Stimulating the immune system with echinacea may be counter-productive to the healing process.

Whether or not to vaccinate your companion involves heated arguments among animal care professionals on both sides of the issue, as well as political, social, economic, and legal interests. At the root of all the confusion lies a pressing question: Should well-informed animal guardians be allowed to decide what is best for their beloved companion animals? We, of course, believe that owners should have that right. Although we cannot advise anyone to break the law in areas where vaccinations are deemed mandatory, we are holistically opposed to vaccinating animals.

HERBS FOR IMMUNE SYSTEM SUPPORT

Many of the diseases and problems discussed in this book are related to the immune system. A few diseases or syndromes are recognized as being directly related to immunity and might be considered autoimmune diseases. When most herb users think of immune system support, immunostimulant standbys such as echinacea immediately come to mind. For many immune-related disorders, however, increased stimulation of immune system functions represents only a small part of a complete herbal therapy, and in some cases, stimulation of immune activities may actually be counterproductive in the healing effort. A good case in point is discoid lupus erythematosus (DLE), a disease that occurs primarily in dogs and less commonly in cats. Discoid lupus erythematosus is a chronic inflammatory condition of the skin (primarily that of the nose, lips, cheeks, and ears) that occurs as the result of a failure in the regulating mechanisms of the immune system, specifically those that prevent the body from attacking its own cells. In other words, the immune army works against the body it is supposed to protect. Animals with DLE typically suffer from pyoderma, seborrhea, and other chronic conditions of the skin, as well as arthritis, kidney problems, and other immune-mediated forms of disease. For obvious reasons, it would be inadvisable to further stimulate the immune system with herbs such as echinacea. On the other hand, many herbs can act as immune moderators, meaning that they help adjust the immune system into balance. Such herbs include astragalus, shiitake and reishi mushrooms, garlic, and ginseng.

The immune system and its variable problems are complex, and no single herb serves as a panacea for immune system dysfunction. Because a great deal of sensationalism has been placed on herbs that have been shown to stimulate immune system functions, many people have been led to believe that an herb such as echinacea is always the first thing to reach for to fight any problem that involves the immune system. Entrepreneurs have made such claims a multimillion dollar affair, but the claims simply aren't true.

Contrary to what many herb product manufacturers might lead you to believe, immune system support does not begin with stimulation. In fact, stimulation should be limited to activating a healthy immune system in times when increased immune response is necessary to repel viral, bacterial, or fungal infection. In some cases of immune-mediated disease, immunostimulants may ultimately do more harm than good. For instance, echinacea and Saint-John's-wort are capable of stimulating reproduction of killer T cells, the search-and-destroy soldiers whose numbers are severely diminished in people or animals with AIDS. On the surface of the problem, stimulation of T cells may sound like a good idea, but by stimulating their reproduction, we may also be aggravating and accelerating the mechanisms that are causing their destruction. Therefore, the best course of action in immune-mediated problems is to support the body in its efforts to reestablish and maintain healthy balance among all aspects of natural immunity.

If stimulating the immune system is indicated, several herbs are available that have immunostimulant qualities. Some herbs, such as echinacea, have strong and specific immune-stimulating activities, making them especially useful when the immune system needs a quick boost. Others, such as garlic, Siberian ginseng, astragalus, licorice, shiitake and reishi mushrooms, and turmeric, offer immune-supportive qualities in addition to a wide spectrum of tonic activities. For instance, astragalus, shiitake and reishi mushrooms, and Siberian ginseng are all adaptogens, meaning that they help increase energy levels and improve the body's ability to respond to stressful situations (such as systemic disease, infection, or emotional trauma). Garlic offers strong antimicrobial, antioxidant, and hypotensive activities in addition to being an immunostimulant device. Turmeric stimulates liver and digestive functions as part of its immune-boosting agenda. Licorice and borage stimulate the adrenal glands and support and protect the liver, making them useful in treating Addison's disease (hypoadrenocorticism) or problems that stem from steroid drug use or excessive X-ray exposure.

In summary, before you pick up echinacea for immune system support, educate yourself. Find out more about your companion animal's condition and read up on echinacea and other herbs mentioned in this book as well as other immune-supportive herbs. You will likely find an herb that is specifically suited to your companion's needs.

ALLERGIES

Allergies occur when antigenic substances (allergens) enter the body and trigger a disproportionately aggressive immune response. Conventional treatment usually involves the use of antihistamine and corticosteroid drugs. These drugs suppress immune system functions so that the uncomfortable symptoms of allergy cannot occur. This action alleviates the symptoms for a while but leaves their actual causes unaddressed. In fact, such drugs may compound the underlying immune system dysfunction that is causing the problem in the first place.

Allergies are a symptom of an immune system disorder that may be related to a nutritional deficiency or excess, steroid or antibiotic therapies, vaccinosis, or metabolic dysfunction. Therefore, the questions to ask in the holistic treatment of allergies are threefold: (1) What substance is causing an immune response, (2) Why is the immune system responding so disproportionately to the substance, and (3) What can be done to help correct this response?

Holistic treatment is focused on moderating immune responses and improving the body's ability to process and eliminate potential allergens. The effort begins with an intensive assessment of the animal's diet, environment, and health care history. As causative factors are identified and dealt with, herbal therapy begins with tonic support of liver, digestive, lymphatic, and urinary functions that are responsible for filtering and eliminating problematic substances from the body. This in turn supports and improves immune activities by helping to remove antigenic substances and metabolic waste products that might be compounding the problem. At the core of this approach are alterative, diuretic, and cholagogue herbs. Burdock, red clover, dandelion root, spirulina, and alfalfa are all worthy candidates for improving liver efficiency and building strong, healthy blood. The oils or stabilized powders of flaxseed, borage seed, black currant seed, and evening primrose seed contain EFAs that play important roles in immune system development and health. Dandelion leaf serves especially well as an effective diuretic agent to aid in the elimination of waste products that are carried out of the body via the urine. Nettle is an excellent tonic for animals who suffer from seasonal allergies, as it lends mild antihistamine relief in addition to strong diuretic and blood-nourishing qualities. The Basic Support Formula under "Skin Problems" is useful for all of these purposes.

Uncomfortable symptoms of allergy can be approached according to the systems involved. In severe cases in which identification of causative factors proves to be a lengthy process, licorice can be used as a less-obtrusive alternative to steroid drugs. The Systemic Detoxifying Formula under "Skin Problems" may be effective. It's important to remember, however, that symptomatic suppression does not amount to a cure. Don't be fooled into action by the joy of seeing your companion feel better—keep looking for answers until a long-term holistic solution is found.

Because an allergy equates to an overactive immune system, immunostimulant herbs (such as echinacea) may be contraindicated. Adaptogenic herbs, those herbs that improve or support the body's response to stressful circumstances such as Siberian ginseng or astragalus may be helpful in re-establishing and maintaining immune system balances in animals who suffer allergies.

Mouth and Nose Problems

MOUTH PROBLEMS

Some animals have problems with their teeth and gums throughout their lives. Others seem to be lucky or in such good health that their gums and teeth remain healthy for life. A healthy, natural, raw food diet is paramount to healthy gums and teeth. For dogs and cats, this means raw, meaty bones and a diversity of enzyme- and nutrient-rich fresh vegetables. Many herbivores have needs that go beyond simple dietary cleansing and nutrition—their teeth need to be continuously worn down by the foods they eat to prevent the teeth from becoming too long and to remove weak and decaying outer layers of enamel. Fresh, whole, fibrous vegetables and grains are an absolute necessity for this process.

Most mouth problems are easily taken care of at home with a few simple herbal preparations. But if your animal is having difficulty chewing and eating or is pawing at his mouth, he may have a minor tooth or gum infection that can progress into a serious condition if not addressed. In cases of gingivitis, bacteria can eventually infect

Antimicrobial Nose Drops

Calendula tincture *
Oregon grape tincture *
Usnea lichen tincture *
2 oz sterile saline

Combine 10 drops of each of the alcohol tinctures with the sterile saline.

*Tinctures are available through most herb retailers

To use for sinusitis, drop or spray the above solution into each nostril, preferably with the animal's head tilted slightly skyward. Expect resistance and sneezing during administration—your companion probably won't like this. Adverse reactions are rare with this formula, but before administering a full dose, check for hypersensitivity by placing a small drop onto the rim of one nostril. If your companion starts sneezing and doesn't stop within a few minutes, he may be sensitive to one or more of these herbs or the alcohol, so don't use the drops.

A drop or two per nostril twice daily is a sufficient dose for cats and similar-sized animals. Dogs need 4–6 drops per nostril (or a short squirt of the sprayer). Horses and other large animals require 10–20 drops per nostril.

the kidneys, causing irreversible damage to these vital organs. If your herbal efforts fail to remedy your companion's bad breath or oral discomfort or if the animal's gums are severely inflamed, bleeding, or discharging pus, get to a veterinarian immediately. A red gum line (along the base of an animal's teeth) may also be indicative of a serious underlying problem that demands professional attention.

Gingivitis and Infections of the Mouth

Gingivitis is an inflammation of the gums that is usually caused by bacterial infection. Symptoms may include bad breath; reddened, swollen, and sometimes ulcerated gums; and pain and difficulty while eating. Gingivitis rarely occurs in healthy animals who receive a balanced, raw food diet. It's therefore important to make sure your companion receives the vitamins, minerals, enzymes, and probiotics he needs to maintain a strong immune system and good oral health. For dogs and cats, nothing compares with raw, meaty bones for maintaining healthy teeth and gums.

Other causes of oral infection include puncture wounds from fights or rambunctious play (puppy and kitten teeth make for dangerous jaw wrestling), abrasions or lacerations from chewing on nonfood items, wood splinters, and dental cavities.

Dietary supplementation of CoQ_{10}, vitamin C, and a variety of antimicrobial herbs may prove useful for reducing infection and activating the healing process in the mouth. Echinacea provides a needed boost to the immune system. To inhibit bacteria or fungi directly, a tincture of certified organic goldenseal, Oregon grape, thyme, sage, rosemary, or better yet, myrrh, can be liberally applied directly to the animal's gums (or any other site of oral infection)

with a cotton swab. If the animal is less than cooperative, a turkey-basting syringe can be used to rinse the animal's mouth—put 20 drops of tincture in 2 ounces of water or give 2 ounces of tea for each 20 pounds of the animal's weight, two to three times daily. To freshen bad breath, parsley leaf can be fed as a tincture, as a cooled tea, or in its whole form. If bad breath is not a problem, dietary supplementation of garlic can also be helpful. Propolis is also excellent for infected gums or mouth ulcers.

NOSE AND SINUS PROBLEMS

Nose and sinus problems are usually due to environmental influences such as bites, stings, allergens, microbial infection, or litter box dust (a major cause of sinus problems in cats). Provided the problem is isolated to the nose and nasal passages and is related to foreign substances, not a tumor or other metabolic disorder, nose and sinus problems can be treated effectively with simple herbal preparations. If the problem is secondary to other disorders, the therapeutic approach varies according to the nature of onset. For instance, sinusitis secondary to seasonal allergies is best approached with dietary adjustment and herbs that support

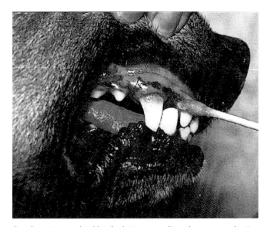

Swab antimicrobial herbal tinctures directly on your dog's gums to treat oral infections.

the various systems involved. Inflammation secondary to an insect sting requires topical (astringent) applications to help relieve uncomfortable symptoms and immunotonic and lymphatic herbs such as echinacea and calendula to support the metabolic processes of removing foreign substances from involved tissues.

Sometimes, abnormal nasal discharge, inflammation, sneezing, or other symptoms may be difficult to link to a cause. In these cases, the diagnostic capabilities and holistic insights of an experienced veterinarian should not be overlooked. If a problem is found to stem from deeper health issues, holistic treatment must begin at those issues and not with the nasal symptoms. This is important: Don't assume anything. Identify the cause of disease before beginning any herbal treatment. If you don't, you may be neglecting your companion's real needs.

For bacterial or fungal infections of the nostrils, sinuses, or outer tissues of the nose, a saline-based preparation of calendula, Oregon grape, and usnea lichen can be effective against a broad spectrum of bacteria and fungi. Externally, this preparation can be liberally applied to all affected areas. For infections inside the nose and sinuses, it can be administered with a dropper or as a nasal spray (empty bottles for nasal spray are available from pharmacies).

Parasite-Related Problems: How to Live with Fleas, Worms, Mites, and Other Things That Suck

If you're like most people who share their homes with companion animals, there's a good chance that this is the first part of the book you've turned to. Parasites are the most common source of torment and frustration shared by animals and their human guardians. From an animal's perspective,

fleas, mites, and other blood-sucking freeloaders are often the causes of sustained torture and misery. To an animal guardian, parasites are evil, disgusting, and invasive. Creatures that latch onto flesh and suck the life fluids from their hosts have earned top billing in our nightmares.

Unfortunately, while we struggle with our hate for such creatures by engaging in a relentless and futile battle to wipe parasites from the face of the planet, we often overlook the deeper reasons they cause so much misery to our animals. After all, tapeworms, fleas, ticks, mites, and other sucking insects have coexisted with animals for millions of years, which implies that there must be natural provisions to allow for a more harmonious coexistence. How did animals cope before humanity developed poisons and vaccines to reduce parasite populations? Did all animals suffer from chronic problems such as flea allergies, digestive dysfunction, or heart disease because they were infested with too many parasites? Of course not. Then why do some animals nowadays live their entire lives virtually undisturbed by parasites, while others with the same level of exposure are constantly tormented by them? To find the answers to such questions, we need to step away from our antiparasitic obsessions long enough to consider the life of a parasite.

HOLISTIC APPROACHES

Parasites, as repulsive as the fact may be, exist inside and on top of every living thing on earth. They even live on each other. In fact, a body (human or otherwise) is home for a teeming biocommunity of millions of interdependent life-forms, many of which happen to be parasites. From a holistic perspective, parasite-related health problems emanate not from the mere presence of these vampires but from the host's inability to deal with them effectively. Some animals may test positive for *Dirofilaria immitis* (heartworm) but never suffer ill health. On the other hand, some animals who appear to be healthy cannot tolerate a single fleabite without getting sick.

Parasites are opportunity seekers that exploit the weaknesses of their host. Their goal in doing so is to reproduce and take control of their environment. If the host is malnourished and poorly equipped to keep parasite populations in check, the parasites will take advantage of the body's inadequate defenses and begin reproducing, eating, and creating waste faster than the body can clean and replenish itself. If the immune system is dysfunctional and responds too aggressively to the parasites, an "allergic response" occurs.

The most effective and holistic approach to parasite infection is to keep your animal well nourished and healthy. An animal with a strong, properly functioning immune system presents an inhospitable living environment for parasites and is less likely to suffer from parasite-related allergies. But there's still an important question to be asked before the holistic picture is complete: What happens to this scenario when we give in to our hatred and fear of parasites and opt to use preventive drug measures in our pets? Any answer to this question is likely to raise controversy. Antiparasitic drugs represent a multibillion-dollar industry in the U.S., and many veterinarians support manufacturers' claims that modern dewormers, skin-absorbed flea control agents, and other internal measures are effective and generally safe. On the other side of the issue, though, holistic practitioners and naturally oriented animal guardians are concerned about the serious long-term effects associated with such

drugs. Of course, we're among those on this side of the issue, and here's why.

To start with, anything that can poison a parasite cannot be good for the host. From a holistic standpoint, anything that bypasses or interferes with natural body functions is likely to create its own state of imbalance in the body. For instance, chemical wormers (aside from being potentially toxic to animals) are not 100 percent selective in what they kill, meaning that beneficial microbes, such as those that play important roles in digestion and nutrient absorption, might be compromised. In addition to this possibility, most antiparasitic agents come with their own long lists of potential side effects, including seizures, liver failure, or even death. Ivermectin, a drug commonly used to treat and prevent heartworm infection, may not only cause central nervous system depression but also act as an immunosuppressant. That is, while it works to kill heartworms it also makes the body more vulnerable to countless other diseases.

The holistic herbalist does not see parasites as a cause of disease but as symptoms of a deeper imbalance. Parasites themselves are viewed as what they really are—tough, adaptable, ancient life-forms that will likely inhabit the earth long after humankind is gone. They are part of nature. Therefore, effective natural solutions to parasite-related disorders are not found through fervent and dangerous attempts to destroy them but from learning to coexist with them.

In our minds (and remember, we're herbalists, not veterinarians), stopping a symptom with chemicals that can harm the patient does not constitute preventive or curative medicine—it only represents a dangerous, short-term intervention that may actually compound the animal's health problems. Indeed, some forms of parasitic infection can be serious, even life threatening. The benefits of antiparasitic drugs are their convenience and their effectiveness at bringing symptomatic relief to an animal who is already suffering. But what are the potential costs to the animal? To find answers, check the back label or product information sheet for a list of side effects of the next antiparasitic drug you consider for your companion. Regardless of the danger issues, you owe your animal the opportunity to stay healthy and naturally free from parasite-related problems. This, of course, is what holistic animal care is all about.

NUTRITION AND OTHER PREVENTION CONSIDERATIONS

As we've stated before, the most effective treatment and prevention for all problems related to parasites is to make sure your companion gets the nutrition he needs. Without a complete natural diet, your animal's resistance and ability to adjust to parasites is greatly diminished. Equally important is the need to identify and correct any element of diet, environment, or activity that may be causing added stress on one or more body systems. If, for instance, your dog has an allergy to the wheat he receives in his daily meals, his immune system will already be compromised when new parasites enter his body. Likewise, if he has undergone long-term drug therapies, his immune system may be in a depressed state and his defenses may be low. Remember that parasites are opportunity seekers.

Digestive enzymes and probiotic bacteria supplements can be of help in maintaining a healthy balance between potentially harmful "digestive bugs," and those that lead the preventive fights for good health. A full array of vitamins and minerals is necessary to keep the blood healthy and the immune system operating at its peak potential. Omega-3 and omega-6 EFAs, along with the proper balance of antioxidant vitamins (especially C, A, and E) and minerals, are necessary for healthy, resilient skin that offers less opportunity for enterprising mites, fleas, and parasitic fungi. In addition to vitamin C's roles as an essential nutrient and antioxidant, it has been shown to lend allergy relief through the antihistamine qualities it possesses. Exercise is also important, as is a clean environment. The harder you work at helping your animal stay healthy, the less time and money you'll spend on treating parasite-related problems after the fact. As is the case in all forms of medicine, prevention truly is the cure.

FLEAS

Animals who are hypersensitive to fleas may suffer a severe reaction from a single bite—so severe that they pull their hair out and chew bloody patches from their skin. Conventional approaches to flea-contact dermatitis typically start with medicated shampoos, flea control devices, and corticoid ointments and then lead to internal corticosteroid drug therapies if conditions worsen. Anyone who has watched a companion suffer from a flea allergy knows how easy it is to look past the dangers of prednisolone. The problem is, prednisolone and other corticosteroid drugs don't just suppress uncomfortable symptoms but they also suppress the immune system. Add to this the possible long-term side effects of water retention, hypertension, liver damage, thyroid dysfunction, obesity, and heart attack, and suddenly the corticosteroid option doesn't sound so kind.

To approach the flea dilemma from a holistic standpoint means to embrace a perspective that includes the animal as a whole body in crisis. We must ask ourselves why fleas are bothering our animals in the first place rather than focus solely on their elimination. Effective flea control starts inside your pet and in his living environment. Holistic therapy does not begin with shampoos, coat dips, rinses, or sprays; it begins by strengthening the host and by making your animal's living quarters less hospitable to fleas. It's important to remember that flea problems are always secondary to something else, and it's that "something else" that makes your companion an attractive "bed and breakfast" for fleas. Healthy animals with healthy coats and properly functioning immune defenses generally don't have many fleas. And even if healthy animals do pick up a few fleas, their systems are able to handle the bites without the excessive histamine responses that cause all of the itching.

To help your healthy animal deal with parasites comfortably, feed him small amounts of garlic as a supplement to a proper diet. Contrary to what many believe, though, garlic should not be fed in quantities that cause that garlic odor to exude from the animal's skin. This is not only a waste of garlic but potentially harmful to your animal.

Dietary supplementation with brewer's yeast and vitamin B complex have been popular for years as antiflea measures, the theory being that these supplements adjust body chemistry in a way that makes the animal less appealing to fleas. The effectiveness of such measures is questionable, and many animals are allergic to brewer's yeast (especially if it is low grade), but nevertheless, these supplements are worth a try.

If your animal has an autoimmune deficiency, immunostimulants such as echinacea, Saint-John's-wort, or astragalus may be of help. However, immunostimulants should be used with caution or may be contraindicated in animals with severe allergies or other diseases that are associated with an overactive immune system or with immune functions that are working against the body (such as lupus and FIV).

In addition to garlic, alterative herbs such as burdock root, dandelion, and red clover serve as useful dietary adjuncts by helping the body eliminate waste and allowing natural defense systems to work more freely in coping with fleabites. Nettle may be sprinkled onto your animal's food to lend nutritive support and a mild antihistamine action that may reduce the severity of an allergic response. Giving ½–1 teaspoon of the dried herb for each pound of food fed is a good starting dosage range. If your animal won't eat dried nettle, you can steep it in hot water or salt-free meat broth, which you can then add to your companion's food. Oxeye daisy (*Chrysanthemum leucanthemum*), a common waste-area weed, is also said to have mild antihistamine qualities that don't really block histamine

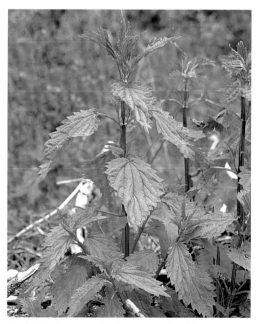

Nettle (dried or steeped in hot water or broth) can reduce an animal's allergic response to fleas.

Herbal Flea Repellent Powder

Combine the following dry ingredients:

1 part diatomaceous earth
2 parts feverfew flowers
2 parts mullein flowers
2 parts yarrow flowers, leaves, and stems
1 part sage or thyme

Sprinkle and brush into your animal's coat daily

but may help slow its release.

If fleabite allergies are severe, itching is persistent, and the skin is red and inflamed, licorice can be used as an internal anti-inflammatory remedy.

Externally, fleas and their effects can be addressed several ways. The animals' living environment can be sprinkled with diatomaceous earth, the sandlike remains of ancient marine organisms. Its activity against parasites is strictly mechanical, as each tiny particle has sharp points and edges that penetrate the bodies of fleas to cause their miserable deaths. Because of its gritty, penetrating nature, diatomaceous earth should not be applied to dry, irritated, hypersensitive skin, and it should never be allowed to contact eyes or other mucous membranes. Care also needs to be taken when spreading the substance onto carpets since walking around can stir up the dust and may cause silicosis, a form of pneumonia related to breathing the dust of silica and other sands. Otherwise it's generally quite safe. In fact, it's approved by the FDA for both internal and external use in livestock animals

and has been used safely in the natural care of companion animals for years.

Some pet owners may have heard that borax products are good flea exterminators, but borates can be quite toxic and may cause death if misused, according to Dr. Michael W. Dryden of the American Veterinary Medical Association (AVMA). One of the manufacturers of borax states that borax is not intended for application to carpet and upholstery.

Frequent vacuuming, washing your animal's bedding, and regularly steam-cleaning your carpet also helps reduce flea populations in the environment. Some products made with nematodes are available to "infect" and kill fleas where they live in your house and in the lawns around the house. All of these measures are available through natural pet-product retailers.

To help eliminate fleas from your animal's coat and to soothe and heal his itchy skin, several herbs come to mind. Flowers of feverfew, pyrethrum daisy, or oxeye daisy (or just about any other flower from the *Chrysanthemum* genus) contain compounds known as pyrethrins. Pyrethrins are well known to have paralytic activities in fleas. In fact, pyrethrins and their synthesized derivatives are common in many brands of flea spray. In their natural form, pyrethrins are safe and can be quite effective. Pyrethrins used in the form of a crude herbal preparation, however, won't always kill fleas but may only paralyze them temporarily. This means you should take additional measures to assure that fleas are out of your life forever.

Making a pyrethrin flea rinse is as simple as plucking a few handfuls of feverfew flowers, putting them into a cup, and steeping them in enough hot water to cover them. Briskly stir the mixture every couple of minutes until the mixture is cool enough to pour over your pet. You can strain the tea away from the flowers or just pour the entire mixture over your

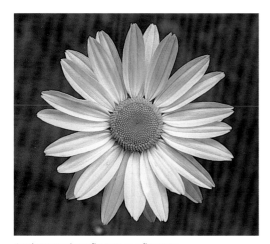

Apply oxeye daisy flowers as a flea rinse.

to 60 percent limonene). For the best results, harvest the seeds while they are green and juicy, and make a tea rinse immediately. Good-quality dried seeds can be used as a second source. Other limonene-bearing "umbels" include dill (leaf and seed) and fennel (seed).

Another herb that has been regaining popularity in recent years as an antiflea device is Canadian fleabane (*Conyza canadensis*). Until recently, Canadian fleabane (also called horseweed) was known by herbalists primarily as a urinary astringent. Its common name has caught the attention of several natural pet-product manufacturers, who claim that it is one of nature's greatest allies against fleas. Current research has concluded that Canadian fleabane contains flea-killing limonene as well. A much stronger source of limonene is essential oil of bitter orange, available through most stores that carry aromatherapy oils. This essential oil is very concentrated—just 6–10 drops diluted into 8 ounces of water is said to be an effective rinse against fleas. Simply moisten the animal's skin and coat with the mixture daily.

pet, but use the rinse right away—the active compounds break down and lose potency shortly after the tea is made. Be sure to soak the animal all the way down to the skin, and allow the rinse to air dry on your companion until the fur is damp but not dripping. Then, at a location that is as far away from the house as possible (remember, many of the fleas will recover with a hunger), rinse the animal with a strong stream of water while combing his coat, and look for paralyzed vampires.

Other flea-killing plant compounds include rotenone and limonene. Rotenone is readily available in the flowers of mullein (*Verbascum thapsus*), an Asian weed that occurs in waste areas throughout most of North America and Europe. The flowering tops are best if used fresh in the form of a strong decoction, but the dried blossoms (available through herb retailers) can be used too, again in the form of a cooled tea. When using mullein flowers or any other form of rotenone, be sure to keep the herb away from fish tanks or any amphibians—although it's safe for mammals, it is quite toxic to aquatic life forms. Limonene is a volatile oil found in citrus and many of the culinary herbs belonging to the parsley (Umbelliferae) family. A good source of limonene is contained in celery seeds (up

Garlic and Mullein Ear Oil

Combine the following:

1 part garlic oil
1 part mullein oil
10–20 drops of vitamin E oil for each 1 oz of the garlic and mullein oil mixture

For instructions on how to make an herb oil, turn to the "Basics of Herbal Preparations" in chapter 1.

To help relieve itching and promote healing, a calendula rinse is a good choice, as is aloe juice, which can be diluted with 4 parts water (e.g., 1 cup of aloe juice to 4 cups of water). Peppermint or lavender may help bring relief as well. If scratching has left oozing, infected scabs, yarrow, rosemary, or thyme can be generously added to the rinse. One advantage of using yarrow is that it adds its own insect-repellent qualities to the effort. If inflammation is severe and scratching has lead to hair loss, an astringent skin rinse may be indicated. Also, many good herbal flea and coat shampoos are on the market. These can be useful for bringing soothing relief. Don't shampoo your animal too often, though, or you might dry out the skin and cause added irritation. When using shampoos, also remember that their overuse can result in microbial imbalances on the surface of the body. Your animal's skin supports a natural community of interdependent organisms, many of which serve antiparasitic or cleansing purposes. To let them do their jobs it's probably best not to shampoo your animal more than once or twice a week during a crisis.

By now you might be wondering why we haven't mentioned North American pennyroyal (*Hedeoma pulegioides*). Well, we won't argue about the effectiveness of pennyroyal at deterring fleas. In fact, it's one of the best antiflea herbs around, which is why it is included in dozens of commercial flea preparations. The problem with it is that the volatile oils (composed mostly of an oil called pulegone) contained in pennyroyal can be toxic to animals, with the list of potential side effects beginning with nausea, vomiting, and abortifacient properties and ending with elevated blood pressure and possible kidney and liver damage. While most flea dips, sprays, and

powders that contain pennyroyal include relatively dilute concentrations of the volatile oil, a cumulative risk may exist to animals who lick off these topical preparations. Cats can be very sensitive to pennyroyal, and those with preexisting kidney disease (a widespread, chronic problem in cats) might even die from it. In our minds, such risks are unnecessary in the presence of safer, more holistic flea control measures. One such measure is the Triple-Punch Herbal Flea Rinse.

Triple-Punch Herbal Flea Rinse

1 part feverfew flowers
1 part mullein flowers (keep away
from aquatic animals!)
1 part yarrow flowers, leaves,
and stems
1 part celery seeds (freshly ground)
3 parts calendula flowers

Make a tea rinse of the herbs by covering the mixture with boiling water and allowing it to stand until cooled. To add even more "punch" to the formula, 6–10 drops of Bitter Orange essential oil can be added to each 8 ounces of rinse.

Herbal flea powders usually aren't as effective as rinses, but they are handy for animals and people on the go. The key to success in making a powder is to be sure that all of the herbal ingredients are as fresh as possible. Pyrethrin-bearing plants lose much of their potency after they are dried, and aromatic herbs such as lavender or yarrow lose their flea-repellent pungency eventually.

The best you can hope for with a homemade flea powder is "flea discouragement." It's unlikely that you will succeed in eliminating or repelling every biting flea without taking other measures as well. To keep your flea powder as fresh and active as possible, make it in small, frequent batches. An electric coffee grinder or a mortar and pestle can be used to grind your herbs into powder.

MITES

Mites are an excellent example of just how common parasites are. These tiny, often microscopic, arachnids are everywhere and on everything. A healthy human body carries millions of them. In fact, all living land animals carry mites—even fleas and mites have mites!

When you're finished scratching, it's important to know that relatively few of the parasitic varieties of mites cause problems. Those that do cause problems burrow under the top layers of the skin to cause hair loss, skin disfigurement, and painful lesions on the skin and in the ears. In dogs, cats, horses, and other mammals, various species of skin mites are commonly referred to as mange. In instances of human infection, we usually refer to them as scabies.

Various species of mange are differentiated by the specific nature of the infections they cause. Sarcoptic mange (*Sarcoptes scabiei*) is the most contagious (some species can be transmitted to humans) and often the most severe form of mange, characterized most frequently by crusty, reddish brown lesions that usually appear first on the head and neck, between the legs, or in the "armpits" of the victim animal. Demodectic mange, or red mange (genus *Demodex*), is a far less contagious mite that infects hair follicles, often causing hair loss and a foul-smelling bacterial infection of the skin. Both chorioptic mange (genus *Chorioptis*) and psoroptic

mange (genus Psoroptes) are common in cattle, horses, sheep, and goats and produce similar symptoms. *Otitis externa*, or otodectic ear mange, occurs in dogs and cats and is characterized by inflammation and brown, waxy discharge from the ears. Rabbits are susceptible to ear mange as well. Occurrence of ear mites in horses and other large animals is relatively uncommon.

All of the mange-causing mites have one thing in common: they are all opportunity-seeking parasites that prefer a defenseless host. Therefore, prevention in the form of a well-balanced natural diet that provides immune system support should begin before an infection occurs.

Fortunately, herbal measures can be quite effective against the various forms of mange. The foremost herb to consider is garlic. Mites don't tolerate sulfur compounds, and garlic contains hundreds of them (which is why garlic smells like it does). For ear mites or localized mite infestations on birds and mammals, garlic oil can be applied to the affected areas twice daily. In addition to its direct intervention with mites, garlic oil helps minimize bacterial infection. When using garlic oil, however, make sure that it's not too concentrated or it may cause irritation. Another good ear mite herb is mullein flower oil. Mullein flowers possess antiparasitic and antibacterial activities that seem well suited to infections of the ear, especially when combined with garlic oil. Vitamin E oil can be added to this combination to help promote healing. The olive oil used as a base for both of these oils also lends soothing and healing qualities to the skin.

For mange infestations that are localized close to the eyes of an animal, you will probably want to purchase or make an ointment or salve preparation. This minimizes the risk of the herb contacting the eyes.

Other herbs to consider for mite infections are lavender, yarrow, Oregon grape, goldenseal (provided it is from cultivated sources), and licorice. Any of these herbs can be used in oils, salves, or ointments as well, or they can be made into a skin rinse (a good option for infections that are generalized over larger portions of the animal's body). Licorice serves as a good alternative for animals who are sensitive to topical applications of garlic. If you have access to it, neem leaf (*Azadirachta indica*), from a tree found in India and Pakistan, can make an effective skin rinse against many forms of mange.

For birds who are crawling with mites, a pinch of Oregon grape or lavender can be infused into their birdbath. For lizards with mite infections, a wet towel wipe of weak Oregon grape, yarrow, or lavender tea might help.

LICE

Several species of lice can infest both mammals and birds. They can generally be divided into two categories: those that suck blood from their hosts (*Anopleura*) and those that bite their victims (*Mallophaga*). Regardless, the term lousy is derived from the concept of louse infestation, and the repulsiveness the word conveys describes the situation accurately. Louse infestation is a common problem for animals who live in cramped or unclean living quarters. The problem is characterized by irritated, itchy skin and frequent scratching.

Lice are tough critters and can be hard to beat with herbs. The most effective and time-honored herb approaches for lice include toxic heavyweights such as tansy (*Tanacetum vulgare*) and even water hemlock (*Cicuta* spp.), either of which can kill an animal host. On the safer side of the herbal spectrum are licorice, yucca, wormwood,

sage, yarrow, yellow dock, lavender, and bee balm. All of these herbs can be used singly or in combination in the form of a daily skin rinse. A daily sprinkling of diatomaceous earth onto the animal's coat may be effective, too.

INTESTINAL WORMS

Worms are often viewed as parasites at their most disgusting worst, but again this is largely because we have a big problem with the thought of things crawling around inside our bodies. Sorry if this gives you the "crawlies," but worms are a natural fact of life. We all have them in one form or another.

Animal guardians tend to overreact to the possibility of worms with the precautionary use of chemical wormers. As we mentioned earlier, such practice is contrary and counterproductive to the purposes of holistic health care. We are not saying that worms cannot be life threatening but that the health risks associated with preventive drug therapies may outweigh the actual need for them, especially in healthy animals who are not likely to be exposed to roundworms, whipworms, or hookworms.

The most common type of intestinal parasites are known as cestodes, or tapeworms. Tapeworms can be transmitted by fleas, feces, or food sources. In rural areas, dogs and cats often become infected by eating rodents. Tapeworms may live in an animal's digestive tract for quite a while, sometimes indefinitely, before they are detected, and they are seldom harmful to the host animal. Usually, we won't even know that our companions have tapeworms until a fecal analysis is done or until we see the worms' body segments in the animals' stools. The segments (put your sandwich down!) look very much like grains of rice. The potential of tapeworms to cause harm to an animal is relative to the general health of the animal and the extent of the tapeworm infestation. In other words, if an animal is generally healthy, a moderate population of intestine-dwelling tapeworms is usually harmless. And if the animal is holistically healthy, has a strong immune system, properly balanced intestinal flora, and is being fed a good diet, tapeworm infestations are likely to be a temporary issue. For instance, we live on 60 remote acres in the Montana Rockies, where our two dogs roam freely around the house. Both occasionally eat a ground squirrel or two (sometimes in the form of carrion), and we expect both of them to have tapeworms by the end of summer. But because they are healthy, most if not all of the worms (as confirmed by fecal analysis) are gone from their bodies after a couple of months of infestation. The opportunity seekers just can't find a stronghold, or they don't like the accommodations.

It's our contention that in most instances, the reason tapeworms are approached with chemical interventions is not always because a real and urgent need to eliminate them exists but because we can't deal with their less-than-appealing nature. Yes, they're disgusting. But are we really helping an animal when we use unnecessary, potentially toxic measures to expel them? We don't think so.

Roundworms, hookworms, whipworms, and threadworms present a much greater risk to your companion because these worms can cause severe intestinal damage and can leave the digestive tract to infest the blood and other organs. Once these parasites leave the digestive tract, they can be difficult to treat.

To help your dog or cat keep intestinal populations in check and to encourage earlier expulsion by less invasive, more natural means, garlic can be fed in moderation on the animal's food. Fennel, grated raw carrot, shredded coconut, and cooked grains also might be of benefit if added to the animal's diet. (Feed as much as the animal wants to eat.) Fresh, raw, unsalted pumpkin seeds help expel worms and generous portions can be fed as a wholesome treat to any animal. The seeds may need to be ground up and added to your pet's food. (You can grind a small batch ahead of time and keep it in a jar in the freezer until you're ready to use it.) Diatomaceous earth is effective at reducing intestinal parasite populations and can be fed at the following recommended rates (approved by the FDA)—large dogs over 55 pounds can have up to 1 tablespoon per day, small dogs and cats can have 1 teaspoon per day. Goats, sheep, cattle, horses, and other large animals can be fed in portions

Antiworm Food Supplement

Combine the following dry ingredients:

- **2 parts unsalted, raw pumpkin seeds** (ground or whole)
- **1 part garlic powder**
- **1 part fennel seed**
- **1 part yucca root**

Feed the mixture as part of your companion's diet at a dosage of 1 teaspoon per pound of food fed daily. Feed five days on and two days off each week until worm populations are reduced to acceptable levels. If this formula proves to be ineffective, try adding 1 part Oregon grape root powder or 1 part wormwood.

up to 1 percent of their daily dry rations; and chickens and most birds can receive up to 5 percent. Oregon grape may be given internally to birds, dogs, cats, horses, and other mammals as a low-alcohol tincture or decoction. A dose of 12 drops per 20 pounds of the animal's body weight (or just a few drops for birds), twice daily for up to one week is appropriate. After one week, give the animal's system a break for two or three days before continuing the twice-daily doses. Chamomile has mild worm-expelling properties, and pineapple weed (*Matricaria matricarioides*), a wild and weedy cousin of chamomile, is believed to possess much stronger activities against roundworms and whipworms.

Other worming agents include black walnut and wormwood. Black walnut hull is an effective worming agent, but it must be used with care because of the potentially irritating tannin constituents it contains. Black walnut should not be used in or around horses, as it may be toxic to them. Wormwood, of course, is a classic dewormer, but it should not be used for long periods and not at all in animals with liver disease. Even more dangerous are tansy and rue. In our opinion, these herbs should be avoided altogether because they're too harsh on the liver.

Herbs that are rich in soaplike saponin constituents such as yucca, valerian, and licorice are sometimes effective as worming agents. Yucca also helps by optimizing absorption of nutrients in the small intestine, an attribute that might be useful in cases of severe infection in which nutrient absorption is hindered by the presence of too many hungry parasites.

Many herbal wormers contain laxative or emetic herbs such as senna, cascara sagrada, aloe, or turkey rhubarb. The idea behind their inclusion is to flush out the parasites by stimulating bowel movement and loosening the stool. In holistic reality, this approach adds stress to the body, causes discomfort to the animal, may cause dehydration and nutrient depletion, and may lead to laxative dependency if used for too long a period. The overall effectiveness of expelling worms is outweighed by the invasiveness of the therapy. If constipation is associated with a worm infestation, marshmallow, plantain, or slippery elm can be used to lubricate the digestive tract without pulling needed fluids from the body, and hepatics such as yellow dock, Oregon grape, or a small pinch of turmeric can be fed to increase bile production and improve digestion. Slippery elm or plantain may be beneficial in cases of worm-related diarrhea because these herbs contain astringent qualities that gently regulate the passage of fluid into the intestine. A safe, general worming remedy that can be added to your companion's food can be found on page 273.

GIARDIASIS

Giardiasis is a digestive disease caused by cyst-forming impregnation of protozoa of the *Giardia* genus in the mucosal lining of the intestines. The result is nausea, vomiting, diarrhea, and other flulike symptoms for several weeks. The most common means of infestation comes from ingestion of water that has been contaminated by the fecal matter of fish and other animals. Animals are much more resistant to Giardia than humans are, but they are still susceptible. As with all parasites, severity of infestation depends on the overall health of the host. Symptoms range from loss of appetite to diarrhea, vomiting, weight loss, dehydration, and general debility.

Herbal interventions are moderately successful at best. Tinctures are the best form of application here because their

A Remedy for Giardiasis

Combine the following tinctures:

2 parts Oregon grape
2 parts licorice
2 parts cleavers
1 part garlic

This formula can be fed to dogs, cats, birds, horses, and other large herbivores at least one hour before feeding, at a dosage of about ¼ teaspoon (1 milliliter) per 20 pounds of the animal's body weight, twice daily for up to ten days. If positive results aren't seen within ten days, it's time to call your holistic vet. Low-alcohol tinctures are best because of their relative ease of administering, but alcohol tinctures can be used provided they are diluted to half-strength with water, which means you will have to give the animal twice the liquid volume.

high concentrations of readily available constituents are needed against these tough little beasties. Of particular interest are Oregon grape, goldenseal (from cultivated sources), and other herbs that contain the active alkaloid constituent berberine. Berberine, being water soluble, highly assimilable, and able to withstand the digestive acids that destroy many other types of antibiotic agents, finds it way deep into the digestive tract to work its wonders, especially when given in concentrated extract form over periods of several days. Garlic may lend antiprotozoa support as well. Licorice is a good adjunct, lending antimicrobial, anti-inflammatory, and healing properties to the effort. Cleavers helps drain lymph-engorged tissues that surround the cysts.

HEARTWORM

The term *heartworm* is really a misnomer, as the parasitic worm (*Dirofilaria immitis*) that causes the disease usually infects the pulmonary arteries, not the heart itself.

Heartworm is generally passed by mosquitoes, who pick up the parasite from the bloodstreams of dogs (less frequently from cats and ferrets) while the worms are in their prelarval stage. While inside the mosquito, the infant parasites called microfilaria mature into infective adults that are deposited into other host animals. After two to four months, the parasites penetrate blood vessel walls and travel to the pulmonary arteries, where they reproduce if conditions are right. While the worms are in the pulmonary arteries, the body launches an immunologic attack against them. If the worms have already reproduced to numbers that the immune system cannot effectively control, an allergic response ensues, and the pulmonary arteries and surrounding lung tissues may become severely inflamed, causing a life-threatening situation. Animals with advanced stages of heartworm infestation may exhibit chronic coughing; labored breathing; diminished physical stamina and a low tolerance to stress; weight loss; and heart failure.

Unfortunately, the scenario becomes even more frightening when we consider conventional treatment of the disease, which involves the use of thiacetarsamide, an intravenously administered arsenic derivative that poisons the parasites at great expense to the host animal's liver. In our opinion and that of several holistic veterinarians, the deworming medication ivermectin and other preventive measures for heartworm can also be detrimental to an animal, which brings us to an especially important point in the prevention of the disease.

In some areas of the U.S., heartworm is a real and constant threat to companion animals. But in many areas of North America, it is more of a fear-induced paranoia than an actual danger. In Montana, for instance (where we live), heartworm is almost unheard of. Unfortunately, horror stories about heartworm lead many people to medicate their animals anyway. We believe that people should rationally weigh the pros and cons as well as the need of administering a preventive heartworm treatment to their animal companions.

Another problem arises from the blood and antigen tests that are performed to detect heartworms. In these tests, 30 percent of infested dogs do not test positive, meaning that the disease may progress unchecked. Likewise, a positive test for heartworm does not necessarily mean that the parasites will become problematic, especially if the host animal is healthy.

Natural prevention of heartworm begins with identifying just how much "at risk" your companion is. If you live in a high-risk area, your animal's coat should never be cut. Allow it to grow to full length and serve its natural function as an antimosquito barrier. Areas where mosquito populations are especially high (such as swamps, sloughs, and other breeding grounds) should be avoided, and perhaps a tightly knit cotton or breathable nylon garment is in order for shorthaired dogs. (Several clothing catalogs for dogs are available.) Proper nutrition and tonic immune system support will build and maintain your companion's resistance to the parasite. In addition to a full array of supplemental vitamins and minerals, garlic can be added to an animal's diet to strengthen the immune system. When venturing into higher-risk areas, echinacea can be preventatively administered for two or three days before the excursion and continue for three days after.

If your animal does contract heartworm, don't panic. Instead, continue supporting the immune system and call your holistic veterinarian to determine the next step of action. There are many options. Among them may be black walnut hull tincture (made from unripe green hulls instead of dried ones). As of 1999, we had been contacted by several individuals who claim that black walnut hull may be effective at controlling the parasites. Given what we know about this herb and the parasite, we remain skeptical but hopeful that clinical use will validate this claim.

Pregnancy and Lactation

One of the most frequently asked questions we hear as animal herbalists is, What should I be giving to a pregnant animal? Our response is often a cause of disappointment: Aside from the elements of good nutrition, as little as possible.

During pregnancy and lactation, a mother's body is in a state of continual hormonal fluctuation. Her nutritional demands change as her body experiences a roller-coaster ride of metabolic events that are incomparable to any other experience. It is a period when her body must maintain delicate checks and balances while responding to unprecedented demands. These are times when the proactive efforts of an animal herbalist really pay off. Having received a good natural diet, a healthy living environment, and complementary measures of health-supporting vitamin, mineral, and herb supplements throughout her life, the pregnant animal is physically and mentally prepared to undertake the rigors of childbirth and motherhood. This is a time when the body should be allowed to work its natural wonders without interference from introduced stimulation, suppression, or irritation. With this in mind, the bigger and better question is, What herbs shouldn't be used in pregnant or lactating animals?

HERBS TO AVOID

Many herbs should not be given to pregnant or lactating animals. Herbs that contain considerable amounts of volatile oil constituents such as juniper, any of the aromatic mints, and parsley seed should not be used during pregnancy because the oils are capable of crossing the placenta to the fetus. Volatile oils may also infiltrate a mother's milk, so these herbs should be avoided during lactation as well. Herbs that stimulate or suppress hormone production should also be avoided—these include licorice, wild yam, and yucca root. Herbs that are high in tannin constituents such as uva ursi, white oak bark, black walnut hulls, and slippery elm may cause uterine contractions and miscarriage. Herbal laxatives that contain anthraquinone constituents such as senna, cascara sagrada, turkey rhubarb, and yellow dock should be avoided as well. If your companion becomes constipated during pregnancy, try lubricating her digestive tract by feeding marshmallow, flaxseed, or psyllium husks. Chickweed can also serve as a safe and effective laxative in pregnant animals.

Herbs that contain large percentages of bitter alkaloids such as Oregon grape and goldenseal may have abortifacient activities and should not be used. Red clover, feverfew, and ginkgo all inhibit platelet aggregation in the blood and may contribute to excessive hemorrhage during or after birthing.

In summary, if you're not sure about the safety of an herb during pregnancy, assume that it's contraindicated and don't use it!

TONIC SUPPORT

Contrary to what many herbalists regard as tradition, we do not use most of the "classic birthing and pregnancy herbs" (such as blue cohosh) during this fragile time. Instead, our approach is strictly nutritive. Raspberry leaf tea has been long regarded as an excellent uterine tonic for pregnant humans and animals, but it should not be given during the first few weeks of pregnancy. Nor should it be fed in large amounts, as there is a small risk that its astringent activities may trigger abortion in sensitive animals (especially cats). In our opinion, nettle leaf and spirulina are both better choices as uterine tonics because they contain higher concentrations and broader assortments of essential and trace minerals and vitamins. This means they can be fed more conservatively, and the risk (as low as that risk may be) of inducing uterine contractions is thereby reduced.

HERBS AND LACTATION

Healthy animals who receive all necessary elements of nutrition during motherhood should have no problems with milk production or quality. If a nursing mother is not providing her young with enough milk, it's probably because of a nutritional deficiency, hormonal imbalance, or another dysfunction. Fennel seed, borage, dill, and yucca root are all said to increase milk production in nursing mothers, but these herbs are useful only to healthy animals who need more milk to feed a big, hungry litter. If your dog or cat has given birth to a small- or average-sized litter and is having trouble feeding her young, then deeper problems need to be addressed before you start trying to induce milk production. Forcing a mother's body to perform beyond its capacity with estrogenic herbs may only worsen an already serious situation. In many cases, switching an animal from a commercial diet to one that offers a diversity of whole, raw foods makes a world of difference. Moderate quantities of supplemental vitamins, minerals, probiotics, and EFAs can be of tremendous help as well because lactation can deplete an animal's reserve supply of vital nutrients. In cats, this depletion can cause a life-threatening deficiency of taurine, an amino acid that is critical to the heart.

Respiratory Problems

COUGHING AND SNEEZING: NATURAL HEALING MECHANISMS

Occasional coughing or sneezing is part of a body's normal health maintenance program. Most animal guardians know that when dust particles, pollen, or other foreign matter enters the trachea, spasms are triggered to expel the material from the body. Yet many people try to suppress coughing and sneezing rather than allow the body to do its job because the conventional Western mind-set dictates that anything that is socially offensive or that causes discomfort must be suppressed. To tend to an animal's holistic health needs, we must learn to control our urge to interfere with the body's natural functions. Suppressing activities such as sneezing, coughing, and discharging mucus deprives the body of its natural healing mechanisms and may actually contribute to the underlying disease by prohibiting expulsion of pathogenic microbes and other foreign substances.

Instead of suppressing disease symptoms, the holistic healer's efforts are centered on assisting the body to cleanse and heal itself. In the respiratory tract, this entails supporting and encouraging the productivity of coughing, sneezing, and expulsion of mucus. Most animals do not produce mucus as readily as humans do. Therefore, herbs and other remedies that serve as cough suppressants or discourage expectoration (such as wild cherry bark) should be reserved for special circumstances, such as when a continuous, unproductive cough has deprived an animal of sleep for several days. Even then, such remedies should be used in moderation as adjuncts to herbs that support productive coughing.

Many respiratory ailments can be treated at home with some simple herbal preparations. But if your companion's coughing or sneezing continues or worsens, or if you have any doubt whatsoever about its cause, you should have your friend examined by a holistic vet. A persistent cough can mean minor throat irritation caused by chewing on a stick, or it can be a symptom of a life-threatening situation such as heartworm, pneumonia, cardiopulmonary disease, or a serious viral infection.

ASTHMA

Asthma is characterized by a sudden onset of bronchial inflammation and respiratory distress. Animals with severe asthma may begin an attack by wheezing, sneezing, and coughing, which may quickly progress to obstructed airways, labored breathing, and a life-threatening crisis. According to most veterinarians, dogs do not suffer from asthma, but this disease is known to occur frequently in cats and many other animals.

Many people regard asthma as a cause of respiratory distress, but in most cases it's really only a symptom of a deeper immune-mediated disorder. Asthma usually occurs as part of a severe allergic reaction. Therefore, holistic treatment does not focus solely on suppression of asthma attacks but also on proactive correction of the dysfunctional mechanisms that trigger the attacks. (For more information on long-term holistic treatment, see "Allergies" in the "Immune System Care" sections of this chapter.)

Symptomatic herbal treatments for non-life-threatening cases of asthma are essentially the same as those used for kennel cough and other forms of bronchitis (see below). Lobelia may be useful for suppressing asthma attacks in cats, especially if a tincture is administered at the first signs of onset. Lobeline, the active constituent of lobelia, is potentially toxic (it has central nervous system effects similar to those of nicotine), so it should be administered only under the direction of a holistic veterinarian.

BRONCHITIS AND KENNEL COUGH

The term *bronchitis* refers to inflammation of one or more of the large air passages of the lungs. Causes are variable, ranging from inhalation of dust and other airborne irritants to viral, bacterial, or fungal infection; tumors; or cancer. An accumulation of mucus in the bronchi and a deep, rumbling cough are usually associated with bronchitis.

Bronchitis that is secondary to bacterial, fungal, or viral infection is often accompanied by elevated body temperature and mucus discharge. If your companion is coughing up fluid, take an unpleasant moment to examine it. If it's pink, frothy, blood streaked, or bright yellow, get your companion and a specimen of the discharge to a veterinarian immediately. Respiratory infections or bleeding progress rapidly and need to be treated aggressively.

Kennel cough is a generic term for a dry, hacking cough that occurs in dogs and sometimes cats. It is caused by viral (such as canine adenovirus II, parainfluenza) or bacterial infection (such as *Bordetella*

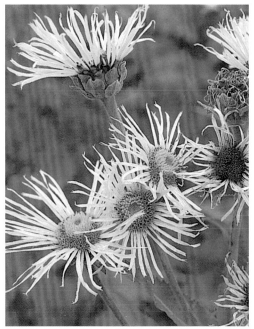

Elecampane can decrease the symptoms and shorten the duration of bronchitis and kennel cough.

bronchiseptica) and is generally self-limiting in that it rarely progresses beyond minor inflammation of the trachea. No discharge, fever, respiratory edema, or other symptoms are associated with kennel cough—just coughing. This is an important point to remember because if your animal is exhibiting symptoms in addition to a hacking cough, you may be facing a condition more serious than kennel cough.

Once diagnosed, kennel cough and most other types of bronchitis can be treated safely at home. If other animals in the home are susceptible to infection, take preventive measures to keep them healthy. We administer immune-supportive herbs to our animals before, during, and after suspected exposure to infectious bronchitis. Dietary supplementation of fresh chopped garlic is a good preventive measure because garlic has excellent immunotonic qualities and antibacterial and antiviral principles that are exhaled through the lungs. Astragalus or organically grown echinacea are also well suited for boosting your companion's immune system against kennel cough before or during an infection. Eucalyptus essential oil can be placed into a vaporizer with some water and left within a few feet of your companion's resting quarters. (Don't use this method in conjunction with a homeopathic prescription, as it may antidote the remedy.) The vapor helps open the animal's respiratory passages and provides a continuous measure of antimicrobial intervention.

Coltsfoot, grindelia, mullein leaf, and elecampane offer antiviral, antibacterial, expectorant, and antispasmodic qualities that can help shorten the duration of your companion's ailment. Yarrow is also strongly antimicrobial and helps increase pulmonary efficiency by dilating blood vessels of the lungs. Slippery elm, plantain, and marshmallow each lend soothing relief to

An Herbal Formula for Asthma, Kennel Cough, and Bronchitis with Dry Cough*

Combine the following low-alcohol (glycerin) tinctures:

> **1 part coltsfoot**
> **1 part grindelia or elecampane**
> **1 part mullein leaf**
> **1 part yarrow**
> **1 part marshmallow**

* This formula eases spastic coughing, fights bacterial infection, and soothes inflamed membranes.

This combination can be added to a small amount of honey and fed to dogs or cats two or three times daily until the illness has run its course. An appropriate dose is 0.25–0.5 milliliters for each 20 pounds of the animal's body weight. Additionally, a twice-daily dose of echinacea or astragalus is recommended for immune support. If the coughing is associated with nervousness or hyperexcitability, bugleweed, skullcap, valerian, hop, or a small measure of wild cherry bark can be added to the twice-daily regimen.

An Herbal Formula for Wet Coughs

> **1 part coltsfoot**
> **1 part goldenrod**
> **1 part yarrow**

If your companion's cough involves copious amounts of thick, hard-to-expel mucus, this formula serves to reduce inflammation of mucous membranes, reduce and thin mucous secretions in the bronchi, and help to make the cough less violent and more productive.

This formula can be added to a small amount of honey and fed to dogs or cats two or three times daily until the illness has run its course. An appropriate dose is 0.25–0.5 milliliters for each 20 pounds of the animal's body weight.

sore and inflamed membranes of the trachea and bronchi. Goldenrod is especially helpful in cases in which bronchial inflammation is yielding excessive mucus that the body cannot effectively expel (e.g., bronchial pneumonia).

PNEUMONIA AND PULMONARY EDEMA

Pneumonia is a condition in which lung volume and pulmonary efficiency is reduced by the presence of fluid (edema) or a solid mass (tumor). Pneumonia can originate from bacterial, viral, fungal, or protozoan infection; allergy; cancer; injury, or systemic dysfunction. Pneumonia is a life-threatening situation that can be progressive. Treatment varies according to the cause and symptoms.

The term *pulmonary edema* refers to the presence of fluid in the lungs. With few

A Tonic Formula for Animals with Pneumonia

Combine the following glycerin-based herb tinctures:
   2 parts echinacea
   1 part astragalus
   1 part coltsfoot
   1 part yarrow

This formula can be added to dandelion leaf tea and fed two or three times daily until the disease has run its course. The dose for dogs, cats, and other small animals is 0.25–0.5 milliliters for each 20 pounds of the animal's body weight. Horses and other large herbivores can receive 20–30 milliliters.

exceptions (such as drowning), pulmonary edema is secondary to other disorders, such as congestive heart failure, inhalation of toxic chemicals, or damage of lung tissues.

In cases of pneumonia or pulmonary edema, pulmonary (lung) efficiency is reduced so the blood does not receive the oxygen it needs to supply tissues throughout the body. In other words, the body progressively suffocates as the condition worsens. Symptoms at onset include reduced physical stamina; coughing, panting, or gasping for air; and diminished mental capacity. As the situation worsens, the tongue and mucous membranes of the eyes begin to turn blue from lack of oxygen, the animal becomes weak and lethargic, and the brain and other vital organs begin to die. Even if you have only a hunch that your animal may have pneumonia or a condition involving pulmonary edema, the first course of action is to consult a veterinarian immediately to rule out the possibility of a life-threatening situation. Don't hesitate. Pneumonia can be aggressive in animals, especially those who are aging or weakened by chronic illness.

Conventional approaches usually involve the use of furosemide or other strong diuretics to help move fluid out of the lungs, as well as antibiotic therapies directed toward any bacteria or fungi that might be involved.

Once the nature of the problem has been identified and the animal's condition has stabilized, herbs can be used to strengthen the immune system and support the body in its efforts to regain well-being. Large doses of a strong, dark dandelion leaf tea (as much as you can get the animal to drink) serves as a strong diuretic to help with the elimination of fluid from the lungs. If the animal won't drink the tea, use a salt-free meat or vegetable broth instead of hot water or sweeten the tea with honey. Unlike the aforementioned furosemide, dandelion helps replace potassium and other nutrients that are usually lost through increased urination.

Dandelion leaf tea should be fed continuously. Provide as much as the animal will take throughout the therapy. Echinacea and garlic can be used to boost your companion's immune system, and astragalus or Siberian ginseng may increase his body's ability to function under the added stress. Coltsfoot and elecampane are both good choices for stimulating respiratory function, inhibiting bacterial reproduction, and helping with the elimination of mucus from the bronchi. Inhalation therapy using a vaporizer and eucalyptus oil (as mentioned for bronchitis) can also bring relief. Yarrow and cayenne can both increase pulmonary circulation and increase oxygen delivery to the blood. Used in combination with the diuretic qualities of dandelion leaf, these two herbs may be especially useful for racehorses who suffer acute respiratory bleeding and pulmonary edema as a result of strenuous exercise. Cayenne can also be used as part of this program as a respiratory stimulant and to assist the activities of the other herbs—one small gel cap daily for dogs and cats and five to ten large gel caps daily for horses.

In animals who are suffering pulmonary edema secondary to congestive heart failure or other cardiopulmonary problems, hawthorn, ginkgo, or bugleweed may be indicated. Other herbs worth considering in a wide variety of respiratory problems include horehound (excellent, but hard to administer because of its bitterness), thyme, rosemary, and lovage.

Skin Problems

Skin is something we tend to take for granted. After all, we see it all the time. It covers our dogs, cats, horses, birds, and our own bodies. And unlike treatments for a diseased organ that is hidden deep and mysteriously within the body, our approaches to skin disorders are often as shallow as we perceive the skin itself to be.

The skin regulates body temperature as well as peripheral blood and lymph circulation and provides frontline protection from harmful influences that exist outside the body. The skin also helps with the elimination of systemic wastes that are not effectively eliminated through the urinary and digestive tracts. Therefore, what might appear to be nothing more than a superficial annoyance such as a skin disorder might indicate a serious underlying disease. Animals don't complain as much as people do and are unable to express the discomforts of a deep-seated disease. That means the causes of a chronic skin problem may go unnoticed until they progress to a point where an animal is noticeably suffering from a condition such as arthritis, liver disease, kidney failure, or even cancer. Compounding the problem is the difficulty of accurately identifying the underlying causes of many skin-related disorders—the list of possible causes is almost unlimited. As a result, many conventional therapies amount to nothing more than relief of surface symptoms.

In conventional veterinary medicine, skin problems are most often treated as conditions occurring on the outside of the body, and a common course of therapy typically involves topical creams, salves, rinses, or shampoos. When these external measures fail, corticosteroids, antihistamines, or other drugs are usually prescribed to depress the immune system and thereby squelch the uncomfortable symptoms. While this approach to skin disease can ease an animal's discomfort quickly or even make the disease appear to go away, the underlying causes of the disease may never be considered, much less acted upon. As a result, they may progress to other, more serious problems. In human dermatology, eczema or psoriasis present excellent examples. Both are viewed by Western medicine as symptomatic manifestations of various systemic or external causes such as hormonal imbalances; systemic dysfunction; or viral, fungal, or bacterial infection; but the reasons the body allows such problems to occur remain largely unknown. In the absence of curative answers, only the symptoms are addressed.

The principles of holistic herbal medicine do not allow healers to employ solutions that address only the surface manifestations of disease. While it's true that finding a cure for chronic skin disorders is as difficult for holistic healers as it is for conventional research scientists, we are gifted with a special weapon: a holistic perspective that enables us to help the body find a cure for itself. The holistic herbal approach to skin disease reaches beyond symptoms to accept the fact that the body has mysterious but powerful abilities to heal itself. Fully understanding these abilities is not absolutely necessary. The function of the herbalist is not to substitute the body's natural methods of treating disease with new methods but to assist the body in healing itself naturally. This applies to all forms of skin disease. Whether the problem is a contact dermatitis that can be quickly relieved with an application of herbal salve or a more complex condition that emanates from within the body to create chronic seborrhea, the approach is to assist the body's efforts to heal while trying to identify and address the underlying causes.

Writing comprehensively on herbal approaches to animal skin problems would entail writing an entire book—perhaps even multiple volumes. So instead we present some generalized herbal treatments with strong emphases on the holistic principles by which they are most effectively applied, for a few of the most common skin problems in companion animals.

SKIN PROBLEMS OF INTERNAL ORIGIN

Chronic, or recurring, skin conditions that cannot be attributed to elements outside the body usually indicate systemic disease. Generally speaking, if an animal's body system cannot effectively eliminate waste or if foreign bodies or toxins cannot be effectively dealt with by a strong immune system, the body tries to push the problem outward, away from the vital organs. When the body resorts to such measures, it is usually because one or more of the organs or body systems that monitor and respond to foreign bodies and systemic waste have somehow become dysfunctional. The liver, kidneys, and immune and lymph systems become overburdened, the skin is asked to take actions it cannot take, and a "skin problem" erupts in the form of an oily, flaky coat; irritated, itchy skin; subcutaneous cysts; excessive hair loss; pus-filled eruptions, and so forth.

Treating skin conditions that are secondary to systemic disorders is difficult. Persistent skin conditions such as seborrhea (dry or greasy, flaky or scaly skin) or pyoderma (pus-filled eruptions) may be attributable to any number of deep-seated factors, including dietary deficiencies, food or environmental allergies, immune system disease, or a microbial infection that may or may not be evident upon analysis of the skin itself. In such cases, the entire system must be evaluated, systemic deficiencies must be identified and corrected, and the search for direct causes must continue throughout the therapy, even if the symptoms are under control. The golden rule to remember is this: The outward symptoms of many types of chronic skin disease represent only a small part of the holistic picture. We cannot expect to find curative solutions unless we focus our efforts beyond the symptoms to identify and address the underlying causes. This rule applies to all forms of skin disease, from an allergic response to fleabites to chronic hair loss.

SKIN PROBLEMS OF EXTERNAL ORIGIN

Skin problems that are triggered from outside the body are often, but not always, easier to identify and quicker to correct than those that emanate from within. For example, the cause of recurrent urticaria (an inflammation of the skin surface characterized by small, itching welts) may be quickly identified and eliminated when it is discovered that Rover has been sleeping in a patch of stinging nettles growing along the backyard fence. In this case, the holistic approach might be to neutralize the stinging acids with a dandelion flower or nettle tea rinse. A problem such as dermatophytosis, or ringworm, a parasitic fungal infection of the skin in dogs, cats, horses, and many other animals (including humans), presents the holistic caregiver with a more complex scenario. Ringworm is passed directly from an infected environment to the animal host. And like most parasites, including fleas and various skin-burrowing mites (sarcoptic mange, barn itch, demodectic mange, to name a few), ringworm is more likely to infect diseased or immunocompromised animals than those with healthy disease resistance. Therefore, to holistically treat an animal suffering from ringworm, we must take the animal's environment and his general state of health into consideration. Ringworm can be largely prevented by keeping the living environment clean, but infection must also be discouraged by maintaining the health of the potential host.

This brings us right back to our main point: Before other causative factors can be addressed, the overall health of the individual must be fully evaluated and supported.

HOLISTIC APPROACHES

It's important to keep in mind that herbs alone are seldom curative solutions to chronic forms of disease. In holistic medicine, most skin problems are viewed as indicators of systemic dysfunction within the body. Rather than working in ways that exclude natural body functions (as many drugs do) to suppress the symptoms of disease, herbs serve best as functional adjuncts to a variety of other corrective measures. Nutrition; the animal's age; his physical, psychological, and neurological conditions; genetic predispositions characteristic to his breed; and the quality of his living environment must be taken into account as equal parts of a holistic health picture.

Feeding the Skin

Your effectiveness at treating conditions such as flaky skin and a dull coat is gauged by how deeply you are willing to look into your animal's whole body, lifestyle, and environment. To begin the healing process, some careful measures must be taken to assure that the skin is properly fed. Start with a critical assessment of your companion's diet, looking not just at the diversity and types of food ingredients but at the quality of each ingredient as well. The skin is an organ that must continually regenerate itself to survive the constant effects of aging and bombardment from environmental elements. To do so it must receive a unique array of special nutrients and nutritional adjuncts, many of which will not be found in a typical commercial diet. At the top of this special-requirement list are antioxidant vitamins (A, C, and E), minerals, proteins, and especially EFAs, which can be administered to an animal through supplementing his diet.

Essential fatty acid supplements might include flaxseed powder or oil, fish oil, or wheat germ oil. Vitamins A, C, and E are needed for their regenerative and antioxidant effects, and digestive enzymes are also required. In terms of herbs, horsetail and gotu kola may help regenerate and strengthen skin structure; and nutritive herbs such as spirulina, nettle, alfalfa, and red clover can provide trace minerals and antioxidant vitamins. Fresh burdock root is available at many health food stores and can be grated (raw) directly into your animal's food. Burdock is considered a specific alterative for chronic skin problems. It is safe and nutritious and gently supports an animal's liver and gallbladder. Feed your animal as much as he likes.

The quality of protein you are feeding also plays a vital role here—low-grade proteins (such as soy-based fillers and most meat by-products) are difficult for animals to metabolize, and instead of being received as nutritive protein, they are treated as hard-to-eliminate wastes. By feeding your animal a diversity of high-quality, fresh foods and the proper nutritional supplements, you are equipping him with the components he needs to maintain healthy skin. Without the proper nutritional components, the skin becomes weak and vulnerable to the effects of the environment, its related body functions become compromised, and the entire system falls out of holistic balance.

Piecing Together a Puzzle

Once you are sure that your companion is getting the nutritional components needed for healthy skin and coat, consider the potential sources of any chronic problem. Does your animal have a food allergy? This can often be determined by removing food ingredients from the diet one at a time. For a dog or cat, start by changing the type of meat your animal is eating—especially if he is eating beef or a food that is made from mostly one type of meat. Next, try weeding out grains and yeast one at a time. Start by eliminating soy, then try wheat, then yeast.

While you are ruling out food allergies, also consider anything else that may be compromising your companion's immune system. It is the immune system's job to react to invading microbes or harmful substances. If the system is compromised and cannot react correctly or effectively, it may overreact, causing an allergic response.

Is your companion hypersensitive to fleabites? Is the animal subjected to frequent vaccinations (a major cause of many skin and immune system problems, in our opinion), protracted antibiotic therapies, or any environmental toxins that may be depressing or stimulating immune functions? Find out the answers. Any of these factors may contribute to a chronic skin problem.

After you have an idea of what might be entering your companion's body to trigger the problem, then start looking for telltale signs of which organs or body systems might be affected. Is your animal friend suffering from constipation or diarrhea, and does his skin, coat, or breath smell bad? If so, the digestive system and liver probably need herbal support. Is the urine concentrated and strong smelling, or does it have blood in it? Are urinary infections or stones a problem? In these cases, you need to optimize urinary efficiency and perhaps relieve inflammation in the urinary tract and kidneys.

It's impossible to ask yourself too many questions when looking for clues to the causes of a chronic skin problem. Just remember to conduct your investigation throughout the body, focusing on the organs and systems responsible for elimination of waste: the liver, kidneys, gallbladder, stomach and intestines, immune system, and lymph system. If you're having problems doing this yourself, ask your holistic vet for help.

HERBAL THERAPIES

Since most forms of skin disease are related to poor elimination of systemic waste or immune system deficiency, a great deal can be accomplished by supporting the liver, kidneys, lymphatic system, immune system, and digestive functions with herbs. You should begin tonic herbal therapy while you are trying to pinpoint the actual causes of disease. Using tonic herbs to gently support the body's cleansing systems helps the body to heal itself. Oftentimes, tonic alterative herbs change the course of systemic dysfunction, and the body regains its ability to deal with whatever was triggering the skin problem. In these cases, the animal's body finds its own cure, even though you never identify a cause.

The herbs of choice for treating skin problems are stimulatory tonics and alternatives that can be used safely over a long period as daily dietary supplements. Burdock has long been regarded as a specific alterative for treating chronic forms of dermatitis. Cleavers improves lymph circulation, thus helping to remove waste and toxins from body tissues. It is also a diuretic and is mildly astringent, so it reduces inflammation that may exist in the urinary tract while encouraging elimination. Dandelion (root and leaf) is diuretic and nutritive and serves as a safe and reliable liver stimulant. It increases bile production and gently stimulates the gallbladder and the kidneys to help improve digestion and aid in the elimination of both solid and urine-carried wastes. Red clover helps burdock

work and adds antioxidant and immune supportive qualities to a broad spectrum of vitamins and minerals. It is generally considered to be a blood purifier because it helps improve blood structure, which in turn allows for better transport of waste products and toxins from the body. Garlic offers immune system support, liver support, antimicrobial activities, and antioxidant properties. All these herbs are ingredients in the following formula for skin problems.

As the symptoms and mechanisms of a chronic skin problem become more defined, herbs can be used to provide added support to specific body systems in need. Herbs can also be used to relieve uncomfortable symptoms. The ingredients of the Basic Support Formula (see box on page 287) can then be adjusted to suit special needs. For instance, for a dog suffering from seborrhea attributed to food-borne heavy metals (a condition your holistic vet must diagnose), a short-term regimen of yellow dock can be added to the formula to help to quickly eliminate toxic buildups of metals or chemicals in the body. For an animal with a skin disorder associated with chronic constipation, Oregon grape may be useful to quickly increase bile production from the liver and improve digestion and elimination of waste, while marshmallow may also benefit the animal by lubricating the colon.

When using herbs to relieve the symptoms of disease, it's important to keep your perspective holistic. Remember, symptoms are valuable evidence of what's going on within an animal's body—don't suppress them unless you are finished using them to determine corrective measures for the underlying problem. For instance, if you use licorice to relieve your companion's inflamed skin without improving his diet, the goal of finding a curative solution will never be reached. Dermatitis—a symptom—may be

Basic Support Formula

Combine the following:

2 parts burdock root
2 parts cleavers *
1 part dandelion, in equal proportions of root and leaf
1 part red clover (flowering tops)
1 part fresh organic garlic powder

*Tincture, tea, or the pressed juice of the fresh herb must be used

Flaxseed oil, evening primrose oil, borage seed oil, fish oil, or a prepared multi-EFA supplement should be fed to the animal with this formula.

This formula can be used in several forms. A combination of the dried ingredients (except cleavers) can be fed directly to an animal or sprinkled onto his food daily at a rate of 1 tablespoon per 40 pounds of the animal's body weight. The cleavers has to be added in the form of a liquid preparation because it oxidizes quickly and loses its potency when dried. Therefore, ¼ teaspoon (1 milliliter) of a glycerin-based cleavers tincture or 2 tablespoons (30 milliliters) of strong cleavers tea should be fed in place of the dry herb for each 40 pounds of an animal's body weight. For cats, ferrets, rabbits, birds, and other small animals, the dosage is prorated according to the animal's estimated weight. A parrot, for example, needs only a few drops of the tincture each day.

Another option that is particularly good for horses, goats, llamas, and other herbivores is to administer the Basic Support Formula as fresh herbs. For these large animals, a few heaping handfuls of the herb mix should suffice each day. For rabbits and other small vegetarians, ½ cup of the mixture can be fed. If the animal eats a portion of the serving and then stops, it might mean that he has received all he needs. Take the remainder away. Cats, dogs, and other carnivores can be fed a raw mixture too, but keep in mind that they may have problems swallowing the cleavers—especially if it is *Galium aparine*, the species most commonly used for herbal medicine. *Galium aparine* has a clinging nature that causes it to stick in the throats of animals who are not accustomed to eating live weeds. While this situation is not life threatening, it can cause some gagging and coughing. You may choose to feed your animal a species of *Galium* that does not share this characteristic, such as Northern bedstraw (*Galium boreale*—a common weed), or a garden variety such as sweet woodruff, (*Galium odoratum*) which does not have a sticky nature.

It's important to remember that the intent of this formula is to assist organ functions and to optimize the body's absorption of needed nutrients. Providing a high-quality, natural diet is therefore paramount. It's also important to keep in mind that tonic herbs, being noninvasive, work only at the body's natural pace. Therefore, a tonic herbal therapy may take several days or even weeks to show results. Be patient, and allow your companion's body an opportunity to heal itself.

temporarily relieved with licorice, but the underlying causes cannot be addressed unless we look at the entire problem holistically.

SEBORRHEA

Seborrhea is a term that is widely used for any form of skin-related disease characterized by dry or greasy, inflamed or itchy skin. Seborrhea may stem from any number of possibilities. At the top of the list are poor food quality and nutritional deficiency, followed by flea- or food-related allergies, vaccinosis, and excessive antibiotic use. Bacterial, fungal, viral, or parasitic (mite) infection and immune system dysfunction are also possible causes.

Conventional treatment of seborrhea typically begins with the use of medicated shampoos and topical steroid and antibiotic preparations. In cases in which clinical diagnosis identifies skin infections, these measures can bring quick relief, but they usually do not address the reasons the skin became infected in the first place. Antibiotic and corticosteroid therapies are often used in cases of seborrhea that do not respond to topical treatment. From a holistic standpoint however, such measures compound the situation by inducing their own levels of systemic imbalance. Antibiotic and steroid therapies may make the symptoms disappear, but the underlying cause continues to go unchecked; the disease may be pushed deeper into the body and result in a much more serious disorder.

The holistic approach begins when we realize that seborrhea is not really a disease itself but a term used for a variety of skin-related disorders. There is no standard herbal treatment to use for every kind of seborrhea. All forms of chronic skin disease, however, have two things in common: all are connected to diet and all are less likely to occur or progress in animals who have

Astringent Healing Skin Rinse

Combine the following:

1 part juniper or uva ursi leaf decoction*
1 part calendula flowers, steeped into a strong tea
1 part peppermint

*See "Basics of Herbal Preparations" in chapter 1 for instructions on making a decoction

Combine all ingredients, herb material and all, and allow the mixture to stand until cooled. Strain the cooled fluid through a sieve, then soak the animal's skin and coat (avoid the eyes) with the solution. Let the animal drip dry.

If the animal insists on licking off the solution, you can use the rinse as a fomentation—wrap an old towel or cloth (preferably undyed and unbleached) around the affected body parts, then thoroughly soak the towel with the cooled solution. This prevents the animal from licking off the solution and enables you to keep the solution on your companion animal for several hours.

healthy waste elimination and strong immune systems.

Diet should be critically evaluated and improved to optimize the animal's resistance to disease. Supplemental EFAs (e.g., flaxseed), digestive enzymes, minerals, and vitamins (especially vitamins E, A, and C) should be provided, and the possibility of food allergies should be considered.

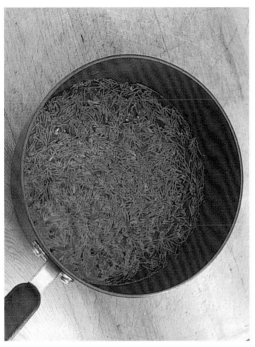

First make a decoction of the juniper or the uva ursi leaves.

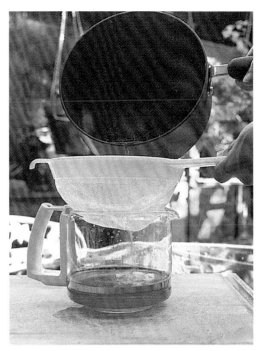

Strain the cooled fluid through a sieve.

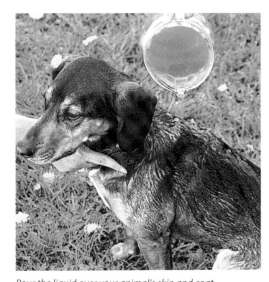

Pour the liquid over your animal's skin and coat.

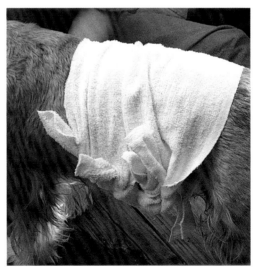

If your animal licks the rinse off his skin, use the rinse as a fomentation instead.

At the same time you are adjusting diet, treatment should begin with herbs that offer tonic support to the immune system and all organs involved in food metabolism and waste elimination. The Basic Support Formula serves as a good starting point. The animal's entire health history should be evaluated to find clues to possible causes. Animals who have been subjected to prolonged antibiotic therapies may respond well to immune-modulating herbs such as astragalus or echinacea.

To relieve itching and inflammation on the surface of the body, herbs with astringent and wound-healing properties are indicated. In dogs or cats with itchy skin that exhibits little or no change of appearance, a liberal application of oatmeal may be applied to affected areas—cook the oatmeal into a loose, wet consistency and allow it to cool before putting it on your animal. A peppermint or lavender skin rinse is another option to help relieve itching. If the itching is associated with minor redness, a daily skin rinse of cooled chamomile, plantain, or calendula tea may bring relief. Completely soak the animal with the tea and allow him to drip dry. If open scratches, scabs, or sores are visible, try combining calendula and comfrey, with sage, bee balm, thyme, or yarrow tea in equal proportions. When cooled and used in a rinse, this mixture accelerates the healing process and helps inhibit bacterial infection.

If your companion's condition is severe—the skin is flaky and red and scratching or chewing is continuous—stronger astringents may be needed. A decoction of uva ursi, juniper leaf, or rose bark are strong astringents that should serve well here. When using strong astringents on animals, proceed with caution. Dogs, cats, rabbits, ferrets, and other small creatures have skin that is often quite sensitive. Before soaking your animal with a fluid that is intended to tighten the skin, test it first—put a small amount on a portion of the animal's body to make sure that there will not be any adverse reaction. One example of a basic astringent skin rinse can be found in the box on page 288.

Birds have especially tender skin, and rinses consisting of strong astringents should be avoided in most cases. Sage, bee balm, or peppermint tea often work well in a birdbath. (Sage may help eliminate mites as well as

Echinacea and Oregon Grape Clay Poultice

Combine the following:

4 oz green or bentonite clay
(powder)*
½ oz echinacea tincture
(alcohol based)
½ oz Oregon grape tincture
(alcohol based)

*Be sure to use only supplement-grade clay (available at health food stores)

Thoroughly combine the three ingredients, adding just enough distilled water to make a thick paste. Then apply the poultice to the affected areas and leave it on to dry, if possible. If licking, rolling, scratching, or other attempts at removal are a problem, wrap the area with a cloth or a piece of gauze. Leftover poultice can be put into an airtight container and stored in the refrigerator almost indefinitely. If it dries out, just add more water or tincture to soften it.

relieve itching.) Add a dilute concentration of the tea to a bowl of clean, chlorine-free water (just enough to tint the water) and place it in the cage. Most birds enjoy taking an occasional bath, especially if they're itchy!

If an established bacterial infection is evident (an area is swollen and red, and sores are discharging pus), internal doses of echinacea tincture can be coupled with external applications of echinacea and Oregon grape (or organically farmed goldenseal) powder, tincture, salve, or ointment at the sites of infection. This boosts immune system response to the infection while adding direct antibacterial intervention. Another effective option for treating isolated infections of the skin is an echinacea and Oregon grape clay poultice, which is discussed in detail below.

In cases in which itching and inflammation are severe, internal doses of licorice may bring relief by boosting production of corticosteroids in the body and lending direct anti-inflammatory activities to the effort. But licorice may not be a good choice in chronic, perhaps inherited skin disorders that require continuous long-term treatment because of its possible side effects. In these cases, herbal treatment is limited to nutritional support and topical relief measures.

If the animal has a fever, a good possibility exists that the infection has moved into the body, meaning it's time to call your veterinarian immediately.

PYODERMA

The term *pyoderma* refers to infections of the skin that are characterized by the presence of subsurface pus. Most often, pyoderma is caused by foreign bodies such as splinters, insect bites or stings, fleas, or mites that have entered the skin and caused infection. In these cases, basic first aid or antiparasitic measures usually solve the problem. But in cases where pyoderma is secondary to systemic disease or dysfunction, its presence may indicate a serious, even life-threatening, condition. The possible causes range from a minor nutritional deficiency or allergy to inherited or acquired metabolic dysfunctions, autoimmune disease or deficiency (including lupus, pemphigus, vasculitis), viral infection (including FeLV and FIV), hormonal imbalances, parasitic infections, long-term steroid therapies, and even cancer. The potential seriousness of pyoderma-related illnesses is testament to the value and importance of requiring a full holistic examination of your companion, his diet, and his environment.

Diet and nutrition, as you may have guessed, are the first factors to consider in treating any pyoderma-related disorder of internal origin. Herbal therapies should start with tonic support. The Basic Support Formula (see page 287) offers a good start. In severe cases, perhaps where acnelike pustules erupt on the chin of a cat and begin to spread to other parts of the body, a safe but aggressive systemic detoxification therapy might be indicated. This might include diuretic herbs such as dandelion leaf; liver stimulants such as yellow dock, Oregon grape, and turmeric; and blood-cleansing alternatives such as red clover and alfalfa. Liver-regenerating herbs such as milk thistle and licorice may be useful as well, especially in cases in which chemical-induced liver damage is a suspected cause. Marshmallow root may help to ease the movement of waste through the colon. Psyllium husks added to the animal's food as per the supplement manufacturer's directions may also assist with the passing of waste.

In addition to supporting the liver, kidneys, and digestive system, it's important to thoroughly evaluate and support the animal's immune system. Clinical blood and urine tests may be useful here, as will the experience of a holistic veterinarian. If a determination is made that the immune system needs stimulation, echinacea or astragalus may prove beneficial. If immune deficiency is compounded by viral infection, liver damage, or inflammation, licorice may serve as a useful adjunct. It's important to note, however, that immune system stimulation may not always be a good idea in the treatment of autoimmune disease in which the body's immune system is working against itself, such as with lupus erythematosus. Again, you are advised to consult your veterinarian before proceeding.

External discomforts can be relieved with the same astringent and anti-inflammatory herbs that are used for seborrhea. Aloe gel or a plantain or chickweed poultice may bring soothing relief as well. For cases in which pyoderma is limited to just a few isolated areas of the body, an herb-clay poultice can be especially effective at relieving itching, inhibiting bacteria and fungi, and pulling infection toward the surface of the body. When applied to the skin, the green or bentonite clay used for the poultice (or paste) naturally pulls fluid and waste products toward itself, while lending its own itch-relieving astringent activities and a diversity of mineral nutrients to the skin. As pathogenic microbes are drawn toward the clay, they are confronted with antimicrobial herb constituents that inhibit their reproduction.

This clay poultice is an excellent first aid remedy for venomous and nonvenomous bites and stings as well. Be aware that the bentonite clay sold at hardware and feed stores often contains harmful bacteria and other impurities. Alcohol tinctures are preferable to glycerin because they add astringency to the formula and serve as preservatives in a poultice that is saved for future use.

CONTACT DERMATITIS

Contact dermatitis is caused when an irritating substance, organism, or allergen contacts or damages the outer surface of the skin. The onset of symptoms can be immediate or delayed for hours or even days.

Contact dermatitis can appear in many forms—from what appears to be a hot, pink-flushed spot of skin to raised wheals, blisters, and ulcers that cover the animal's body.

In dogs and cats, the most common form of contact dermatitis occurs as the result of fleabites. Treatment in these cases begins with examining why the animal is so hypersensitive to the bites and then continues by working to make the environments of these pesky critters less hospitable.

Symptomatic relief can be provided by applying astringent skin rinses (see "Seborrhea"). A skin rinse of grindelia is considered a specific remedy for dermatitis caused by contact with poison ivy or poison oak. Jewelweed (Impatiens capensis), a plant native to eastern and central North America, has also been long regarded as a remedy for poison ivy. The tea of this herb is taken internally by humans, but its safety and effectiveness in animals are unknown. Alterative and diuretic herbs such as burdock root and dandelion leaf may be fed in tea or whole form to help the body eliminate antigenic compounds that may be contributing to the itch and inflammation.

SEBACEOUS CYSTS

Sebaceous cysts are lesions involving the ducts leading from sebaceous glands to their associated hair follicles. They are generally caused by obstruction of the ducts and appear as semisolid, freely moving lumps beneath the skin.

A natural raw food diet is the best prevention. If an animal does get a sebaceous

A Systemic Detoxifying Formula for Dogs, Cats, Horses, and Goats

Combine the following:

2 parts dandelion leaf
2 parts yellow dock root
2 parts red clover
1 part licorice root
2 parts marshmallow

For dogs and cats, a glycerin-based tincture is the best form of application for this detoxifying formula. Yellow dock is bitter, and the sweet flavor of vegetable glycerin aids in administration. Feeding about ¼ teaspoon (1 milliliter) of the combined tincture twice daily for each 20 pounds of an animal's body weight is usually sufficient to stimulate elimination. For best results, feed the tincture directly into the animal's mouth. If this isn't possible, try diluting the tincture with water. As a last resort, add it to the animal's food. This formula should not be used continuously for more than seven days.

Horses, goats, sheep, llamas, and other large herbivores can be fed this formula in fresh or dried, whole-herb form—if they'll eat it. Horses will probably need 3–6 cups of the herbs each day, whereas goats, sheep, and llamas may need only 1½–3 cups. If direct feeding is not possible, try feeding everything but the yellow dock, then administer this bitter herb later in the form of tincture (prorate the tincture's dosage to the amount the animal would receive in the formula).

The idea behind this detoxifying formula is to stimulate gentle elimination of waste from the liver and digestive organs, not to drain your animal. If vomiting occurs, discontinue use immediately. Stools should be soft but not watery and gushing on passage. Likewise, the animal should not show any signs of gastric discomfort such as griping, distention, or odd sounds coming from the stomach. If this occurs, reduce the dose by one-half or discontinue use—the digestive system is stimulated enough and a different approach is warranted. On the other hand, if your animal has been constipated and is not finding relief from this formula, then the dosage can be increased in increments of 10 percent per feeding until stools appear soft or until the equivalent of one and one-half times the original dose is reached. After that, if results are not seen within two days, discontinue use—this formula is probably not going to work for your animal.

This detoxifying formula should not be given continuously for more than ten days without the supervision of a qualified practitioner. It should not be used in pregnant animals or in those with a history of urinary stones or preexisting kidney disease. All of this is because of the oxalic acid contained in yellow dock. When used over a long period of time, oxalic acid can be irritating to the urinary system, and it may contribute to the formation of kidney or bladder stones.

cyst, administering some herbs that help the body eliminate more easily might be in order. Herbs that assist lymphatic drainage, such as cleavers, red clover, calendula, and burdock may help.

Urinary Problems

You may notice that your companion is drinking more and urinating less, urinating in unusual places, or straining while urinating. Blood or other discharge may be visible in the urine, redness and inflammation may be evident at or around the animal's urethra, or urine may be dark or especially odorous. If discomfort is evident when the lower abdomen or the area immediately behind the rib cage is gently palpated with fingertips, your companion may have an infection or inflammation of the bladder or kidneys. While these are all physical signs of a urinary tract disorder, holistic care of an animal's urinary system requires a level of attentiveness beyond mere recognition of such symptoms.

The urinary system is a delicately balanced arrangement of organs and body chemistries that serve a critical purpose of eliminating potentially toxic compounds from the body. The elimination process begins with the kidneys, which are responsible for separating waste material from the blood and delivering it via the ureters to the bladder. The bladder then holds the urine until it is released from the body via the urethra. This system sounds simple but is actually complex when we consider the special nutritive, chemical, and structural requirements of the individual organs. The kidneys are fragile, oxygen-dependent organs with a low tolerance to stress. They work in concert with the digestive tract, liver, and circulatory system, and they are easily damaged if the relationships between these systems become compromised. For instance, if the liver is

deficient in its job of removing dietary and systemic waste via the digestive tract, the kidneys and urinary tract suffer from the stress of handling waste products that they are not designed to handle. The result can be kidney failure, stones, inflammation, or infection. Adding to the holistic complexity of this system is the fact that it is largely made up of smooth-muscle structures, unique vascular arrangements, and mucous membranes that require a special diversity of nutrients and precise chemical balances to remain healthy and functional.

The most effective way to treat or prevent urinary system illness is to recognize your animal's needs before physical symptoms of disease are obvious. Sometimes our companions have strange ways of telling us that they don't feel well. They may start spraying the wall or our favorite clothes. Such behavior may be related to an emotional problem, but it may also mean that our friends are trying to tell us that something is seriously wrong physically. Don't ignore or write off sudden bad behavior as neurosis—the situation could be quite serious.

Effective holistic treatment of urinary disease starts with a critical assessment of the animal's diet. Usually infection, stones, or kidney failure is the progressive result of a nutritional excess, deficiency, or metabolic imbalance. It's well known among clinicians and researchers that animals who receive a balanced natural diet seldom suffer from urinary system ailments.

When using herbs to treat urinary problems, teas and tinctures are the best forms of preparation. The goal is to get the active constituents of a plant into the urine, and the best way to do this is to bypass as much of the digestive system as possible with a liquid solution fed on an empty stomach. Following are some of the more common treatments for urinary ailments we face as animal caregivers.

BLADDER AND KIDNEY STONES (UROLITHIASIS)

Like most forms of urinary disease, stones (sometimes called gravel or crystals) are the by-products of metabolic dysfunction or poor diet. They are associated with the body's inability to effectively metabolize calcium, magnesium, ammonium, or other minerals. Many of the minerals that form stones are essential nutrients in a balanced diet, but they must be received by a healthy balanced body in a readily usable form. It's important to know that excess minerals that the body cannot use must be eliminated through the digestive and urinary tracts.

Stones are formed when urine pH levels or other chemical factors cause the minerals to bind and form crystals, which in turn build upon each other to create solid structures known as uroliths. Uroliths are most likely to occur in the bladder, but they sometimes form in the kidneys. Exposure to cadmium is also known to increase the formation of stones. The most common source of cadmium exposure for animals is cigarette smoke.

To remain clean and free of harmful bacteria, the urinary tract must continually flush itself. If an animal's urethra is blocked by one or more uroliths, uremia, a potentially life-threatening condition, can result. If a ureter is blocked, kidney damage may occur and progress quickly after the onset of symptoms. Even if the animal's condition appears stable and nonprogressive, urolithiasis creates an environment in the urinary system in which impeded waste elimination may lead to infectious growth of harmful bacteria and fungi. Urolithiasis is especially common in cats, but dogs and other animals may suffer from stones as well.

Balanced nutrition is paramount in the

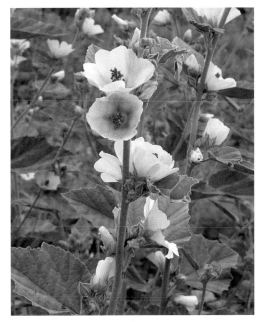

Marshmallow has many qualities that make it a first-choice herb for treating kidney and bladder stones.

effective treatment and prevention of urinary stones. A positive change in diet often equates to a long-term cure. Many types of urinary stones dissolve when urine chemistry is corrected through a change of diet. However, some types of stones such as calcium oxalate uroliths must either be eliminated through the urethra via urination (an often long and painful process) or be surgically removed (depending on the size and number of the stones).

The holistic herbal approach toward urinary system infection or stones must always start with a thorough dietary evaluation. After that, the primary objectives are to assist the body in eliminating the stones, to help moderate urine pH (which is normally slightly acidic) with diuretic and demulcent herbs, and to inhibit infection and reduce the painful inflammation that makes urination difficult by treating with with antimicrobial and anti-inflammatory herbs.

In all cases (whether the stones are in the kidneys or the bladder), our approach begins with a thick, alcohol-free liquid preparation of marshmallow. The slippery oily mucilage of a cooled marshmallow tea or glycerite provides a protective lubricating barrier on swollen mucous membranes, thus assisting with the passage of stones. Marshmallow also has mild astringent qualities and antimicrobial properties that join to reduce inflammation and help inhibit bacterial growth in the healing process. Plantain serves similar purposes but is less mucilaginous than marshmallow and has a slightly higher astringency. This makes it appropriate in cases in which the urethral inflammation from the passage of gravel is causing pain and strain during urination. Gravel root is another traditional option worth considering.

In cases in which minor urinary bleeding is present and bladder or kidney inflammation persists, couch grass and corn silk serve as good anti-inflammatories. If significant bleeding is occurring in the bladder but clinical evaluation has determined that kidney function remains strong and kidney inflammation is not evident, stronger hemostatic and astringent herbs such as horsetail, uva ursi, and yarrow can be added to marshmallow to help stop the hemorrhage. If the kidneys are inflamed, however, these herbs may be contraindicated, and couch grass or shepherd's purse make better options.

Diuretic herbs such as dandelion leaf and cleavers are indicated in cases in which urination has not been severely obstructed because they help to dilute the urine and assist the body in its efforts to flush stones and bacteria out of the urinary tract. Keep in mind that if urination is obstructed, strong diuretics may compound the situation because the increased urine volume may cause added pressure upon the kidneys.

If urine backs up into the kidneys, a life-threatening infection can result. See your veterinarian immediately.

Antimicrobial herbs should be used as a preventive measure against infection, especially in circumstances in which urination is inhibited. Echinacea serves this purpose well. Oregon grape or certified organic goldenseal is useful for fighting bacteria and serve as effective anti-inflammatory agents in the bladder as well. If overly acidic urine is part of the problem, mullein leaf tea may help bring pH levels back toward normal. Mullein leaf also has diuretic and antimicrobial properties.

URINARY SYSTEM INFECTIONS (CYSTITIS)

Bacterial infection of the urinary tract is the most common infectious disease of dogs. At least 10 percent of all dogs seen by veterinarians for any reason have a urinary tract infection. Symptoms may include fever, lethargy, backache, painful urination (dysuria), frequent urination, and blood in the urine (hematuria). Causes are varied, but from a holistic perspective the underlying question is always the same: Why was the animal's body unable to effectively ward off the infection in the first place?

In many cases, this question leads us back to diet, but other causes include immunological deficiency or bacterial, fungal, or protozoan infection from bad water or food. Bladder stones, injury, or tumors may also be contributing factors. In all cases, the focus of symptomatic herbal treatment is fundamentally the same—to assist the body at repelling the infection-causing entities, relieve inflammation and discomfort, dilute urine, and encourage urination.

Urinary tract infections may be caused by various forms of bacteria, fungi, or parasites that have entered the body through the mouth or urethra. Feline lower urinary tract disease, or FLUTD (formerly known as feline urinary syndrome, or FUS), is a nonspecific inflammatory problem that occurs in the bladder and urethra of cats. It is a chronic form of cystitis characterized by high pH (excessively alkaline) urine. Tiny, sharp-edged, struvite crystals form in the lower urinary tract and adhere to the walls of the bladder and urethra, causing inflammation and blockage. If left unchecked, they can develop into larger stones and cause severe and obstructive inflammatory disease of the entire urinary system. A cat with FLUTD has an urge to urinate frequently, but because urine output is greatly diminished by inflammation and accumulated crystals, he may be able to force out only a few drops at a time. This is a very dangerous situation—if urine backs up in the ureters and into the kidneys, irreversible kidney damage can result quickly.

Diet must be closely scrutinized as a primary cause of FLUTD. Because cats are carnivores, they should receive a large part of their daily water intake in the form of juicy raw meat. The process of metabolizing raw meat is essential to the maintenance of healthy feline urine pH levels. When cats must subsist on a dry-food diet, their systems must perform metabolic tasks that are beyond their natural design. Urine pH levels may become severely imbalanced, setting the stage for stone formation and bacterial reproduction. In fact, studies conducted at Cornell University strongly suggest that free-feeding dry foods may predispose cats to FUS. We along with a large percentage of veterinarians agree. Also, setting mealtimes is better than free-feeding. A cat or dog who is able to snack and nibble all day long is more likely to get a urinary infection, especially if the food is out of a bag or can.

The best advice for preventing FLUTD is this: If for whatever reason you cannot feed a raw food diet to your cat, avoid dry kibble and feed a premium-quality, all-natural canned food to prevent your cat from developing urinary problems. If your feline friend is already suffering from FLUTD, adjust or change his diet and take him to a vet to determine whether his kidneys have been compromised. If they haven't, the problem can be symptomatically approached as a case of cystitis with astringent anti-inflammatory herbs such as uva ursi or pipsissewa combined with the soothing mucilaginous properties of marshmallow and the disinfectant qualities of echinacea, garlic, Oregon grape, or yarrow. If kidney involvement is evident, herbs with high concentrations of tannins or strong volatile oils should be avoided. In such cases, corn silk, couch grass, plantain, nettle, shepherd's purse, or raspberry leaf serves as a safer astringent.

Some people and animals find relief from cystitis with cranberry juice or cranberry powder (emptied from capsules) mixed in their food. Cranberry helps keep bacteria from adhering to the walls of the urethra and bladder. But research has found that cranberry juice is effective only at preventing bladder infections, not curing them. In one study, drinking 4–6 ounces of a commercial cranberry juice daily significantly prevented infections in a nursing home population. Another study used doses ranging from 5 to 20 ounces a day (in humans), so for dogs or cats, an ounce or so of cranberry juice or ¼ teaspoon of the powder should serve as a nutritious, vitamin C–rich preventive measure against infection.

The symptomatic herbal approach to any form of urinary system infection centers on the use of herbs that directly inhibit reproduction of the invading microbes. In most cases, Oregon grape,

A Basic Formula for Urinary Infections and Stones*

Make a strong tea or combine low-alcohol tinctures of the following ingredients. If possible, administer the formula on an empty stomach, and encourage your companion to drink plenty of water.

> **3 parts marshmallow root**
> **1 part couch grass**
> **1 part nettle**
> **1 part echinacea**
> **1 part Oregon grape**

*This formula helps to soothe, lubricate, and reduce inflammation of urinary tract tissues, thus helping with the elimination of stones. The echinacea and Oregon grape help to reduce or prevent infection.

For dogs, feed 1 teaspoon (5 milliliters) of the cooled tea, twice daily, for each 30 pounds of body weight. Or feed 1–2 milliliters of the low-alcohol combination tincture twice daily. For cats, feed ½ teaspoon (2.5 milliliters) of the cooled tea, twice daily, for each 30 pounds of body weight. Or feed 0.5–1 milliliter of the low-alcohol tincture twice daily. Horses and other large animals can be given 200 milliliters of the cooled tea, fed twice daily with a turkey baster or similar device. Or you can give 20–30 milliliters of the low-alcohol tincture twice daily.

uva ursi, garlic, raspberry leaf, or echinacea serves this purpose well. But always look at the whole health picture and never stop asking yourself why the infection occurred in the first place. For example, animals with chronic gingivitis sometimes develop serious kidney infections as a progressive result of a bacterial imbalance that originated from poor dental health or immune system deficiency. Again we are brought back to diet. In carnivores, raw bones serve to keep the teeth clean and the gums healthy; in herbivores, it's raw, fiber-rich vegetables. The point is this: if your companion is suffering from a urinary infection, don't expect to find a long-term solution exclusively through the use of herbs. A holistic caregiver must look deeper than the symptoms to find and eliminate the root causes of disease.

See the box on this page for a useful preparation for urinary system infection and stones.

KIDNEY FAILURE

Given the fragility of the kidneys and the extraordinary amount of hard work they do, it's easy to understand why they are often the first body structures to wear out in the later years of an animal's life. However, an alarming percentage of young and middle-aged animals succumb to kidney failure as well.

Kidney failure is often caused and is always compounded by a poor-quality or unbalanced diet. One contributing factor is the overabundance of phosphorus in many commercial brands of dog and cat food. Some brands contain five to nine times the required amount. While excess phosphorus is seldom an issue for animals with strong, healthy kidneys, it can be problematic to animals with preexisting kidney damage, especially if they are receiving a diet that does not contain a necessary balance of readily usable calcium. In these cases, the kidneys may not be able to effectively eliminate the phosphorus, which then accumulates in the kidneys and results in the eventual formation of stones or degeneration of kidney tissues. A variety of other problems, such as diabetes, immune system dysfunction, long-term drug therapies, vaccinosis, chronic liver disease, and digestive problems, often develop as the kidney damage progresses. The worst part of this grim picture is that the entire degenerative process can remain undetected until the damage has progressed into an irreversible state of disease.

Pinpointing the exact causes of kidney failure can be difficult. The kidneys are fragile and slow to heal, and in cases of progressive kidney degeneration, time is of the essence. Therefore, holistic treatment of kidney failure must begin with preventive dietary measures. If it's too late for preventive measures, the problem is best approached as early as possible.

If your companion is urinating excessively, drinking a lot of water, or has suffered from one or more urinary tract infections or a bout with stones, take him to a holistic veterinarian for a thorough examination. If kidney damage is found, chances are your companion will be placed on a reduced-protein, natural-food diet that is designed to moderate urine pH levels. This helps alleviate some of the kidney's workload, allowing the body to direct more energy toward the healing process. Herbal therapy can then commence with tonic herbs that improve renal blood circulation (ginkgo, hawthorn), reduce inflammation of nephritic (kidney) and other urinary tract tissues (couch grass, marshmallow, corn silk), and gently increase urine output (nettle, dandelion, alfalfa, goldenrod). If infection is part of the problem, nonirritating antimicrobials (Oregon

grape, goldenseal) can be added as well. But extra care must be taken to assure that the herbal therapy does not further irritate the animal's condition. Avoid herbs that contain large amounts of aromatic volatile oils (juniper, yarrow, members of the mint family) and those with considerable amounts of tannins (uva ursi, white oak bark, black walnut hulls), especially if the kidneys are inflamed.

Most traditional herbal approaches to kidney failure are centered on increasing

A Basic Herb Formula for Early Stages of Kidney Failure

Combine the tea or low-alcohol tinctures of the following:
- **1 part hawthorn**
- **1 part ginkgo**
- **1 part echinacea**
- **1 part marshmallow**
- **1 part dandelion leaf**

For dogs, a good starting dose is 1 teaspoon (5 milliliters) of the cooled tea or 1 milliliter of the combined tincture per 20 pounds of the animal's body weight, twice daily, preferably given between meals and with plenty of drinking water. For cats, start with 1 teaspoon (5 milliliters) of the cooled tea or 1 milliliter of the combined tincture, twice daily, preferably given between meals and with plenty of drinking water. Horses and large herbivores can receive 25 milliliters of the combined tincture diluted in 8 ounces (240 milliliters) or more of water, twice daily, preferably between meals.

diuresis (urine output) and decreasing inflammation. But we have found better success when equal attention is placed on improving blood circulation in the kidneys.

A Holistic Herbal Approach to Kidney Failure: The Tilford Theory

The fact that the kidneys are second only to the brain in terms of circulatory dependency is often overlooked when treating kidney failure. If the blood flow to the kidneys is blocked by damaged or inflamed tissue, the kidneys will die from lack of oxygen.

We have received several reports from veterinarians and pet owners who have seen promising results in the treatment of early to midstage kidney failure in dogs and cats from use of a formula that combines anti-inflammatory, immunostimulant, and, most important, circulatory tonic herbs. The theory behind this approach is that the kidneys are critically oxygen dependent and made up of hundreds of blood vessels. They are sensitive to blood-pressure disorders, vascular atony, and poor circulation. Through the use of hawthorn, increased renal circulation is achieved without elevating blood pressure. At the same time, ginkgo dilates and improves tonicity of nephritic blood vessels, improves blood return from the extremities, and helps reduce blood pressure in congested tissues. The mucilage content of ginkgo also serves to reduce inflammation throughout the urinary tract and provides a protective lubricating barrier for the passage of wastes. A small amount of garlic or echinacea helps keep bacteria and fungi in check, marshmallow helps soothe and reduce inflammation, and dandelion leaf or the fresh juice of parsley helps to increase urine output. Other herbs worth investigating in cases of kidney failure include alfalfa, astragalus, goldenrod, and couch grass.

URINARY INCONTINENCE

Urinary incontinence is fairly common in aging animals, spayed females (especially dogs), and in females who have lost bladder tone as a result of multiple pregnancies. Urinary incontinence can also be triggered by nervous system dysfunction, emotional disorders, inflammatory disease, or nutritional deficiency.

Identifying the exact cause of urinary incontinence can be challenging, and successful herbal treatment usually depends on just how well the caregiver knows and understands his or her companion. Did the problem begin suddenly, or has there been an occasional drop or two of urine in your companion's bed from time to time in the past? If the latter is true, a gradual degeneration of bladder tone could have been reversed early on. Does your animal appear to be stiff after exercise, do her hind

A Tonic Formula for Urinary Incontinence

Combine the following:

1 part oatstraw
1 part plantain
1 part corn silk
1 part nettle root or saw palmetto
1 part horsetail

We like to use this formula in the form of a glycerin tincture because it's easy to administer, but a tea is equally effective. A good starting dose is 12–20 drops of the glycerite or 1 teaspoon of the strong tea for each 20 pounds of the animal's body weight, twice daily.

legs wobble when she stands after exercise, or does she seem to be holding her rump lower when walking? If any of these are even slightly evident, then your companion may be developing arthritis, hip dysplasia, or some other cause of nerve impairment that may be affecting the tone and function of urinary tract muscles. This illustrates just how important a pet care diary can be. By keeping detailed notes about subtle changes in your animal's appearance, behavior, feeding habits, and physical performance, you can detect trends that point to early stages of disease and that greatly simplify finding curative solutions.

In spayed females, normal hormone production is interrupted when the uterus and ovaries are removed during an ovariohysterectomy. The bladder is composed of smooth-muscle groups that are functionally interdependent with a balance of reproductive hormones, so when hormone production is altered, the bladder loses tone and urine dribble results. Reversing this kind of incontinence is difficult because there is no way that herbs can replace hormones that should be naturally produced by the body. Oatstraw and wild yam (Dioscorea villosa) contain estrogenic (phytoestrogens) compounds. Theoretically, these herbs might help stimulate whatever hormone production is left intact, and to some extent they might mimic natural hormone production enough to serve as a partial remedy for incontinence. Although these herbs are safe in moderate doses, this approach is unreliable and may affect only certain animals. The better approach toward hormone-related urinary incontinence applies to all forms of urinary incontinence: strengthen and support the structure and function of the bladder sphincters and urinary smooth-muscle tissues with long-term use of tonic herbs. Choices include corn silk, raspberry leaf, horsetail, saw palmetto, nettle root, couch grass, uva ursi, agrimony, marshmallow, and plantain. Oatstraw can also be included for the aforementioned purpose and as a nutritive diuretic.

Urinary incontinence is sometimes caused by neurological disorders, especially in older animals who suffer from senility and general debility. Oftentimes, epileptic animals have a problem with incontinence too. In these cases, we can look toward cerebrotonics such as ginkgo and gotu kola to help bring relief. These herbs work to improve synaptic (nerve impulse) transmission and blood circulation in the brain. Skullcap or valerian might help moderate brain activities that are believed to trigger epileptic episodes and may also be instrumental in treating incontinence of neurological origin. If emotional or behavioral disorders are part of the problem, Saint-John's-wort might be indicated.

Glossary

A

abortifacient: a substance that can cause abortion

acupoints: part of traditional Chinese medicine; points on the body that are sights where pressure is applied as in acupressure or needles are inserted under the skin as in acupuncture

adaptogen: a nontoxic substance that is believed to increase stamina and overall energy levels in the body, especially in stressful conditions

aerial parts: the aboveground portions of a plant

allopathy (*see* homeopathy): the use of drugs or other means to antidote a disease or symptom in a manner not necessarily cooperative with the body's natural functions.

alterative: an herb or other agent that gradually alters an existing condition in the body. A blood alterative is often referred to as a blood cleanser because it alters the entrance of toxins and waste materials into the bloodstream, in most cases through stimulation of liver function.

alternate: describing leaves arranged along either side of a stem at various points but never directly opposite each other across the stem

amebiasis: the state of being infected with amoebas, single-celled organisms that (in most cases) are introduced into the body via raw food or drinking water

amine: an organic compound containing nitrogen

amoebicidal: kills certain types of amoebas

analgesic: a pain-relieving substance

anaphylactic: of, relating to, or causing anaphylaxis or anaphylactic shock

anaphylactic shock: severe and sometimes fatal immediate hypersensitivity (usually the result of allergy) that can result in the inability to breathe

anesthetic: a substance that reduces painful sensitivity. Unlike general analgesics, anesthetics are often applied locally. An injection of Novocaine at the dentist is a local anesthetic.

anodyne: soothes pain

annual: a plant that blooms, distributes its seeds, and then dies during its first and only year of growth. Annuals depend solely on seeds for reproduction.

anther: the pollen-bearing organ at the end of the stamen that is responsible for the distribution of pollen. The anther is usually yellow or orange and is the part bees seek out.

antibacterial: effective against bacteria

antibody: any of a variety of molecules that are synthesized by the body for the purpose of combating antigens (toxins or other foreign substances)

anticancer: used to fight or capable of stopping the spread of cancer

anticatarrhal: a substance capable of assisting the body in eliminating excess mucus from the upper respiratory tract through anti-inflammatory actions on the mucous membranes that are responsible for the secretions

antidermatitic: active against various skin problems

antiemetic: helps alleviate vomiting

antigenic proteins: chemical compounds of protein molecular structure that trigger an inflammatory response upon contacting or entering the body

antihydrotic: capable of preventing or inhibiting perspiration

anti-inflammatory: decreases inflammation

antilithic: prevents the formation or aids in the elimination of gravel, or stones, in the urinary system

antimicrobial: helps the body to resist, inhibit, or destroy pathogenic microbes. In holistic medicine, this term generally describes actions that assist the body in fighting bacteria, fungi, or viruses at their original point of infection.

antioxidant: a substance that controls or eliminates free radicals or reduces cellular oxidation in the body

antiparasitic: anything that expels, repels, kills, or inhibits reproduction of parasites

antiplatelet: a compound that inhibits platelet activity in the blood, usually resulting in anticoagulant activity

antipyretic: an agent capable of reducing fever

antirheumatic: an agent capable of relieving the symptoms of rheumatic conditions such as rheumatoid arthritis

antiseptic: a substance that kills or inhibits the growth of pathogenic microbes. In holistic medicine, this term describes substances that interfere with bacterial infections regardless of the body's natural abilities to do so. In this context, antiseptic herbs are applied as allopathic remedies.

antitussive: capable of suppressing coughs

anthelmintic: kills or expels worms

astringent: capable of tightening the soft tissues of the body. Astringent herbs are used to stop bleeding, reduce inflammation, and stop diarrhea.

awn: a slender, stiff bristle, usually occurring at the end of a plant stem

axil: the junction where a petiole or peduncle joins the stem of a plant

axillary flowers: flowers presented at the leaf axils

B

bacteriostatic: specifically acting to inhibit the multiplication of bacteria

basal: referring to the base of something. Basal leaves are found at the extreme lower end of a plant. They are usually the first true leaves to appear after germination.

biennial: a plant that blooms only during its second year of growth and then dies

biotin: a water-soluble dicyclic monocarboxylic acid considered to be part of the vitamin B complex

bitter: stimulates salivation and improves digestion

bitter tonic: a substance that stimulates digestive functions, first in the mouth and later in the stomach and liver. Bitter tonics are traditionally used to aid digestion.

bracts: modified or reduced leaflets usually associated with the flower of a plant; often located beneath the petals

C

candida: any of a yeastlike genus (*Candida*) of fungi that inhabit the vagina or digestive tract (or both) that under certain conditions may cause candidiasis, an acute or chronic fungal infection

capsaicin: the primary active component of cayenne pepper (*Capsicum* spp.). Capsaicin may represent as

much as 48 percent of the fruit's chemical makeup.

carcinogen: a substance or agent that promotes the formation or growth of cancer

cardiac tonic: an agent capable of strengthening the heart muscle or stimulating heartbeat (or both) in a manner beneficial to body functions

cardiotonic: tending to strengthen the heart

carminative: aids in the expulsion of gas from the digestive tract

carrier (for an herb): a compound or group of compounds that serve to transport the medicinally active components of a plant to various portions of the body

catarrh: excessive secretion of thick phlegm or mucus from inflamed mucus membranes (see anticatarrhal)

cathartic: a strong laxative

cerebrovascular: of or involving the veins, arteries, and capillaries of the brain

chambered fruits: fruits with a seed-bearing structure that contains more than one seed-containing chamber

chlorophyll: a green pigment found in plants that enables them to photosynthesize

cholagogue: a substance that stimulates bile production in the liver

choleretic effects: stimulation of bile production in the liver

Crohn's disease: a chronic granulomatous inflammatory disease of unknown cause involving the gastrointestinal tract; also called regional enteritis or ileitis

coagulant: a substance capable of promoting blood clotting, converting blood from a liquid to a semisolid state

compound: a leaf composed of multiple small leaf segments, often pinnately arranged pairs of leaflets

conifers: trees and shrubs that bear their flowers and fruits in the form of scaly, conelike structures; includes all members of the fir, pine, and cypress families

constituent: a single element or a compound ingredient that is part of a whole. A medicinal constituent in a plant is an element or compound that makes the plant medicinally useful.

contraindication: any condition, especially any condition of disease, that renders some particular line of treatment improper or undesirable. Herbs can be contraindicated for use in certain situations.

counterirritant: an irritant that distracts attention away from another irritant. Usually applied externally. A deep-heating, mentholated muscle ointment is a counterirritant to the discomfort of aching muscles.

coumarin: a principle with a bitter taste and an odor resembling that of vanilla beans, derived from tonka bean, red clover, and other plants and also prepared synthetically. Coumarin contains a factor that inhibits the hepatic synthesis of vitamin K–dependent coagulation factors, and a number of its derivatives are used as anticoagulants in the treatment of disorders in which there is excessive or undesirable clotting.

cultivar: a variety of a plant species originating and continuing in cultivation and given a name in a modern language

cystitis: inflammation of the bladder

cytokines: a generic term for nonantibody proteins released by certain cells on contact with specific antigens. Cytokines act as intercellular mediators, as in the generation of an immune response.

D

deciduous: seasonally losing leaves once a year at the end of the growing season

decoction: an herbal preparation made by simmering plant material in water until maximum extraction of active constituents is achieved. This process is usually used for roots, barks, and seeds that are not water soluble enough for use in simple infusions (teas).

demulcent: a substance that provides a protective coating and is soothing to irritated tissues in the body

dermatitis: inflammation of the skin

diaphoretic: a substance capable of stimulating perspiration

digestive tonic: a substance that aids the digestion

disk: the central circular portion of a flower head

diuresis: the process by which the body eliminates waste and excesses through kidney function and subsequent urination

diuretic: a substance that stimulates diuresis

E

edema: usually a fluid-filled swelling

elliptical: relating to an oval shape with opposite ends that are equal in diameter; not egg shaped but like a flattened circle

emetic: a substance that induces vomiting

emmenagogue: a substance that promotes menstruation

emollient: a substance that soothes, protects, and softens the skin; the external counterpart to a demulcent

estrogenic: affects estrogen production in the body

exogenous growth hormones: hormones that the body does not produce but receives via food or other external sources

expectorant: a substance that helps expel mucus from the respiratory tract

F

febrifuge: fever reducing

flavonoid: a chemical compound found in various forms in several plants. Flavonoid constituents are responsible for a wide range of medicinal actions and are generally responsible for the pigmentation of various red, yellow, or purple fruits. Also known as a bioflavonoid.

flower essence: usually made from flower petals that are floated on top of spring water in a crystal bowl in the sunshine for a specified period of time, after which the water is filtered off, bottled, and brandy is added as a preservative. Also called flower remedy.

fodder crops: cultivated plants that are used as livestock feed

fomentation: treatment by a warm and moist application; similar to a poultice

formic acid: an acid compound that is known to cause a burning and tingling sensation as well as blistering when applied to skin or other body tissues. Formic acid is primarily responsible for the well-known sting that is induced by red ants.

fungicide: a substance that helps kill fungi

G

galactagogue: anything that stimulates milk production

genitourinary: having to do with the genital and urinary organs

glabrous: having a surface that lacks hairs, a characteristic of certain plant stems and leaves

grand mal seizures: the spasms and convulsions produced by a severe epileptic episode; an "epileptic fit"

H

Heinz-body anemia: a condition that causes deformation of red corpuscles, diminishing the blood's capacity to collect and transport oxygen and nutrients throughout the body

hematoma: a localized collection of blood, usually clotted, in an organ, space, or tissue due to the break in the wall of a blood vessel

hemostatic: stops bleeding. Most herbal hemostatic substances work by astringent actions.

hepatic: relating to or associated with the liver

hepatotonic: strengthens liver function

hepatotoxic: toxic to the liver

hips: the swollen, ripened, seed-producing portion of a rose flower head

homeopathy: a modality of healing founded by Samuel Hahnemann in the late 1700s. The science of homeopathy involves a meticulous diagnostic investigation of an individual's physical, behavioral, and historical state of being, after which a remedy is tailored to the specific needs of the individual. Homeopathic remedies are composed of organic or nonorganic compounds that are diluted from their original strength hundreds or even thousands of times. The goal of homeopathic medicine is to effect a desired physical or psychological response by stimulating body systems at very low, perhaps even molecular levels. Often, a "like versus like" approach is employed, such as when the homeopathic remedy Arsenicum, an extremely dilute preparation of arsenic, is used to counter a disease that produces symptoms similar to those of arsenic poisoning.

homeostasis: a maintained state of health in which all checks and balances between interdependent elements of mind, body, and spirit are functioning harmoniously

hybridize: to genetically alter a plant species in such a way that inhibits or eliminates the plant's abilities to reproduce by natural means

hydroquinones: reduced form of quinone, containing two hydroxyl groups (sometimes used as an antioxidant)

hyperlipidemia: elevated concentrations of lipids in plasma; elevated blood fats

hyperthyroidism: overactive functioning of the thyroid gland

hypothyroidism: depressed thyroid function

hypotension: low blood pressure

hypotensive: capable of reducing blood pressure

I

immune modulator: an herb that acts to help the immune system by optimizing it's ability to adjust to stressful circumstances. Often used synonymously with the term *immunostimulant*, immune modulator is becoming more common in herbalists' vocabulary as more is learned about how certain immune-supporting herbs work in the body.

immunostimulant: an herb that strengthens the body's resistance to infection by stimulating and increasing immune system responses. In herbal medicine, this term specifically refers to the medicinal support of infection-fighting antibodies in the bloodstream and overall tonification of the lymph system.

immunotonic: an herb that strengthens the immune system

infusion: a preparation made by pouring boiling water over herbs and allowing them to steep; a tea

interleukin: a generic term for a group of multifunctional cytokines that are produced by a variety of lymphoid and nonlymphoid cells and whose effects occur at least partly within the lymphopoietic system

isoflavone: a flavone compound (e.g., flavonoids) with molecular structures that contribute steroidal properties to a plant

K

ketogenic diet: a high-fat diet that is believed to help in certain cases of epilepsy in humans

kinesiology: the study of body motion. In holistic medicine, kinesiology is used as a diagnostic tool involving the observation and analysis of physical responses to touch, questioning, or other stimuli; the manner in which the body responds to the stimuli is used to determine the existence and nature of illness.

L

lignan: an organic cellulose-like substance that acts as a binder for the cellulose fibers in wood and certain plants and adds strength and stiffness to cell walls

linear: long and narrow. Referring to leaf characteristics, a linear leaf is too narrow to be considered narrowly lance shaped and instead resembles a blade of grass.

loam: rich soil composed of clay, sand, and organic matter

lobed: referring to leaf characteristics, a lobed leaf has margins (outer edges) that are deeply indented in two or more places but not as deeply as a palmate leaf (e.g., maple leaves).

lymph system: the system of the body responsible for the cleansing of tissues and the production of various antibodies and white blood cells

lymphocytes: any of the mononuclear, nonphagocytic leukocytes found in the blood, lymph, and lymphoid tissues that are the body's immunologically competent cells and their precursors

M

marc: the solid plant material that remains of an herb preparation after the liquid (tincture, extract, etc.) has been pressed off

margin: the outer edges of a leaf

MAOI: see monoamine oxidase inhibitor

medicinal action: any of a variety of terms used to describe the effect that an herb, or other substance that may be considered therapeutic, has on or in the body

menstruum: the solvent used to extract plant constituents in making an extract or tincture; a solvent medium

microbe: a microscopic organism, including various bacteria, viruses, fungi, and protozoa

modality: the employment of, or the method of employment of, a therapeutic agent or a set of ideas or principles

monoamine oxidase inhibitor (MAOI): any of a variety of chemical substances that inhibit the activities of monoamine oxidase (MAO), an enzyme that is thought to regulate the production of certain antidepressive or antihistamine chemicals in the body. By blocking the activities of MAO with an MAOI, the body's production of seratonin, epinephrine, or histamine is increased to bring about antidepressive effects or other therapeutic results.

monocyte: a large, nongranular white blood cell with a single round or egg-shaped nucleus

montane: of or relating to mountainous terrain

mucilage: a sticky, oily substance often used in herbal medicine to soothe and protect irritated tissues

mucilaginous: of, relating to, or secreting mucilage. Mucilaginous herbs are generally used as emollients or demulcents.

N

navicular syndrome: inflammation of connective tissues of the navicular joint (in the forefoot) of a horse; also known as navicular disease

nephritic: of or relating to the kidneys

nephritis: inflammation of the kidney

vine: a substance that affects the nervous system

noxious weed: a plant species that many people generally hate and want to eradicate

nutritive: nourishing

O

opposite: leaves arranged directly across from each other at regular intervals along the stem of a plant

ovate: oval shaped

oxalate: a salt of oxalic acid. Calcium oxalate stones are a type of urinary calculi. (See struvite)

oxytocic: induces contractions

P

palmate: resembling the shape of the human hand with fingers extended. A palmate leaf has margins deeply indented nearly to its base. (See lobed)

pathogen: any disease-causing microorganism

pathogenic microbes: microscopic organisms that act negatively on or in the body; harmful, infectious bacteria, fungi, and viruses are all pathogenic microbes.

pedicel: flower stem

peduncle: the stemlike structure that holds the fruit or flower of a plant, commonly known as a pedicel

perennial: a plant that returns from its rootstock year after year. Perennials reproduce by seed and root reproduction.

peristalsis: the involuntary wave-type motion of the alimentary canal contracting to propel waste through and out of the body

petals: the bractlike inner segments of a flower; usually the most colorful part of the flower

petiole: the stemlike structure of a plant leaf that connects the leaf to the stalk, branch, or true stem of the plant; sometimes referred to as a leaf stem

pH: a numerical measurement of acidity or alkalinity. Relating to soil, a pH level of 7.0 is regarded as neutral; lower numbers indicate increasing acidity, higher numbers indicate increasing alkalinity.

phytoestrogenic principles: chemical components of a plant that are similar to estrogen produced in an animal's body, or that mimic or stimulate estrogen functions in the body

pinnate: a compound leaf pattern in which leaflets are arranged in opposing pairs along two sides of an axis

pipette: a small piece of apparatus used to insert a rectal suppository; or a dropper used for drawing fluid

polysaccharide: a carbohydrate, which on hydrolysis yields a large number of monosaccharide. Polysaccharides are present in many species of plants, often serving as medicinally active components (e.g., the polysaccharide constituents of *Echinacea* spp. are partly responsible for the immunotonic activities of the plants).

potentiate: to make stronger, quicker to act, or more effective

potentiating adjunct: an herb substance that can be added to an herbal medicine to make the

herbal medicine stronger, quicker to act, or more therapeutically effective

poultice: an herbal preparation made by mashing plant materials with a liquid (usually water) to form a wet paste

probiotics: friendly bacteria or enzymes that serve to support natural digestive functions within the body

psychotropic drug: a drug that affects the mental state of the subject receiving it

pulegone: a flea-killing insecticidal chemical compound most notably found in pennyroyal (*Mentha pulegium*)

purgative: an extremely, perhaps violently, strong laxative with uncontrollable effects. Purgatives generally cause abdominal cramping and near-incontinent conditions. They are usually reserved by herbalists for use only in dire circumstances.

R

rabies miasm: the chronic result of rabies vaccinations; it is believed to be passed down through successive generations

ray: the extended bladelike petal of a ray flower

rhizome: an underground plant stem that extends itself horizontally and produces shoots above and roots below. Crabgrass is an excellent example of a rhizomatous plant.

riparian habitat: an ecosystem in proximity to a consistent source of water (such as floodplains, stream banks, lakeshores, and marshes)

rosette: a cluster of leaves that emerges in an overlay pattern resembling the shape of a rose flower

rotenone: an insecticidal compound found in the flowers of mullein (*Verbascum thapsis*) and in the leaves and flowers of various other plants

rubefacient: a substance that reddens and heats the skin when applied topically

S

saponin: a glycoside (soaplike) plant compound. Although many types of saponins have medicinally useful properties, many may be irritating to the digestive tract and cause toxic reactions if ingested.

sepal: a modified leaf (usually green) that encloses

a flower bud. Some plants have sepals that are more conspicuous than their flowers.

sialagogue: any substance that increases the secretion of saliva

simple: referring to leaf characteristics, a simple leaf has margins that are void of any serrations, divisions, or lobes. A simple leaf is a basic leaf.

stratification: a germination process by which a seed must be subjected to a prolonged period of cold (often freezing) temperatures and moisture to break its dormancy

Streptococcus: a genus of gram-positive, spherically shaped bacteria in microscopic chains. Most forms of *Streptococcus* are normally present and harmless in the body, while others, such as *Streptococcus pneumoniae* (bacterial pneumonia), are potentially deadly.

stomachic: a stimulant or tonic for soothing the stomach

struvite: a urinary calculus composed of pure ammoniomagnesium phosphate, forming the hard crystals known to minerologists as struvite

styptic: an agent that causes bleeding to stop by making tissues contract rapidly; essentially the same as an astringent

symbiosis: a relationship in which two dissimilar organisms live together for mutual benefit

T

taproot: a plant root that extends vertically downward into the soil (e.g., carrot or parsnip)

terminate: referring to flowers that are the absolute end-tips of plant stems; also referred to as terminal

tincture: an herbal preparation made by soaking plant material in a liquid solvent (called a menstruum) to extract active medicinal constituents. Commonly referred to as herbal extracts, tinctures may be made from menstruums of alcohol, glycerin, or vinegar.

titer: the quantity of a substance required to produce a reaction with a given volume of another substance, or the amount of one substance required to correspond with a given amount of another substance. In veterinary medicine, titer analysis is sometimes used to measure an animal's resistance to an antigen—such as rabies virus. By testing an animal's blood for natural resistance

to viral or bacterial infection, vaccination can often be avoided.

tonic: a general term for a nourishing substance that invigorates and increases the tone and strength of tissues and improves the function of one or more body systems

tonicity: a property of the strength and resiliency of a body tissue

U

umbel: an umbrella-shaped flower. True umbels consist of tiny florets, each extending an equal distance from a common point to form dense clusters. In this book, the terms *umbel* and *umbel-like* are used loosely to include flowers that appear umbrella shaped regardless of the "true" criteria.

uremia: more correctly referred to as azotemia. An excess presence of urea, creatinine, and other nitrogenous end products of protein and amino acid metabolism in the blood; may point to chronic renal failure.

urolithiasis: a condition marked by the formation of urinary calculi, or stones

urolith: urinary calculus or stone

uterine stimulant: an agent that is capable of stimulating contraction of the uterus

uterotonic: strengthens the uterus

V

vaccinosis: sickness resulting from cumulative effects of years of vaccines

vasoconstrictor: an agent that is capable of tightening the walls of blood vessels; opposite of vasodilator

vasodilator: an agent that is capable of dilating or widening blood vessels; opposite of vasoconstrictor

vetch: a common name for several plants in the pea family

vulnerary: used to promote the healing of wounds

W

wildcrafted: harvested from a wild, not cultivated, source

wort: an old term for *plant*

References

Abdullah, T. H., D. V. Kirkpatrick, and J. Carter, "Enhancement of Natural Killer Activity in AIDS with Garlic." *Deutsche Zeitschrift für Onkologie 21* (1989): 52–3.

Acker, Randy, DVM, and Jim Fergus. *A Field Guide: Dog First Aid*. Belgrade, Mont.: Wilderness Adventure Press, 1994.

Aizenman, B. E. "Antibiotic Preparations from Hypericum Perforatum." *Mikrobiolohichny Zhurnal* (Kiev) 31 (1969): 128–33 (CA 70: 118006e).

Ali, M. S., et al. "Isolation of Antitumor Polysaccharide Fractions from Yucca Glauca." *Growth* 42, no. 2 (1978): 213–23.

Allard, M. "Treatment of Old Age Disorders with Ginkgo Biloba Extract: From Pharmacology to Clinic." *In Rokan (Ginkgo Biloba): Recent Results in Pharmacology and Clinic*, ed. E. W. Fünfgeld, 180–211. New York: Springer-Verlag, 1988. (Original source: Presse Médicale 15, no. 31 [Sept. 25, 1986]: 1540–5.)

Allport, Richard B. *Heal Your Cat the Natural Way*. New York: Reed International Books, 1997.

———. *Heal Your Dog the Natural Way*. New York: Reed International Books, 1997.

Al Makdessi, S., et al. "Myocardial Protection by Pretreatment with Crataegus Oxyacantha: An Assessment by Means of the Release of Lactate Dehydrogenase by the Ischemic and Reperfused Langendorff Heart." *Arzneimittel-Forschung* 46 (Jan. 1996): 25–7.

Almquist, H. J. "The Early History of Vitamin K." *American Journal of Clinical Nutrition* 28 (1975): 656–9.

American Botanical Council. Oats. German Commission E Monographs, in *Bundesanzeiger* (Cologne, Germany), Oct. 15, 1987.

Anderson, Nina, and Howard Peiper. *Are You Poisoning Your Pets?* Garden City Park, N.Y.: Avery, 1998.

———. *Super Nutrition for Animals*. Garden City Park, N.Y.: Avery, 1996.

Animal Protection Institute. *What's Really in Pet Food*. Sacramento, Calif.: Animal Protection Institute, 1997.

Aonuma, S., T. Minuma, and M. Tarutani, "Effects of Coptis, Scuttellaria, Rhubarb, and Bupleurum on Serum Cholesterol and Phospholipids in Rabbits." *Yakugaku Zasshi* 77 (1957): 1303–7.

Association of American Feed Control Officials. "Feed Ingredient Definitions." In *Official Publication of AAFCO*. Atlanta: AAFCO, 1997.

———. "Minimum Feeding Protocols: Dog and Cat Maintenance Claims." *In Official Publication of AAFCO*. Atlanta: AAFCO, 1997.

Bai, M. X., et al. "Effects of Alanyl-Glutamine on Gut Barrier Function." *Nutrition* 12 (Nov./Dec. 1996): 793–6.

Bamberger, Michelle, DVM. *Help! The Quick Guide to First Aid for Your Cat*. New York: Howell Book House, 1993.

Bauer, R., and H. Wagner, "Echinacea Species as Potential Immunostimulatory Drugs." In *Economic and Medicinal Plant Research*, ed. H. Wagner and N. R. Farnsworth, 5:253–351. New York: Academic Press, 1991.

———. "Echinacea—der sonehut—Stand der forshung." *Zeitschrift fur Phytotherapie* 9 (1988): 151–9.

Beath, O. A. "The Composition and Properties of the Yucca Plant." *Kansas Academy of Science* 27 (1914): 102–7.

Belaiche, P., and O. Lievoux, "Clinical Studies on the Palliative Treatment of Prostatic Adenoma with Extract of Urtica Root." *Phytotherapy Research* 5 (1991): 267–9.

Belfield, Wendell O., DVM, and Martin Zucker. *The Very Healthy Cat Book: A Vitamin and Mineral Program for Optimal Feline Health*. New York: McGraw-Hill, 1983.

Bergner, Paul. *The Healing Power of Garlic*. Rocklin, Calif.: Prima, 1996.

Bicks, Jane R., DVM. *Dr. Jane's 30 Days to a Healthier, Happier Cat*. New York: Berkeley Publishing Group, 1996.

Billinghurst, Ian, BVSc, BScAgr, Dip. Ed. Give Your Dog a Bone: *The Practical Commonsense Way to Feed Dogs for a Long Healthy Life*. Ian Billinghurst, New South Wales, Australia 1993.

Bissett, Wichtl. *Herbal Drugs and Pharmaceuticals*. Boca Raton, Fla.: CRC Press, 1994.

Block, Eric. "The Chemistry of Garlic and Onions." *Scientific American* 252, no. 114 (1985): 3–25.

———. "The Organic Chemistry of Garlic Sulfur Compounds." Speech, First World Congress on the Health Significance of Garlic and Garlic Constituents, Washington D.C., 1990.

Boucard-Maitre, Y., et al. "Cytoxic and Antitumoral Activity of Calendula Extracts." *Pharmazie* 43 (1998): 220.

Bourre, J. M., et al. "Fatty Acids of the Alpha-Linolenic Family and the Structures and Functions of the Brain: Their Nature, Role, Origin and Dietary Importance—Animal Model." *Corps Gras Lipides* 2 (1995): 254–63.

———, et al. "Structural and Functional Importance of Dietary Polyunsaturated Fatty Acids in the Nervous System." *Advances in Experimental Medicine and Biology* 318 (1992): 211–29.

Bravetti, G. "Preventative Medical Treatment of Senile Cataract with Vitamin E and Anthocyanosides: Clinical Evaluation." *Annali di Ottalmologia e Clinica Oculistica* 115 (1989): 109.

Bray, Dr. Robert E. "Enteroliths: A Potential Problem with Horses." Article prepared for Equi-Tech Conference, Los Angeles, Nov. 1993.

British Herbal Medicine Association. *British Herbal Pharmacopoeia*. London: British Herbal Medicine Association, 1983.

Brown, N. D., and J. Donald. *Herbal Prescriptions for Better Health*. Rocklin, Calif.: Prima, 1996.

Buchanan, R. L. "Toxicity of Spices Containing Methylenedioxybenzine Derivatives: A Review." *Journal of Food Safety* 1 (1978): 275–93.

Buhner, Stephen Harrod. *Herbal Antibiotics: Natural Alternatives for Treating Drug-Resistant Bacteria*. Pownal, Vt.: Storey Books, 1999.

Buist, R. "The Malfunctional 'Mucosal Barrier' and Food Allergies." *International Clinical Nutrition Review* 3 (1983): 1.

Bult, H., et al. "Modification of Endotoxin-Induced Haemodynamic and Haematological Changes in the Rabbit by Methylprednisolone, F(ab´)2 Fragments and Rosmarinic Acid." *British Journal of Pharmacology* 84 (1985): 317–27.

Caprioli, J., and M. Sears. "Forskolin Lowers Intraocular Pressure in Rabbits, Monkeys, and Man." *Lancet* 1 (1983): 958–60.

Carlisle, E. M. "Silicon as an Essential Trace Element in Animal Nutrition." In *Silicon Biochemistry*, 123–39. Ciba Foundation Symposium 121. Chichester, N.Y.: Wiley, 1986.

Cassady, J. M., et al. "Use of a Mammalian Cell Culture Benzo(a)-pyrene Metabolism Assay for the Detection of Potential Anticarcinogens from Natural Products: Inhibition of Metabolism by Biochanin A, an Isoflavone of Trifolium pratense L." *Cancer Research* 48, no. 22 (1988): 6257–61.

Castelman; Michael. *The Healing Herbs: The Ultimate Guide to the Curative Power of Nature's Medicines*. Emmaus, Pa.: Rodale Press, 1991.

Chadha, Y. R., ed. *The Wealth of India*. New Delhi: Publications & Information Directorate, CSIR, 1985.

Chakarski, I., et al. "Clinical Study of a Herb Combination Consisting of Humulus lupulus, Mentha Piperita, Cichorium Intybus in Patients with Chronic Calculous and Noncalculous Cholecystitis." Probl. Vatr. Med. 10 (1982): 65–9.

———. "Treatment of Chronic Colitis with an Herbal Combination of Taraxacum Officinale, Hypericum Perforatum, Melissa Officinalis, Calendula Officinalis, and Foeniculum Vulgare." *Pharmazie* 43, no. 3 (March 1988): 220.

Chandler, R. F., et al. "Ethnobotany and Phytochemistry of Yarrow, *Achillea Millefolium.*" *Economic Botany* 36 (1982): 203–23.

———. "Herbal Remedies of the Maritime Indians: Sterols and Triterpenes of *Achillea Millefolium L.* (Yarrow)." *Journal of Pharmaceutical Science* 71 (June 1982): 690–3.

Chariot, E., and R. Charonnat. "Therapeutic Agents in Bile Secretion," *Annals of Medicine* 37 (1935): 131–42.

Chen, M. F., et al. "Effect of Glycyrrhizin on the Pharmacokinetics of Prednisolone Following Low Dosage of Prednisolone Hemisuccinate." *Endocrinologia Japonica* 37 (June 1990): 331–41.

Chung, Hsi I., et al. "Effects of *Astragalus Membranaceus* on Enhancement of Mouse Natural Killer Cell Activity." *Clinical Laboratory Immunology* 4 (Aug. 1984): 484–5.

Collier, H. O. J., et al. "Extract of Feverfew Inhibits Prostaglandin Biosynthesis." *Lancet* 2 (1980): 922–73.

Collin, M. A., and H. P. Charles, "Antimicrobial Activity of Carnosol and Ursolic Acid: Two Antioxidant Constituents of *Rosmarinus Officinalis.*" *Food Microbiology* 4 (1987): 311–5.

Day, Christopher. *The Homeopathic Treatment of Small Animals: Principles and Practice.* Saffron Waldon, England: C. W. Daniel, 1992.

Deal, C. L., et al. "Treatment of Arthritis with Topical Capsaicin: A Double-Blind Trial." *Clinical Therapeutics* 13, no. 3 (1991): 383–95.

De Bairacli Levy, Julliette. *Cats Naturally: Natural Rearing for Healthier Domestic Cats.* New York: Faber & Faber, 1991.

———. *The Complete Herbal Handbook for the Dog and Cat.* New York: Faber & Faber, 1991.

———. *Herbal Handbook for Farm and Stable.* New York: Faber & Faber, 1991.

Derbentseva, N. A., and A. S. Rabinovich, "Isolation, Purification, and Study of Some Physicochemical Properties of Novoimanin (a Hypericum Derivative)." In *Novoimanin Ego Lech. Svoistva, ed. A. I. Solov'eva,* 15–8. Kiev, USSR: Naukova Dumka, 1968.

Desai, K. N., H. Wei, and C. A. Lamartiniere. "The Preventive and Therapeutic Potential of the Squalene-Containing Compound, Roidex, on Tumor Promotion and Regression." *Cancer Letters* 101, March 19, 1996, 93–6.

Didry, N., and M. Pinkas. "Antibacterial Activity of Fresh Leaves of *Tussilago* sp." *Bulletin de la Societe de Pharmacie de Lille* 38 (1982): 51–2.

———, et al. "Components and Activity of *Tussilago Farfara,*" *Annales Pharmaceutiques Francaises* 40 (1982): 75–80.

Dong, D. C., L. F. Zhou, and J. X. J. Chen. "Changes in Proteinuria, Renal Function, and Immunity after Treatment with Injections of a Solution of *Astragalus Membranaceus.*" *Chung Hsi I Chieh Ho Tsa Chih* 7 (July 1987): 388, 403–4.

Dorland's Illustrated Medical Dictionary, 28th ed. Philadelphia: W. B. Saunders, 1994.

Dorosz, Edmund R., DVM. *Let's Cook for Our Cat.* Fort Macleod, Alberta, Canada: Our Pets, 1993.

———. *Let's Cook for Our Dog*. Fort Macleod, Alberta, Canada: Our Pets, 1993.

Duke, James A. Handbook of Medicinal Herbs. Boca Raton, Fla.: CRC Press, 1985.

Duncan, Karen L., William R. Hare, and William B. Buck, "Malignant Hyperthermia-Like Reaction Secondary to Ingestion of Hops in Five Dogs." *JAVMA* 210, no. 1 (1997).

Eaton, S. A., et al. "Digital Starling Forces and Hemodynamics during Early Laminitis Induced by an Aqueous Extract of Black Walnut (*Juglans Nigra*) in Horses." *American Journal of Veterinary Research* 56 (Oct. 1995): 1338–44.

El-Olemy, M. M., J. J. Sabatka, and S. J. Stohs. "Sapogenins of *Yucca Glauca*." *Phytochemistry* 13 (1974): 489–92.

Fairbairn, J. W., and F. J. El-Muhtadi, "Chemotaxonomy of Antraquinones in Rumex." *Phytochemistry* 11 (1972): 263–8.

Foster, Steven. "Echinacea: The Cold and Flu Remedy." *Alternative Complementary Therapies* 1, no. 4 (1995), 254–7.

———. *Herbal Renaissance: Growing, Using, and Understanding Herbs in the Modern World*. Layton, Utah: Gibbs Smith Books, 1993.

Fox, Michael W., DVM. *The Healing Touch: The Proven Massage Program for Cats and Dogs*. New York: Newmarket Press, 1991.

Frazier, Anitra, with Norma Eckroate. *The New Natural Cat: A Complete Guide for Finicky Owners*. New York: Penguin Books, 1990.

Frohne, D. "Untersuchungen zur Frage der Harndesinfizierenden Wirkungen von Barentraubenblatt-Extrakten." *Planta Medica* 18 (1970): 23–5.

———, and H. J. Pfander. *A Colour Atlas of Poisonous Plants*. London: Wolfe, 1984.

Fujihira, K. "Treatment of Cataract of Ba-wei-wan." *Japan Society for Oriental Medicine* 24 (1974): 465–79.

German Institute of Research for Drugs and Medical Devices. *Commission E Monographs*. Austin, Tex.: American Botanical Council, 1998.

Gerstenfeld, Sheldon L., VMD. *The Cat Care Book: All You Need to Know to Keep Your Cat Healthy and Happy*. Reading, Mass.: Addison-Wesley, 1989.

———. *The Dog Care Book: All You Need to Know to Keep Your Dog Healthy and Happy*. Reading, Mass.: Addison-Wesley, 1989.

Gfeller, Roger W., DVM, and Shawn R. Messonnier, DVM. *Handbook of Small Animal Toxicology and Poisonings*. St. Louis, Mo.: Mosby, 1998.

Gisvold, O., and E. Thaker. "Lignans from Larrea Divaricata." *Journal of Pharmaceutical Science* 63 (1974): 1905–7.

Goldstein, Martin, DVM. *The Nature of Animal Healing: The Path to Your Pet's Health, Happiness, and Longevity*. New York: Knopf, 1999.

Gracza, L., et al. "Biochemical-Pharmacological Investigations of Medicinal Agents of Plant Origin, I: Isolation of Rosmarinic Acid from Symphytum Officinale and Its Anti-Inflammatory Activity." *Archiv der Pharmazie* (Weinheim) 318 (1985): 1090–105.

Grainger, Janette, and Connie Moore. *Natural Insect Repellents for Pets, People, and Plants*. Austin, Tex.: Herb Bar, 1991.

Greaves, J. D., and C. L. A. Schmidt. "Nature of the Factor in Loss of Blood Coagulability of Bile Fistula Rats." *Proceedings of the Society of Experimental Biology and Medicine* 37 (1937): 43–5.

Greene, James. *The Herbal Medicine-Maker's Handbook*. Forestville, Calif.: Simpler's Botanical Co., 1990.

Grieve, Maud. *A Modern Herbal*. Vols. 1 and 2. New York: Dover Publications, 1971.

Grosjean, Nelly. *Veterinary Aromatherapy*. Essex, UK: C. W. Daniel, 1994.

Gupte, S. "Use of Berberine in Treatment of Giardiasis." *American Journal of Diseases of Childhood* 129 (1975): 866.

Habersang, S., et al. "Pharmacological Studies with Compounds of Chamomile IV: Studies on Bisabolol." *Planta Medica* 37 (1979): 115–23.

Haggag, M. Y., et al. "Thin Layer and Gas Chromatographic Studies on the Essential Oil from *Achillea Millefolium*." *Planta Medica* 27 (1975): 361–6.

Hara, H. "Experimental Study on the Effect of CoQ_{10} Administration to Isoproterenol-Induced Cardiomyopathy of Rats." *Kurume Medical Journal* 28 (1981): 125

Harris, C., et al. "Efficacy of Acemannan in Treatment of Canine and Feline Spontaneous Neoplasms." *Molecular Biotherapy* 3, no. 4 (1991): 207–13.

Hawcroft, Tim. *First Aid for Birds*. New York: Howell Book House, 1997.

———. *First Aid for Horses*. New York: Howell Book House, 1997.

Hayes, Karen E. N., DVM. "Don't Let DOD Derail Your Foal." *Modern Horse Breeding*, May 1992.

Heinerman, John. *Heinerman's Encyclopedia of Healing Herbs and Spices*. West Nyack, N.Y.: Parker Publishing, 1996.

Hendriks, H., et al. "Central Nervous Depressant Activity of Valerenic Acid in the Mouse." *Planta Medica* 51 (1985): 28–31.

Hof, S., and H. P. T. Ammon. "Negative Inotropic Action of Rosemary Oil, 1,8-Cineole, and Bornyl Acetate." *Planta Medica* 55 (1989): 106–7.

Hoffmann, David. *An Elders Herbal*. Rochester, Vt.: Healing Arts Press, 1993.

———. *The New Holistic Herbal*. Longmead, Shaftsbury, Dorset, UK: NIMH; Element Books, 1990.

Hunter, Francis. *Homeopathic First-Aid Treatment for Pets*. Wellingborough, Northamptonshire, UK: Thorsons London, 1988.

Ieven, M., et al. "Screening of Higher Plants for Biological Activities I. Antimicrobial Activity." *Planta Medica* 36 (1979): 311–21.

Ikram, M. "Medicinal Plants as Hypocholesterolemic Agents." *Journal of Pakistan Medical Association* 39 (1980): 38–50.

Irlbeck, N. A. *Nutrition and Care of Animals*. Dubuque, Iowa: Kendall/Hunt Publishing, 1996.

Ito, N., S. Fukushima, and H. Tsuda. "Carcinogenicity and Modification of the Carcinogenic Response by BHA, BHT and Other Antioxidants." *Critical Reviews in Toxicology* 15, no. 2 (1985): 109–50.

Jackson, P., et al. "Intestinal Permeability in Patient with Eczema and Food Allergy." *Lancet* 1285 (1981): 1285–6.

Jain, R. C., M.D. "Onion and Garlic in Experimental Atherosclerosis." Letter. *Lancet* 1, May 31, 1975, 1240.

Jalsenjak, V., et al. "Microcapsules of Sage Oil: Essential Oils Content and Antimicrobial Activity." *Pharmazie* 42 (1987): 419–20.

James, John W., and Frank Cherry. *The Grief Recovery Handbook: A Step-by-Step Program for Moving beyond Loss*. New York: HarperPerennial, 1988.

Janick, J., et al. "Borage: A Source of Gamma Linolenic Acid." *Herbs, Spices, and Medicinal Plants: Recent Advances in Botany, Horticulture, and Pharmacology*, ed. L. E. Crakerand and J. E. Simon, 4:145–86. Phoenix, Ariz.: Oryx Press, 1989.

Johnston, C. S., L. J. Martin, and X. Cai. "Antihistamine Effect of Supplemental Ascorbic Acid and Neutrophil Chemotaxis." *Journal of the American College of Nutrition* 11, no. 2 (1992): 172–6.

Ju, H.S., et al. "Effects of Glycyrrhiza Flavonoid on Lipid Peroxidation and Active Oxygen Radicals." *Yao Hsueh Hsueh Pao*, 24, no. 11 (1989): 807–12.

Jurcic, K., et al. "Zwei probandenstudien zur stimulierung der granulozytenphagozytose durch echinacea-extract-haltige praparate." *Zeitschrift fur Phytotherapie* 10 (1989): 167–70.

Jurisson, S. "Flavonoid Substances of Capsella Bursa-Pastoris." *Farmatsiya* (Moscow) 22 (1973): 34–5.

Kamen, Daniel, D.C. *The Well Adjusted Dog: Canine Chiropractic Methods You Can Do.* Cambridge, Mass.: Brookline Books, 1997.

Kaminski, P., and R. Katz. *Flower Essence Repertory.* Nevada City, Calif.: Flower Essence Society, 1994.

Kendall, Roger V. "Basic and Preventative Nutrition for the Cat, Dog, and Horse." In *Complementary and Alternative Veterinary Medicine: Principles and Practice*, ed. Allen M. Schoen and Susan G. Wynn. St. Louis, Mo.: Mosby, 1997.

Kishimoto, C., et al. "The Protection of Coenzyme Q_{10} against Experimental Viral Myocarditis in Mice." *Japanese Circulation Journal* 48 (1984): 1358.

Kleijnen, J., and P. Knipschild, "Ginkgo Biloba." *Lancet* 340 (1992): 1136–9.

Kovach, A. G. B., M. Foeldi, and L. Fedina, "Die wirkung eines extraktes aus crataegus oxycantha auf die durchstroemung der coronarirkung von hunden." *Arzneimittel-Forschung* 9, no. 6 (1959): 378–9.

Kowaleski, Z., W. Kedzia, and I. Mirska, "Effect of Berberine Sulfate on Staphylococci." *Archives of Immunology and Experimental Therapeutics* 20, no. 3 (1972): 353–60.

Kuroda, K., and K. Takagi, "Studies on Capsella Bursa-Pastoris. 1: Diuretic, Anti-Inflammatory, and Anti-Ulcer Action of Ethanol Extracts of the Herb." *Archives Internationales de Pharmacodynamie et de Thérapie* 178 (1969): 382–91.

Lazarus, Pat. *Keep Your Pet Healthy the Natural Way.* Indianapolis: Macmillan, 1983.

Lenau, H., et al. "Wirksamkeit und Vertraglichkeit von Cysto Fink bei Patienten mit Reizblase und/oder Harninkontinenz." *Therapiewoche* 34 (1984): 6054.

Leung, A. Y. *Encyclopedia of Common Natural Ingredients Used in Food, Drugs, and Cosmetics.* Chichester, N.Y.: Wiley, 1980.

Lin, C. C., et al. "Anti-Inflammatory and Radical Scavenge Effects of Arctium Lappa." *American Journal of Chinese Medicine* 24, no. 2 (1996): 127–37.

———. "Search for Biologically Active Substances in Taiwan Medicinal Plants. 1: Screening for Antitumor and Antimicrobial Substances." *Chinese Journal of Microbiology* 5 (1972): 76–8.

Loeper, J. E., et al. "Fatty Acids and Lipid Peroxidation during Experimental Atheroma. Silicon's Action." *Pathologie et Biologie* 32 (1984): 693–7.

Mabey, Richard. *The New Age Herbalist.* New York: Collier Books, 1987, 60–1.

MacLeod, George. *Cats: Homeopathic Remedies.* Essex, UK: C. W. Daniel, 1990.

———. *Dogs: Homeopathic Remedies.* Essex, UK: C. W. Daniel, 1990.

Makheja, A. M., and J. M. Bailey. "A Platelet Phospholipase Inhibitor from the Medicinal Herb, Feverfew." *Prostaglandins, Leukotrienes, and Medicine* 8 (1982): 653–60.

Mammato, Bobbie, DVM. *Pet First Aid.* St. Louis, Mo.: Mosby, 1997.

Mann, C., and E. J. Staba, "The Chemistry, Pharmacology, and Commercial Formulations of Chamomile." In *Herbs, Spices, and Medicinal Plants: Recent Advances in Botany, Horticulture, and Pharmacology,* ed. L. E. Craker and J. E. Simon, 2:235–80. Phoenix, Ariz.: Oryx, 1986.

Martin, Ann M. *Foods Pets Die For: Shocking Facts about Pet Foods*. Troutdale, Ore.: NewSage, 1997.

McCutcheon, A. R., et al. "Antiviral Screening of British Columbian Medicinal Plants." *Journal of Ethnopharmacology* 49 (Dec. 1995): 101–10.

McFarlane, J. M., and C. D. Metheney, "Effect of Micro-Aid (a Product Containing Yucca) on Canine and Feline Fecal Odors When Added to Six Dog Food and Six Cat Food Diets." MAFGD-4 and MAFGD-5. Distributors Processing, Porterville, Pa., 1988.

McKay, Pat. *Natural Immunity: Why You Should Not Vaccinate*. Pasadena, Calif.: Oscar, 1997.

———. *Reigning Dogs and Cats*. Pasadena, Calif.: Oscar, 1992.

McKinnon, Helen L. *It's for the Animals! Cookbook and Guided Tour of Natural Care and Resource Directory*, 3rd ed. Clinton, N.J.: CSA, 1997.

———. *It's for the Animals! Natural Care and Resources*, 1998. To order, call: (888) 339–4382.

McWatters, Alicia. *A Guide to a Naturally Healthy Bird: Nutrition, Feeding, and Natural Healing Methods for Parrots*. East Canaan, Conn.: Safe Goods, 1997.

Melman, Steven. *Skin Diseases of Dogs and Cats: A Guide for Pet Owners and Professionals*. Potomac, Md.: DermaPet, 1994.

Merchant, S. "Advances in Veterinary Dermatology." *Compendium* 16 (1994): 445.

The Merck Veterinary Manual. 7th ed. Rahway, N.J.: Merck & Co., 1991.

Meruelo, D., and D. Lavie. "Therapeutic Agents with Dramatic Antiretroviral Activity and Little Toxicity at Effective Doses: Aromatic Polycyclic Diones Hypericin and Pseudohypericin." *Proceedings of the National Academy of Sciences of the United States of America* 85 (1988): 5230–4.

Miller, Neil Z. *Vaccines: Are They Really Safe and Effective? A Parent's Guide to Childhood Shots*. Santa Fe, N.M.: New Atlantean Press, 1992.

Mittman, Paul. "Randomized, Double-Blind Study of Freeze-Dried Urtica Dioica in the Treatment of Allergic Rhinitis." *Planta Medica* 56, no. 1 (1990): 44–7.

Miyazawa, M., and H. Kameoka. "Constituents of Essential Oil from Rumex Crispus." *Yakagatu* 32 (1983): 45–7.

Mizobuchi, S., and Y. Sato. "Antifungal Activities of Hop Bitter Resins and Related Compounds." *Agricultural Biological Chemistry* 49 (1985): 399–405.

Montgomery, Mary, and Herb Montgomery. *A Final Act of Caring: Ending the Life of an Animal Friend*. Minneapolis: Montgomery Press, 1993. To order, write: P.O. Box 24124, Minneapolis, MN 55424.

———. *Good-Bye My Friend: Grieving the Loss of a Pet*. Minneapolis: Montgomery Press, 1993. To order, write: P.O. Box 24124, Minneapolis, MN 55424.

Moore, Michael. *Medicinal Plants of the Mountain West*. Santa Fe: Museum of New Mexico Press, 1979.

———. *Medicinal Plants of the Pacific West*. Santa Fe: Red Crane Press, 1993.

Moraleda, G., et al. "Inhibition of Duck Hepatitis B Virus Replication by Hypericin." *Antiviral Research* 20 (1993): 235–47.

Morelli, I., et al. *Selected Medicinal Plants*. Rome: FAO, 1983.

Morita, K., et al. "Chemical Nature of a Desmutagenic Factor from Burdock (*Arctium Lappa Linne*)." *Agricultural Biology and Chemistry* 49 (1985): 925–32.

Morris, T., et al. "Evaluation of the Healing Activity of Hydrocotyle (Gotu Kola) Tincture in the Treatment of Wounds." *Phytotherapy Research* 1 (1987): 117–21.

Moskalenko, S. A. "Preliminary Screening of Far-Eastern Ethnomedicinal Plants for Antibacterial Activity." *Journal of Ethnopharmacology* 15 (1986): 231–59.

Mowrey, Daniel B., PhD. *Herbal Tonic Therapies*. New Canaan, Conn.: Keats, 1993.

———. *The Scientific Validation of Herbal Medicine*. New Canaan, Conn.: Keats, 1986.

Muldner, Von H., and M. Zoller. "Antidepressive wirkung eines auf den wirkstoffkomplex hypercin standardisierten hypericum-extraktes." *Arzneimittel-Forschung* 34 (1984): 918.

Murphy, E. W., A. C. March, and B. W. Willis. "Nutrient Content of Spices and Herbs." *Journal of the American Dietetic Association* 72 (1978): 174.

Nalini, K., et al. "Effect of *Centella Asiatica* Fresh Leaf Aqueous Extract on Learning and Memory and Biogenic Amine Turnover in Albino Rats." *Fitoterapia* 63, no. 3 (1992): 232–7.

Nasyrov, K. M., and D. N. Lazareva, "Study of the Anti-Inflammatory Activity of Glycyrrhizin Acid Derivatives." *Farmakol Toksikol* 43 (July/Aug. 1980): 399–404.

Newall, Carol A., Linda A. Anderson, and J. David Phillipson. *Herbal Medicines: A Guide for Health Care Professionals*. London: Pharmaceutical Press, 1996.

Norsworthy, Gary D., and Sharon K. Fooshee. *Ask the Vet: Questions and Answers for Cat Owners*. Guelph, Ontario, Canada: Lifelearn, 1997.

———. *Ask the Vet: Questions and Answers for Dog Owners*. Guelph, Ontario, Canada: Lifelearn, 1997.

Okpanyi, S. N., and M. L. Weishcer. "Tierexperimentelle Untersuchungen zur psychotropen wirksamkeit eines Hypericum-extraktes." *Arzneimittel-Forschung* 37 (1987): 10–3.

O'Neill, L. A. J., et al. "Extracts of Feverfew Inhibit Mitogen-Induced Human Peripheral Blood Mononuclear Cell Proliferation and Cytokine Mediated Responses: A Cytotoxic Effect." *British Journal of Clinical Pharmacology* 23 (1987): 81–3.

Opdyke, D. L. J. "Parsley Seed Oil." *Food Cosmetics Toxicology* 13 (1975): S:897–8.

———. "Rosemary Oil." *Food and Cosmetics Toxicology* 12 (1974): 977–8.

Orzechowski, G. "Antibiotics from Higher Plants." *Pharmazie in unserer Zeit* 10 (1981): 42–54.

Patmore, Angela, and Tim Couzens. *Your Natural Dog: A Guide to Behavior and Health Care*. New York: Carroll & Graf, 1993.

Peng, S. Y., et al. "Decreased Mortality of Norman Murine Carcinoma in Mice Treated with the Immunomodulator, Acemannan." *Molecular Biotherapy* 3, no. 2 (1991): 79–87.

Petkov, V. "Plants with Hypotensive, Antiatheromatous, and Coronarodilatating Action." *American Journal of Chinese Medicine* 7 (1979): 197–236.

Piekos, R., et al. "Studies on the Optimum Conditions of Extraction of Silicon Species from Plants with Water." *Planta Medica* 27 (1975): 147. *Cited in Herbal Medicine*, ed. Rudolf Fritz Weiss, 238–40. Beaconsfield, England: Beaconsfield Publishing, 1988.

Pinkas, M., et al. "Phenolic Components from Some Species of Grindelia." Annales *Pharmaceutiques Françaises* 36 (1978): 97–104.

Pitcairn, Richard, and Susan Hubble Pitcairn. *Natural Health for Dogs and Cats*. Emmaus, Pa.: Rodale, 1995.

Pizzorno, J. E., and M. T. Murray, "*Hydrastis Canadensis, Mahonia Aquifolium*, and Other Berberine-Containing Plants." In *Textbook of Natural Medicine*. Seattle, Wash.: John Bastyr College Publications, 1985.

Plechner, Alfred J., and Martin Zucker. *Pet Allergies: Remedies for an Epidemic*. Inglewood, Calif.: Very Healthy Enterprises, 1986.

Preininger, V. "The Pharmacology and Toxicology of the Papaveracea Alkaloids." In *The Alkaloids*, ed. R. H. F. Manske and H. L. Holmes, 15:239. New York: Academic Press, 1975.

Priest, A. W., and L. R. Priest. *Herbal Medication*. London: Fowler & Co., 1982.

Puotinen, C. J. *The Encyclopedia of Natural Pet Care*. New Canaan, Conn.: Keats, 1998.

Pyrrolizidine Alkaloids. Environmental Health Criteria series, no. 80. Geneva: WHO, 1988.

Quackenbush, Jamie, MSW, and Denise Graveline. *When Your Pet Dies: How to Cope with Your Feelings*. New York: Simon & Schuster, 1985.

Reader's Digest. *Magic and Medicine of Plants*. Pleasantville, New York: Reader's Digest, 1986.

Recio, M. C., et al. "Antimicrobial Activity of Selected Plants Employed in the Spanish Mediterranean Area, Part 2." *Phytotherapy Research* 3 (1989): 77–88.

Ridker, P. M., et al. "Hepatic Venocclusive Disease Associated with the Consumption of Pyrrolizidine-Containing Dietary Supplements." *Gastroenterology* 88 (1985): 1050–4.

Riedel, E., et al. "Inhibition of Y-Aminobutyric Acid Catabolism by Valerenic Acid Derivatives." *Planta Medica* 48 (1982): 219–20.

Ripperger, W. "Pflanzliche laxatien und cholagogue wirkungen," *Medizinische Welt* 9 (1935): 1463–7.

Samec, V. "Effect of Lycopus Extracts on Thyroid Metabolism and Autonomic Disorders." *Wiener Medizinische Woche* 31 (1961): 513. *Cited in Herbal Medicine*, ed. Rudolf Fritz Weiss. Beaconsfield Publishing, England: Beaconsfield, 1988.

Sanchez de Medina, E., et al. "Hypoglycemic Activity of Juniper Berries." *Planta Medica* 60 (1994): 197–200.

Schmalreck, A. F., et al. "Structural Features Determining the Antibiotic Potencies of Natural and Synthetic Hop Bitter Resins, Their Precursors, and Derivatives." *Canadian Journal of Microbiology* 21 (1975): 205–12.

Schoen, Allen M., DVM. *Love, Miracles, and Animal Healing*. New York: Simon & Schuster, 1997.

———, and Susan G. Wynn, eds., *Complementary and Alternative Veterinary Medicine: Principles and Practice*. Saint Louis, Mo.: Mosby, 1998.

Schultze, Kymythy R. *The Ultimate Diet: Natural Nutrition for Dogs and Cats*. Descanso, Calif.: Affenbar Ink, 1998.

Segura, J. J., et al. "Vitro Amoebicidal Activity of *Larrea Tridentate*." *Boletin de Estudios Medicos Y Biologicos* 30 (1979): 267–8.

Self, Hilary Page. *A Modern Horse Herbal*. Addington, Buckingham, UK: Kenilworth Press, 1996.

Shashikanth, K. N., S. C. Basappa, and V. Sreenivasa Murthy, "A Comparative Study of Raw Garlic Extract and Tetracycline on Caecal Microflora and Serum Proteins of Albino Rats." *Folia Microbiologica* (Praha) 29 (1984): 348–52.

Sheets, M. A., et al. "Studies of the Effect of Acemannan on Retrovirus Infections: Clinical Stabilization of Feline Leukemia Virus-Infected Cats." *Molecular Biotherapy* 3, no. 1 (1991): 41–5.

Shibata, M. A., et al. "The Modifying Effects of Indomethacin or Ascorbic Acid on Cell Proliferation Induced by Different Types of Bladder Tumor Promoters in Rat Urinary Bladders and Forestomach Mucosal Epithelium." *Japanese Journal of Cancer Research* 83 (Jan. 1992): 31–9.

Shipochliev, B. T. "Extracts from a Group of Medicinal Plants Enhancing the Uterine Tonus." *Veterinary Medicine Nauki* 18 (1981): 94–8.

Siegal, Mordecai, and Cornell University. *The Cornell Book of Cats*. New York: Villard Books, 1989.

———, and the School of Veterinary Medicine, University of California at Davis. *UC Davis Book of Dogs*. New York: HarperCollins, 1995.

Sife, Wallace, PhD. *The Loss of a Pet*. New York: Howell Book House, Macmillan, 1993.

Slagowska, A., I. Zgorniak-Nowosielska, and J. Grzybek, "Inhibition of Herpes Simplex Virus Replication by Flos Verbasci Infusion." *Polish Journal of Pharmacology and Pharmacy* 39 (Jan./Feb. 1987): 55–61.

Smart, C. R., et al. "Clinical Experience with Nordihydroguaiaretic Acid-Chapparal Tea in the Treatment of Cancer." *Rocky Mountain Medical Journal* 67 (Nov. 1970): 39–43.

Smith, Carin A., DVM. "Is Your Horse Hypothyroid?" *Horse Illustrated*, Jan. 1994.

Solomons, N. W., and I. H. Rosenberg, eds. *Absorption and Malabsorption of Mineral Nutrients*. New York: A. R. Liss, 1984.

Someya, H. "Effect of a Constituent of Hypericum Erectum on Infection and Multiplication of Epstein-Barr Virus." *Journal of Tokyo Medical College* 43 (1985): 815–26.

St. Claire, Debra. *The Herbal Medicine Cabinet: Preparing Natural Remedies at Home*. Berkeley, Calif.: Celestial Arts, 1997.

Stein, Diane. *The Natural Remedy Book for Dogs and Cats*. Freedom, Calif.: Crossing Press, 1994.

Stewart-Spears, Genie. "Disease Linked to Nutrition." *Chronicle of the Horse*, Jan. 1992.

Strombeck, Donald R., DVM, PhD. *Home-Prepared Dog and Cat Diets: The Healthful Alternative*. Ames: Iowa State University Press, 1998.

Taddei, I., et al. "Spasmolytic Activity of Peppermint, Sage, and Rosemary Essences and Their Major Constituents." *Fitoterapia* 59 (1988): 463–8.

Takagi, K., K. Watanabe, and Y. Ishi, "Peptic Ulcer Inhibiting Activity of Licorice Root." *Proceedings of the 7th International Congress of Pharmacology* 7, no. 2 (1965): 1–15.

Tangri, K. K., et al. "Biochemical Study of Anti-Inflammatory and Antiarthritic Properties of Glycyrretic Acid." *Biochemical Pharmacology* 14 (1965): 1277–81.

Tarle, D., J. Petricic, and M. Kupinic. "Antibiotic Effects of Aucubin, Saponins and Extract of Plantain Leaf—Herbe or Folium Plantago Lanceolata." *Farmaceutski Glasnik* 37 (1981): 351–4.

Tellington-Jones, Linda, with Sybil Taylor. *The Tellington TTouch: A Revolutionary Natural Method to Train and Care for Your Favorite Animal*. New York: Penguin, 1995.

Teng, C. M., et al. "Antiplatelet and Vasorelaxing Actions of the Acetoxy Derivative of Cedranediol Isolated from Juniperis squamata." *Planta Medica* 60 (1994): 209–13.

Thompson, Diana. *"Too Much of a Good Thing."* AERC Endurance News, Oct. 1992.

Tiekert, Carvel G., DVM. "Editor's Comments." A*HVMA Journal* 15 (May/July 1996): 4.

Tilford, Gregory L. *Edible and Medicinal Plants of the West*. Missoula, Mont.: Mountain Press, 1997.

———. *From Earth to Herbalist*. Missoula, Mont.: Mountain Press, 1998.

Tomodo, M., et al. "Hypoglycemic Activity of Twenty Plant Mucilages and Three Modified Products." *Planta Medica* 53 (1987): 8–12.

Tozyo, T., et al. "Novel Antitumor Sesquiterpenoids in *Achillea Millefolium*." *Chemical and Pharmaceutical Bulletin* (Tokyo) 42 (May 1994): 1096–100.

Tyler, Varro E., PhD. Herbs of Choice: *The Therapeutic Use of Phytomedicinals*. Binghamton, New York: Pharmaceutical Products Press, 1994.

———. "Saint-John's-Wort: The Leading Herb for Mild to Moderate Depression." *Natural Pharmacy* 1 (Feb. 1997): 8.

Van Den Broucke Co. "The Therapeutic Value of Thymus species." *Fitoterapia* 4 (1983): 171–4.

and J. A. Lernli. "Pharmacological and Chemical Investigation of Thyme Liquid Extracts." *Planta Medica* 41 (1981): 129–35.

Vandergrift, Bill, PhD. "Helping Horses That Tie Up." *Modern Horse Breeding*, Sept. 1994.

Vest, M. "Vitamin K in Medical Practice." *Vitamins and Hormones* 24 (1966): 649–63.

Vlamis, Gregory, and Helen Graham. *Bach Flower Remedies for Animals*. Forres, Scotland: Words Distributing Co., 1999.

Volhard, Wendy, and Kerry Brown, DVM. *The Holistic Guide for a Healthy Dog*. New York: Howell Book House, Macmillan, 1995.

Walker, Kaetheryn. *Homeopathic First Aid for Animals: Tales and Techniques from a Country Practitioner*. Rochester, Vt.: Healing Arts Press, 1998.

Wargovich, M. J., et al. "Chemoprevention of N-Nitrosomethylbenzylamine-Induced Esophageal Cancer in Rats by the Naturally Occurring Diallyl Sulfide." *Cancer Research* 48, Dec. 1, 1988, 6872–5.

Weiss, Rudolf Fritz, MD. *Herbal Medicine*. Beaconsfield Publishing, UK: Beaconsfield, 1988.

Weng, X. S., et al. "Treatment of Leucopenia with Pure Astragalus Preparation: An Analysis of 115 Leucopenic Cases." Clinical Trial, Wuxi TCM Hospital, Jiangsu. *Zhongguo Zhong Xi Yi Jie He Za Zhi*. 15 (Aug. 1995): 462–4.

Werbach, Melvyn R., MD, and Michael T. Murray. *Botanical Influences on Illness: A Sourcebook of Clinical Research*. Tarzana, Calif.: Third Line Press, 1994.

Weston, C., et al. "Veno-Occlusve Disease of the Liver Secondary to Ingestion of Comfrey." *British Medical Journal* 295 (1987): 183.

White, P. "Essential Fatty Acids: Use in Management of Canine Atopy." *Compendium* 15 (1993): 451.

Wohlfart, R., et al. "The Sedative-Hypnotic Principle of Hops." *Communication: Pharmacology of 2-Methyl-3-Buten-2-Ol. Planta Medica* 48 (1983): 120–3.

Wolff, H. G., DVM. *Your Healthy Cat: Homeopathic Medicines for Common Feline Ailments*. Berkeley, Calif.: North Atlantic Books, 1991.

Wren, R. C. *Potter's New Encyclopedia of Botanical Drugs and Preparations,* ed. E. W. Williamson and F. J. Evans. Saffron Walden, Essex, UK: Daniel, 1988.

Wulff-Tilford, Mary, and Gregory L. Tilford. *Herbal Remedies for Dogs and Cats: A Pocket Guide to Selection and Use*. Conner, Mont.: Mountain Weed, 1997.

Wysong, R. L. *Rationale for Animal Nutrition*. Midland, Calif.: Inquiry Press, 1993.

Yang, G., and P. Geng. "Effects of Yang-Promoting Drugs on Immunological Functions of Yang-Deficient Animal Induced by Prednisolone." *Journal of Traditional Chinese Medicine* 4, no. 2 (1984): 153–6.

Yarnall, Celeste. *Cat Care Naturally*. New York: Charles E. Tuttle, 1995.

Zhang, N. D., et al. "Effects of Astragalus Saponin 1 on cAMP and cGMP Level in Plasma and DNA Synthesis in Regenerating Rat Liver." *Acta Pharmaceutica Sinica* 19, no. 8 (1984): 619–21.

Zheng, G. Q., and P. M. Kenney, "Anethofuran, Carvone, and Limonene: Potential Cancer Chemopreventative Agents from Dill Weed Oil and Caraway Oil." *Planta Medica* 58 (1992): 338–41.

Index

Index